Third Edition

Peripheral Manipulation

G. D. Maitland MBE
AUA, FCSP, FACP(Monog.), FACP (Specialist Manipulative Physiotherapist), MAppSc., APTA

Member of the Order of the British Empire.
Associate of the University of Adelaide.
Fellow of the Chartered Society of Physiotherapy.
Fellow of the Australian College of Physiotherapy.
Visiting Specialist Lecturer for the 'Graduate Diploma in Advanced Manipulative Therapy' within the School of Physiotherapy of the South Australian Institute of Technology, Adelaide.
Master of Applied Science (Physiotherapy).
Honorary Life Member American Physical Therapy Association.

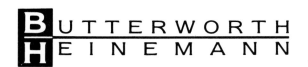

Butterworth-Heinemann Ltd
Linacre House, Jordan Hill, Oxford OX2 8DP

ℛ A member of the Reed Elsevier group

OXFORD   LONDON   BOSTON
MUNICH   NEW DELHI   SINGAPORE   SYDNEY
TOKYO   TORONTO   WELLINGTON

First published 1970
Reprinted 1974, 1976
Second edition 1977
Reprinted 1978, 1979, 1980, 1981, 1983, 1984, 1986, 1987
Third edition 1991
Reprinted 1992, 1993

© Butterworth-Heinemann Ltd 1991

British Library Cataloguing in Publication Data
Maitland, G. D. (Geoffrey Douglas)
    Peripheral manipulation — 3rd ed.
    1. Man. Joints. Manipulation
    I. Title
    616.7′20622

ISBN 0 7506 1031 X

Library of Congress Cataloguing in Publication Data
Maitland, G. D. (Geoffrey Douglas)
    Peripheral manipulation/G. D. Maitland — 3rd ed.
    p. cm.
    Includes bibliographical references
    ISBN 0 7506 1031 X
    1. Manipulation (Therapeutics)   2. Joints — Diseases — Treatment.
    I. Title
    (DNLM: 1. Manipulation, Orthopedic. WB 537 M232p)
    RD736.M25M3 — 1990
    018.T′20622 — 0020   89 — 22345 CIP

Printed and bound in Great Britain by
Thomson Litho Limited, East Kilbride, Scotland

Peripheral Mani[pulation]

Third Edition

†

To my wife Anne
for her continuing patience and encouragement

Preface

There have been many important developments in passive movement since the first edition of this book in 1970. Three outstanding examples are 1, the uniting of 'non-uniting fractures' by passive movement techniques when all other medical and surgical procedures have failed, 2, the marked functional and cosmetic improvement when passive movement is incorporated into the treatment of cleft palate of the new-born child (M. Rocabado), and 3, progression of treatment of abnormal neural and its supportive tissue by David Butler (textbook in press) is of outstanding importance, and it blends well with the concept of this book. These 3 examples alone are sufficient evidence to indicate that treatment by passive movement does something particular to structures attempting to heal which *nothing* else seems to achieve. The work originated by the orthopaedic surgeon Salter for the healing of damaged hyaline cartilage by what is now referred to universally as continuous passive motion has been an important step forward in the scientific proof of the importance of passive movement in treatment. What lies ahead in the scope of passive movement treatment defies the imagination.

The changes in the text of this edition are extensive especially in the chapters associated with examination by passive movement. Emphasis has been placed on *listening* to the person who lives with his disorder, and determining the main functional movements which he can demonstrate will reproduce his symptoms. In the physical examination sections, the text describes 'differentiation tests'. These are used to determine the movements of structures which result in symptoms demonstrated by that patient.

Importance has been placed on communication and its role in assessment. Further emphasis has been given to recording examination and treatment findings. The movement diagrams, which play an invaluable role in tutor-teaching and self-teaching, have been modified as have the representations of passive movement grades and rhythms.

Techniques and treatments have been taken a step further, and the importance which compression can play in a treatment movement is explained.

There are two techniques which are unique in the concept and are portrayed in this text. They are, 1, the shoulder quadrant and its allied close-packed locking position, and 2, hip flexion/adduction. Because they are difficult techniques to perform and teach, serial photographs have been included in this edition as an aid to understanding their subtleties.

I am indebted to many people who have given me encouragement and help. First, my thanks go to my long-standing friend and famous playwright, Richard Beynon, who read through the text making appropriate corrections for me. Unfortunately, in the limited time he had, he was unable to make a literary man out of me. Mark Jones' constructive criticisms and suggested modifications have been very helpful, and Charles Fry of Butterworths has been a long-standing friend, both patient and encouraging. And my wife Anne, who has done so much to help me in this project, as well as throughout my professional life, has again added to all of the previous drawings she has done. Without her help and patience the text could not have been completed. Gisela Rolf, who has so constructively added much to the teaching of the concept and the upholding of high standards, has contributed the audio-visual component. This has been no small task and my thanks go to her also.

G. D. Maitland
Adelaide 1990

Preface to First Edition

Treatment of painful peripheral joints by passive movement has become almost a forgotten art among physiotherapists. In the present era active exercise, combined with heat or cold therapy, is the popular and established approach. Passive movement is not routinely used because in the past its techniques have been used too strongly, causing the patient unnecessary discomfort and sometimes aggravating the condition.

Hesitation on the part of doctors and physiotherapists to use passive movement arises from a lack of understanding of how and when to apply gentle techniques, and of their effectiveness. Physiotherapists, inexperienced in handling painful joints passively, may have inadvertently aggravated the pain and thus wrongly concluded that passive movement should not be used. This condition is unfortunate; when precise physical signs of joint disturbance can be determined, quicker and better results may be achieved using passive movement guided by the signs. Often quite gentle techniques can be used.

Many books have been written about manipulation of peripheral joints. Among these are important contributions by Dr Cyriax[1] and Drs James[2] and John Mennell[3]. Dr Cyriax's work is particularly notable for the presentation of accurate methods of examination. The treatment techniques he outlines are those of the stronger type, some of which require the assistance of physiotherapists. Dr John Mennell[3] continues the work of his father, Dr James Mennell[2], who stressed the importance of accessory movement (or, in his own terminology, 'joint play').

Even with these books, and others written by lay manipulators there are still several facets of the field of passive movement treatment which are not covered. There are occasions when patients are referred for physiotherapy with joint disorders which require techniques not previously described, or when the reasons for choosing particular amplitudes and positions in the range have not previously been described or related to the examination findings of the joint disorders.

The purpose of this book is to present techniques for all peripheral joints, to discuss in detail the relevant parts of examination by passive movement, and to relate the method of applying the techniques to the examination findings.

Most people think of passive movement treatment as a stretching process to increase the range of movement of a stiff joint. However, the application of passive movement to painful peripheral joints is far wider than this. *Its use in the treatment of joint pain, whether the range of movement is limited or not, has not been appreciated.* This subject has not been treated in any other text published and possibly may not have been considered before. For this reason alone the following text is necessary to fill a gap in the physical treatment of joint pain.

Although some of the techniques will be similar to those published by others, many will be different, and some of the moving parts for which techniques are described have not been presented before. Also, some of the movements described for certain joints have not been presented before.

Diagnosis will not be discussed in this book as this is the province of the medical practitioner. However, when he refers a patient, very careful examination of joint movement must be undertaken by the

[1] Cyriax, J. *Textbook of Orthopaedic Medicine.* Vol. II, 7th edn. London; Baillière Tindall (1965)
[2] Mennell, James *Science and Art of Joint Manipulation.* Vol. II. London; Churchill (1952)
[3] Mennell, John McM. *Joint Pain.* Boston; Little Brown & Co (1965) London; Churchill (1964)

physiotherapist. The findings will guide the choice of technique and the style of movement to be used (i.e. small amplitude, large amplitude, avoiding pain or moving into pain), and the range in which it is performed. The findings also act as guides for the assessment of progress.

When any new form of treatment becomes popular, people tend to think only about the new techniques; the idea being that once the techniques are learned, nothing remains but to apply them to patients. If this idea is carried out by numerous people, it follows that standards of treatment fall, results are poor, and consequently the treatment method lapses. This idea of solely learning techniques and applying them indiscriminately is totally inadequate. For this reason considerable space in the ensuing text is given to minute examination detail and to the ways in which the techniques should be applied to the findings. The process may seem tedious at first and may even emphasize the points which seem too trivial to mention. However, this depth of detail is designed to prevent misunderstanding of the reasons for the application of the techniques. Also as a musculoskeletal disorder may present different joint signs at different stages of development of the complaint, it is essential that examination of the joint signs be carried out in detail. Different joint signs require different treatment techniques.

In the chapter on Examination appreciation of the various factors which constitute the joint signs determined by passive movement tests is discussed. In the appendices 'movement diagrams' have been offered as the best method at present available for teaching this appreciation. The 'movement diagram' has also been used in the chapter on Treatment to express more clearly the relationship between passive movement used in treatment and the clinical signs. The concept of a 'movement diagram' was evolved by Miss J-M. Ganne, MCSP, MAPA, DipTP, and further developed in an article jointly written by Miss Jennifer Hickling, MCSP and the author, published in the *Journal of the Chartered Society of Physiotherapy*[4] and the *Australian Journal of Physiotherapy*[5]. Thanks are due to Miss Hickling and to the Editors of both journals for permitting part of the article to be reproduced in this book.

Dr D. A. Brewerton, MD, FRCP, has provided an invaluable medical approach to the many aspects of passive movement treatment, and I am grateful to him for his contribution. Much needs to be said about attitudes to an prejudices against this form of treatment which cannot properly be said by a physiotherapist, and I am very pleased to have Dr Brewerton's willing support and I thank him sincerely. Many amendments regarding presentation were made to the text as it evolved and Mrs J. Trott, Miss Patricia Trott, AUA, Grad. Dip. Manip. Ther., MAPA, MCSP, and Miss M. J. Hammond, AUA, MAPA, MCSP, Dip.TP, have been patient, helpful and encouraging. The illustrations drawn by my wife more than achieve their purpose. They clearly and simply illustrate the text and avoid the distractions often present with photographs. I am especially grateful for her helpfulness and suggestions throughout the project. Without the willing help of the many people who carried out typing, modelling, and drawing of graphs, the book could not have been completed and I extend to them my grateful thanks.

Adelaide   G. D. Maitland
                                                              1970

---

[4] Hickling, J. and Maitland, G. D. Abnormalities in passive movement: diagrammatic representation. *Journal of the Chartered Society of Physiotherapists,* **56**, 105 (1970)

[5] Hickling, J. and Maitland, G. D. Abnormalities in passive movement: diagrammatic representation. *Australian Journal of Physiotherapy,* **XVI**, 13 (1970)

Contents

1

Introduction – The concept

Of those people (both medical and lay) who have an interest in manipulation as a form of treatment, the majority, perhaps as great as 80% or more, automatically think of manipulating the spine. It is this 'manipulation of the spine' that generates the greatest interest and the greatest controversy. This is partly because of the wide variety of symptoms about which patients complain, some of them being quite bizarre, and also because of the apparent 'cures' which are often effected by manipulating the spine. The medical book shops are flooded with books on the subject; some of these are valuable contributions while others are so unacceptable as to be destructive to the application and understanding of such treatment.

The use of manipulative treatment in the management of peripheral joint disorders has a much wider and more diverse application than has manipulation of the spine; and the areas of future growth have far greater and more important implications. Areas such as the management of intra-articular disorders; the reversing of the process of non-uniting fractures; the better management of sporting-type injuries; these are areas that touch but the tip of the iceberg in future development – they are exciting areas which are largely untapped by manipulative therapists – they are areas which, as a responsibility, must be explored, investigated and utilized by the medical and paramedical professions.

To portray all of these areas in one small book is difficult, and certainly it is difficult to provide the full stimulus to those people reading the text on the subject. Nevertheless it is one of the intentions in this book to achieve it sufficiently, such that patients in increasing numbers will become the benefactors.

Before commencing this project it is necessary to clarify a mis-conception. Of those people who are interested in the subject, the greatest majority are interested in the techniques. This unfortunate and narrow line of thought is, of itself, destructive rather than either productive or constructive. The reasoning and planning in the application of the techniques are the *sine qua non,* not the techniques *per se.*

Reference has been made verbally and in the literature to 'Maitland Techniques'. Although some techniques are required to form a basis from which developments can be made, there are no such things as 'any-one's techniques'. It was Dr W. M. Zinn, the Medical Director of Fortbildungszentrum Hermitage, Medizinische Abteilung Bad Ragaz, in Switzerland, who first talked of a 'Maitland Concept of examination, treatment and assessment by passive movement'. It is about using this approach to the subject, rather than the techniques, that the record needs to be put straight.

In the 5th edition of *Vertebral Manipulation* ten points were stated as the essential components of the concept. Following considerable discussion and comments during the Jubilee Congress of the South African Society of Physiotherapy in April 1985, physiotherapists and patients highlighted a different sequence (or relative importance) of these ten components. They considered that the new sequence was more basic or more fundamental to the concept. The text that follows is an expression of what these people considered were fundamental components in the right sequence of priority.

1. Central theme or core

The central theme or core of the concept is a positive personal commitment to understand what the person (patient) is enduring. Within the concept this entails:

1. Making evident, from the outset of the first consultation, a sincere desire to know what HE (the patient) considers is the problem(s) from which he wishes to be freed. This entails knowing, in *his own* use of words, the site and the behaviour of his symptoms in detail. To gain this information, in a way that makes sense medically, while at the same time allowing him to express his worries in his own terminology, requires skills in both relating to people and in deducing all the required appropriate medical details.
2. Being able to read and interpret the verbal and non-verbal information which a patient provides, both from the point of view of the affect which the disorder has on him, and also from the possible 'frame-of-reference' from which he provides them.
3. Being able to use non-verbal messages (within the verbal communication) in such a way as to encourage, in the patient, a feeling of confidence and trust in us, the clinicians.
4. LISTENING to the patient in an *open-minded* and *non-judgemental* manner.
5. BELIEVING him, yet, at the same time questioning him. Believing and listening are very demanding skills requiring a high level of self-criticism.

It is a very sad thing to hear patients say that their doctor or physiotherapist does not listen to them, or listen carefully enough, or listen sensitively enough, or listen in sufficient depth, when they want to discuss their disorder. The following quotation from *The Age*, an Australian daily newspaper, sets out the demands of 'listening' very clearly.

'Listening is itself, of course, an art: that is where it differs from merely hearing. Hearing is passive; listening is active. Hearing is involuntary; listening demands attention. Hearing is natural; listening is an acquired discipline.'
The Age (1982) August 21

Believing the patient is essential if trust between patient and clinician is to be established. We must believe his subtle comments about his disorder even if they may sound peculiar. Expressed in another way, he and his symptoms are innocent (that is, he is giving a truthful report about his disorder) until proven guilty (that is, his report is unreliable, biased, or downright false). In this context he needs to be guided to understand that his body can tell him things about his disorder and its behaviour and that we (the clinicians) cannot know unless he expresses them.

This central core of the concept of total commitment must begin at the outset of the first consultation and be carried throughout the total treatment period to the end.

2. Particular mode of thinking

The next aspect of the concept is the clinician's particular mode of thinking, interpreting, planning and acting, which is used to reach conclusions related to diagnosis, management of treatment, and prognosis of the patient's disorder.

This thinking mode is not used in any other philosophy of manipulative therapy; it is the strength of the concept and the security of the therapist

Thinking in separate compartments

First there is the requirement to think in two distinctly separate compartments. These two compartments, *although separate* and quite different, *are interdependent*. One compartment contains all of the theoretical information, known and speculative, which is of a theoretical nature, and the other contains all of the information of a person's disorder that is of a clinical nature (Table 1.1).

Table 1.1 The two compartment mode of thinking

THEORETICAL	CLINICAL

It is because much of the medical theoretical knowledge (such as diagnosis, pathology, biomedical engineering, etc.) is still incomplete, that it should not be given any opportunity to obstruct the searching for all of the appropriate clinical facts associated with a patient's disorder (that is, its history, its subjective presentation and effects, and its effects on his movements) (Table 1.2). In the day-to-day encounters with patients, such obstruction is a frequent occurrence and the theory DOES spoil the clinical search, thereby affecting the treatment unfavourably. The two-compartment *modus operandi* is therefore a *demand* requirement, so much so that it is helpful to imagine that the two interdependent compartments are separated by a 'symbolic, permeable, "brick wall"' (Table 1.2).

Table 1.2 The symbolic permeable 'brick wall'

Theoretical		*Clinical*
Pathology Biomedical engineering Neurophysiology Anatomy	} Diagnosis	History Symptoms Signs

This mode of thinking also allows for discussions on hypotheses and speculations about patients' clinical presentations without there being any blocking of progress in knowledge and skills. Also it encourages the formulation of sensible research projects directed towards more complete under-standing of the causes of disabilities, particularly painful disabilities. A bonus from the 'brick wall' is that the left-hand compartment allows for the widest of thinking (it in fact encourages it) while knowing that, if that thinking is correct, it must match the right-hand compartment – this right-hand compart-ment can ALWAYS be correct (Table 1.3).

Table 1.3 Freedom for speculation, hypotheses and research

Theoretical		Clinical
Diagnosis		History
Hypothesis		Symptoms
Speculation		Signs
Research		

Use of words

The suggested mode of thinking requires using words in particular ways. To speak or write in wrong terms means that the thought processes required to choose the words must also be wrong. The phrases used show very clearly the way the thought processes are working.

A simple example may help to make this point clear. Imagine a clinician presenting a patient at a clinical seminar, and the patient, on being asked, demonstrates his area of pain. During the ensuing discussion, the clinician may refer to where the patient's pain is by saying 'sacro-iliac pain'. This is a wrong choice of words. To be true to the concept, that is to be true to the separated theoretical and clinical compartments of thinking, the words that should be used in place of 'sacro-iliac pain', are 'pain in the sacro-iliac area'. It would be better still if the clinician demonstrated the area of pain and said 'pain in this area'. To have used the words 'sacro-iliac pain' indicates that the thought processes *could include* the thought that the sacro-iliac joint *is* the *cause* of the pain. Obviously it does not mean that the thought processes *must* include this thinking, but it does mean that it *could*. On the other hand, by using the words 'sacro-iliac area', or *demonstrating* the area of pain, indicates that although the thought processes *may* include the thought that the sacro-iliac joint could well be the source of pain, it is virtually *impossible* for the subconscious thought process to include the thought that the sacro-iliac joint IS the source of the pain. This is an *important* and essential element of the concept. Some readers may believe that *attention to this kind of detail is unnecessary*. Quite the opposite is true; if the correct choice of words is made with care, and with the right mode in mind, then the thinking process must be right. And when this is so, the whole process of examination, treatment and interpretation, must be the best that is possible.

A clinician's written record of a patient's exami-nation and treatment findings shows clearly whether the thinking processes are right or wrong.

Diagnostic titles

Coping with diagnosis and diagnostic titles is difficult. Even within medicine, many diagnostic titles are sometimes inadequate or even incorrect; they may be merely linked to patterns of symptoms or even based on suppositions. Titles are often used quite loosely and even inappropriately. It is often impossible to arrive at a specific diagnosis, yet the treatment required is clearly known. Many people consider that treatment should not be administered unless an accurate diagnosis is available. This is true to some extent; it IS necessary to know whether a patient's symptoms are believed to be arising from a musculo-skeletal disorder rather than an active disease, but it is not always necessary to have a precisely accurate diagnostic title. Provided that the word diagnosis is used in the terms defined in Butterworth's *Medical Dictionary* quoted below, there is no difficulty:

'Diagnosis. The art of applying scientific methods to the elucidation of the problems presented by a sick patient. This implies the collection and critical evaluation of all the evidence obtainable from every possible source by the use of any method necessary. From the facts so obtained, combined with the knowledge of basic principles, a concept is formed of the aetiology, pathological lesions and disordered functions which constitute the patient's disease. This may enable the disease to be placed in a certain recognized category but, of far greater importance, it also provides a sure basis for the treatment and prognosis of the individual patient.'[1]

The title in relation to the two compartments of thinking poses no problems. The mode of thinking requires that the clinician must know the history, the symptoms and the signs very clearly, and while keeping these in mind, full use can be made of the theoretical compartment. In such a manner, as clear an understanding as is possible about the patient's disorder can be achieved.

1. Critchley, M. (ed.) *Butterworths Medical Dictionary,* 2nd edn. Butterworths, London (1978)

Mode of thinking

The mode of thinking in relation to treatment is clearly seen in the choosing of treatment techniques. The choice of technique is made in relation to the patient's symptoms and signs, not to the diagnostic title, though the theoretical compartment *may* influence the vigour and choice of the technique.

Planning the treatments demands logical thinking. The treatment carried out at any one session is chosen with care and it must make sense both logically and medically. Each step in the planning of the whole treatment programme is made on the basis of the same logical medical sense. Prognosis is another aspect of treatment that is determined logically. This is achieved by assessing changes in the patient's symptoms and signs effected by treatment which is, at the same time, related to the theory of the diagnosis. Therefore, full use is made of the two interdependent compartments of thinking to achieve the best end results.

When a serious disorder is present, the diagnosis takes a primary role. However when the presentation clearly shows a mechanical-type disorder, the clinical compartment takes precedence.

3. Examination

The next three aspects of the concept are:

1. EXAMINATION.
2. TECHNIQUES.
3. ASSESSMENT.

They are interrelated and interdependent. To relate them to the concept in their order of importance would place assessment first. However, for assessment to be so important, examination must be accurate and complete and techniques must be effectively chosen and performed. To make assessment clearer to understand, and to help it to remain more firmly in the reader's mind, it will be discussed last. And as *physical* examination techniques are frequently used as *treatment* techniques, examination will be dealt with first.

The usual routine examinations by physical means are standard and are not special to the concept. However, knowing in detail the intensity, behaviour and relationships of pain, stiffness and muscle spasm during the test movements *is* special. Such care reveals to the clinician the evidence of 'through-range-pain', 'end-of-range-pain', 'irritability' and the varieties of 'latent pain', all of which are special and fundamental to the use of passive movement espoused by the concept. There are, however, other examination procedures which are special and which do relate particularly to the concept.

Subjective examination

When questioning the patient about his symptoms, it is basic for the clinician to know, in depth, the particular site(s) and behaviour(s) of these symptoms. One should be able to 'live' these symptoms through a complete cycle, and to 'feel' emotionally and appreciate the effect they have on the patient.

Essential beliefs

It is essential to believe that a patient may:

1. Have one disorder yet have different kinds of pain interacting together in associated areas.
2. Have overlapping areas of pain from different components of the one disorder.

It is also necessary to believe that the patient's body can make these distinctions clear to the patient, but only clear to the clinician by her encouraging the patient to talk about them. These beliefs are an integral part of the central core of the concept.

Behaviour of pain

Pain can behave in many different ways, depending upon the effect that rest, activity and positions have on the disorder. It is necessary to know the behaviour of the patient's symptoms if a reasonable understanding of the state of the disorder is to be determined.

These first two examination requirements are very special to, and peculiar to, this particular concept of treatment.

Objective examination
Accessory movements

Examining accessory movements in both the loose-packed positions and at the end of limited ranges, or in painful positions of a free range of movement, are, in one way, special to the concept. Though other concepts assess the range of accessory movements, assessing the pain responses in relation to the suffered pain is not. Nor is the assessment of the pain response of accessory movements in a painful, yet not limited physiological position. To know which accessory movement most closely relates to the patient's symptoms gives information about the disorder which cannot be gained in any other way. This aspect IS special to the concept.

Combined movements

Although the physical examination of routine physiological movements is not special to the concept the coupling together of these movements into combined movement tests is. Combining accessory test movements with physiological movements is equally special. The formalizing of these tests has been the original contribution of Edwards[2].

Compression tests

There are occasions when, during the objective examination, it becomes evident that the two joint surfaces should be held firmly compressed together when performing a test movement[3]. Only by adding such compression may the evidence of the origin of a patient's symptoms become clear.

Functional reproducing movements

When pain, rather than stiffness–disability, is the patient's problem, he can quite often demonstrate a particular movement, activity or function that will reproduce his symptoms (and it is the using of this that is the aspect related to this concept). Encouraging the patient to so demonstrate the movement, together with the clinician's analysis of it, is another aspect that is special to the concept. Frequently the demonstrated movement may be used as, or give an idea for, the *treatment* movement.

Injuring movement

When a comparable examination movement/pain-response cannot be found, or when a sprain or injury has been the cause of the symptoms, re-enacting the injuring direction of the stress as an examination procedure may divulge the comparable sign. Again, such use in physical examination, which is routine in this concept, is not found in other examination routines.

Differentiation

Differentiation tests are special tests that are used when a passive test movement, causing simultaneous movement of at least two joints, reproduces a patient's symptoms. The method is, when the test movement is at the point in the range of reproducing the patient's pain, further movement is produced in one of the two joints affected, which, at the same time, either reduces the movement in the other joint or retains it at an unchanged degree of stress. This test, which increases the stress at one joint and reduces it at the other, will either increase or decrease the reproduced pain. The test is then performed in the reverse manner. The pain response (that is increase, or decrease) confirms which joint was found to be at fault with the first test.

Range and pain response

It is a mandatory rule in this concept that when testing a movement in any direction of any joint, the recording of the findings must include both the range and the pain response.

A detailed examination of movements seeks to reveal the smallest changes in the behaviour of the pain and the limitation of the range with each direction of movement. For example, does the patient feel pain or discomfort throughout the range or is it painful only to the end of range? ('through-range-pain' and 'end-of-range pain' respectively). Does the behaviour of the pain with the movement match the behaviour of the resistance with that same movement within its available range? Appreciating the fine differences in the behaviour of the abnormal elements of the movement is imperative to the application of treatment.

NEVER THINK OF RANGE WITHOUT THINKING OF PAIN
NEVER THINK OF PAIN WITHOUT THINKING OF RANGE

Effect of over-pressure

When examining a movement of a particular structure, it can only be classed as being normal if a very firm over-pressure can be applied without provoking anything more than the expected normal stretch responses. Under these circumstances when the stretch response is normal and the over-pressure has been of adequate firmness the movement may be recorded with two ticks, as shown below, indicating its normality:

F $\checkmark$ $\checkmark$

The F represents the movement being tested, in this case flexion, and the first tick means that over-pressure has been applied and that the range is normal. The second tick means that the stretch response to the over-pressure has been normal.

Movement diagrams

Movement diagrams are included as part of the concept for two reasons:

1. They formulate a basis from which any clinician can learn more from each clinical experience. To draw a diagram representing the findings on examining a particular movement forces the clinician to analyse the relationships of the pain/stiffness/muscle-spasm which may be present.

2. Edwards, B. C. Combined movements of the lumbar spine. *Australian Journal of Physiotherapy,* **25**, 4 (1979)
3. Maitland, G. D. The importance of adding compression when examining and treating synovial joints. *Aspects of Manipulative Therapy,* 2nd ed., Churchill Livingstone, Melbourne, pp. 109–115 (1985)

2. As a means of communication in the teaching situation, the diagrams provide a tool for learning which can be used in a way which is foolproof.

4. Techniques

The importance of treatment techniques has been discussed, and reference was made to the fact that some people are always looking for new techniques rather than understanding the 'how, when and why' of how they should be modified and used. Techniques, as they apply to the concept proposed in this book, are never-ending and they never SHOULD have an ending. So long as patients present with different symptoms and signs, there will have to be changes in the techniques to free the patients of their symptoms. Although there are basic techniques which must be taught, the concept is that the clinician's mind must be so open as to allow for modification of the techniques until they achieve what they are set out to achieve. The basic treatment techniques must include every movement of which the joint is capable, both the physiological movements and the accessory movements, and all possible combinations of them.

When it comes to selecting techniques for treatment, it is necessary to know firstly, the passive movements, or positions, which provoke or relieve the patient's symptoms. When the symptoms are easily reproduced, the technique chosen may be either the movement that relieves the symptoms or the movement that provokes the symptoms. Similarly the starting *position* in which the technique is performed will be one which either relieves the symptoms or reproduces the symptoms, as indicated above.

There are no set techniques or invariable techniques; there are no times when a teacher can say 'you must *always* do it this way'. The only MUST is that the technique *must* achieve its intention both while it is being performed and after it has been performed. The clinician's mind must always be open; the teacher must never be dogmatic.

| A TECHNIQUE IS THE BRAINCHILD OF INGENUITY |

Primarily the concept demands knowing how to relate (1) the rhythm required for the technique, (2) the position in the range that it should occupy and (3) the amplitude and the strength of the technique to the examination findings.

Because the style of movement to be used as a treatment technique can be of different amplitudes and can be in different parts of an available range, GRADES OF MOVEMENT AND RHYTHMS OF MOVEMENT BECOME ESSENTIAL TO THE CONCEPT. These grades are described on pages 47 and 48. They are essential for three reasons:

1. They form the best basis for teaching and communication.
2. They force the clinician to think in much finer detail about the technique to be performed.
3. They form an effective method of abbreviation when recording treatment. Their use saves time and they also, in forcing the clinician to commit the technique to paper, make the clinician consciously analyse the technique in greater depth.

When actually performing a technique, the clinician must become as involved with the procedure as is the soloist musician when performing with a symphony orchestra.

There are two styles of technique that are particularly unique to the concept. They are essential if the clinician's manual skills are to equip her fully to produce the best results in the treatment of musculo-skeletal disorders. They are as follows:

1. There are techniques that include moving a joint in an oscillatory fashion (two or three per second, plus or minus). These techniques are performed within a range of movement that is neither painful nor affected by any stiffness or muscle spasm.
2. There are times when the adjacent joint surfaces need to be held firmly compressed together while performing a movement technique. This also applies to using accessory movements while the joint surfaces are compressed.

In essence, it is essential to have an open-minded attitude to treatment techniques, being able to innovate and improve freely, unhindered by theory; and to relate the techniques to the functional disturbances.

5. Assessment

Each session of a patient's treatment can be divided into three parts; examination of the patient, treatment techniques, and assessment. It is necessary to know the relative importance that these three parts bear to each other. Though skill in each of the three is important, the degree of the skill required for each is not equivalent. Obviously the best treatment cannot be given without perfectly performed examination techniques and treatment techniques. However techniques are the least important of the three parts. *Continuous analytical assessment* heavily outweighs the others. Clinicians who seek to copy any particular person's techniques merely to use them on their patients, have a totally wrong idea of passive movement treatment, and anyone conducting courses that consist mainly of techniques should be vigorously censured.

Flawless analytical assessment is the vital link of this concept of treatment; it is the keystone, without which the whole concept would collapse.

There are three types of assessments.

The first is the assessments made during the initial examination of the patient; relating the findings to the behaviour of the patient's symptoms; and relating the findings to the diagnosis, its stage if the disorder is a progressive one, and the stability of the disorder at the time of treatment.

The second is 'proving or assessing the value of a technique' in treatment. This entails knowing what the intention of the technique should be while it is being performed, and having an expectation of what changes the technique will effect following its use. Two effective applications of a technique are necessary before it is discarded as being useless for the present stage of the disorder.

The third assessment is an analytical assessment which is used both during a treatment programme and at the completion of the programme. During the programme it is used to provide a clear retrospective picture of the effect of treatment and to know whether the disorder is spontaneously recovering, recovering due to treatment, or a combination of both. Analytical assessment at the completion of a total treatment programme is used to determine the future prognosis of any mode of treatment and the likely recurrences of the patient's disorder.

The mental processes consist of simply thinking logically in a way that includes:

1. Vertical thinking.
2. Lateral thinking.
3. Inductive thinking.
4. Deductive thinking.

The achievements are limited only by the extent of one's lateral and logical thinking.

The body has two capabilities that influence assessments.

The body has an astonishing capacity to *adapt to* changes that are forced upon it by congenital abnormalities, trauma, life-long heavy work and disease. The body also has an enormous capability to *compensate* for damage and disease, and it is these capacities of the body that must be borne in mind when making analytical assessments.

There is also another capacity that the body has, and which can be utilized in assessment. The patient's body can tell him things relating to his disorder that can never be detected by the clinician even by the most thorough objective examination. These are frequently subtle messages which the patient may comment upon, yet feeling that they are almost too trivial to state. Nevertheless they may be priceless. The only way the clinician can elicit these subtleties is to listen to the patient and to encourage him to mention anything that might be relevant, irrespective of how trivial or unimportant it may seem to be to him. The patient who is 'tuned in to his body' will be aware of these subtleties, and the clinician can educate the patient to notice these trivia and to report them. This is an essential way in which the patient can assist in the moment-by-moment subjective assessment of his disorder and its behaviour.

'It is open-mindedness, mental agility and mental discipline, linked with a logical and methodical process of assessing cause and effect, which are the demands of the concept.'

6. Recording

Recording the treatment of a patient must include detailed information yet must be brief.

When recording a treatment session, the first words must include a quotation of the patient's opinion of the effect of the previous treatment. This quotation must be worded in such a way that it is a 'comparison', it must not be just a statement of fact. The second requirement is to record the movements that are affected by the disorder; these too are recorded as *comparisons* with the previous findings.

Before performing a treatment technique, the planning and the reasoning for its selection should be recorded. This forms the third recording requirement.

The treatment and its effect should be recorded next. This entails the record of the treatment technique, its grade, its rhythm, and its symptomatic response while being performed. Once the technique has been completed the patient should then be asked to make a comparison of any changes in symptoms resulting from the technique. This is followed by a re-examination of the affected movements; their state and comparison should be recorded.

Finally, at the end of a treatment session, the clinician should commit thoughts to paper about how treatment may need to be modified at the next treatment session. Such a record not only forces the clinician to analyse thoughts, but also stimulates memory of the last treatment session and thereby makes all of the treatment sessions more complete in terms of knowing the path the treatment is moving along.

7. In summary
1. *The central core*

A sublimation of 'self' and a positive personal commitment to understanding the effects that the disorder has on the patient.

1. Making sense of information which the patient provides.
2. Listening and believing the patient without any pre-judging.
3. Using the patient's own terminology (the clinician adapts herself to the patient rather than continuously expecting the patient to adapt himself to the clinician).
4. Having skill in understanding and using verbal and non-verbal communication.
5. Endeavouring to understand the 'frame-of-reference' from which the patient expresses the effects of the disorder.
6. Knowing what the clinician needs to know.
7. Encouraging a feeling of confidence and trust in us, the clinicians.

2. Mode of thinking

A special mode of thinking in two separate but interdependent compartments, separated by a symbolic permeable 'brick wall' thus allowing for hypotheses, speculations and incomplete diagnoses. The separation into a 'theoretical compartment' and a 'clinical compartment' prevents thoughts relating to the *theory* of a disorder from discovering the patient's disorder in terms of its history, its symptoms and its signs in fine depth of detail. It also allows for incomplete or uncertain diagnoses.

3. Examination

An essential requirement is believing that a patient can have:

1. More than one kind of pain.
2. Different pains in overlapping areas.
3. Different pains with different behaviours.

It is also important to believe that there are fine details of information which the body can tell the patient and that the clinician cannot know about them unless the patient is encouraged to talk about these trivia.

In the objective examination the aspects peculiar to this concept are:

1. Functional movements which the patient can perform to demonstrate the pain for which he seeks treatment.
2. Re-enacting the injuring movement when the disorder has been caused by some traumas.
3. Pain responses to accessory movements performed in loose-packed positions and at the end of range of physiological movements.
4. Pain response in response to 'combined movement' tests.
5. Pain response with movements, both physiologic-

al and accessory, performed while the joint surfaces are held compressed together.
6. Differentiation tests.
7. Test movements requiring over-pressure to establish normality.
8. Never thinking of range of movement without relating the pain response to it, and vice versa.
9. Movement diagrams for purposes of learning and teaching.

4. Techniques

Although it is necessary to have a basis of techniques from which to teach, the clinician must be totally open minded and capable of adapting and modifying techniques to achieve the purposes for which they were chosen in relation to movement and pain.

A TECHNIQUE IS THE BRAINCHILD OF INGENUITY

Grades of movement and rhythms are used for recording purposes. Two styles of technique are peculiar to this concept alone:

1. Performing a movement in an oscillatory fashion within a range of movement where there is no stiffness, muscle spasm or pain.
2. Using compression as a component of a treatment technique. Recording treatment must be complete, in depth, yet brief.

5. Assessment

This is the epitome of the concept. It is used at the initial consultation in a manner to determine the effect of the disorder on the patient as a person, and on the movements of his affected joint areas.

The second application of assessment is in proving the value of a technique. Analytical assessment is used throughout treatment and at the end of treatment.

Such assessment must be made in the light of the fact that the body has an enormous capacity to compensate for injury, disease or congenital abnormalities; it also has the capacity to inform the patient of seemingly trivial details which the clinician must encourage the patient to report so that assessments can be more informed and accurate.

IT IS OPEN-MINDEDNESS, MENTAL AGILITY AND MENTAL DISCIPLINE LINKED WITH A LOGICAL AND METHODICAL PROCESS OF ASSESSING CAUSE AND EFFECT WHICH ARE THE DEMANDS OF THE CONCEPT.

2

Manipulation: Definition and role

Definition

The term 'manipulation' can be used loosely in medicine to mean passive movement of any kind. As used in this text it can be divided into the following categories: (1) mobilization; (2) manipulation.

1. Mobilization

Mobilizations are passive movements performed in such a way (particularly in relation to the speed of the movements) that at all times they are within the control of the patient so that he can prevent the movement if he so chooses. Two main types of movement are:

1. Passive oscillatory movements, two or three per second, of small or large amplitude, and applied anywhere in a range of movement.
2. Sustained stretched with or without tiny amplitude oscillations at the limit of the range.

These oscillatory movements may consist of the joint's accessory movements or its physiological movements. Physiological movements are those that the patient can carry out actively. Accessory movements are movements that a person cannot perform himself but which can be performed on him by someone else. For example, a person cannot perform pure rotation of the shaft of the metacarpal at the metacarpophalangeal joint of his index finger, but somebody else can rotate it for him. Therefore, that rotation of the metacarpophalangeal joint is an accessory movement.

The movements referred to in (1) and (2) above may be performed while the joint surfaces are held

distracted or compressed. Distraction is the keeping apart of the opposite joint surfaces; compression is the squeezing together of the joint surfaces. Both positions are used in treatment. They can be used in conjunction with other directions of movement or used alone; that is, distraction is used as an examination test movement or as a treatment; likewise compression.

2. Manipulation

There are two procedures that can be termed manipulation:

1. Manipulation is a sudden movement or thrust, of small amplitude, performed at a speed that renders the patient powerless to prevent it.
2. Manipulation under anaesthesia (MUA) is a medical procedure performed with the patient under anaesthesia and used to stretch a joint to restore a full range of movement by breaking adhesions. The procedure is not a sudden forceful thrust as mentioned in the preceding paragraph, but is done as a steady and controlled stretch. This procedure can also be performed on the conscious patient.

If adhesions are torn during treatment using the 'mobilizing' technique as described in section 1.2 above then the technique may be classed as a manipulation even though a sudden thrust has not been used.

The 36th edition of *Gray's Anatomy*[1], and particularly the section on arthrology (pp. 420–503), is among the best references relating to current

1. Williams, P. L. and Warwick, R. *Gray's Anatomy*, 36th edn., Churchill Livingstone, London (1980)

knowledge of joint structure and function. Information fundamental to examination of joint disorders and treatment by passive movement is given; the bibliography and diagrams are excellent. It is important that physiotherapists treating joint disorders by passive movement are well versed in musculo-skeletal anatomy, in the principles of movement at each joint, in the neurophysiology related to pain with joint movement, and in the part played by muscle spasm.

Role

Mobilization and manipulation show their best effect when directed at mechanical type problems for which they perform the following main roles.

1. Restoring structures within a joint to their normal positions or pain-free positions so as to recover a full-range painless movement

For example, if a patient tears a meniscus of the knee or the temporomandibular joint, he will have a restricted range of movement which will be painful and limited in range in some directions. Passive movement treatment aims to alter the position of the meniscus so that the range of movement of the joint becomes full and pain free. When pain-free movement has been restored, the next step is to prevent recurrences by exercising to increase the strength, the endurance and the speed with which the muscles can contract to control the movements.

2. Stretching a stiff joint to restore range

Passive movement techniques can be used to stretch a stiff pain- free joint to improve the range until it reaches the stage of being functional once more. The movements used should be those described in *Gray's Anatomy*, that is, treatment movements that include the spin, roll, and slide which are normal for that particular joint. There are other movements described in the text which are used to increase range. They should all be performed as small, strong oscillatory movements at the rate of two or three per second. They will provide the manipulator with more accurate 'feel' of the resistance than would be possible with a sustained stretching technique.

When the patient experiences considerable pain during the stretching, the suggested oscillatory movements must be performed much more slowly; there may even be no oscillation, but rather a slow and gradually increasing movement stretching tight structures. When pain reaches a peak the movement is retained at that position allowing time for the pain to decrease before attempting to take the movement further. It may even be necessary, if the intensity of pain *sharply* increases, to quickly slacken the pressure slightly so as to be able to sustain a holding position with an acceptable degree of pain and to wait for the pain to decrease before attempting to take the movement further.

The following statement is important to make at this stage, because it differs from the opinions and philosophies of other manipulators, yet is primary to the concept of this text: when endeavouring to restore the patient's ability to achieve a certain movement or position (which may require restoration of more than one direction of physiological movement) *two* groups of movements (not just *one*) must be stretched:

1. The first group consists of those physiological movements that are restricted.
2. The second group consists of the accessory movements that exist at the limit of the related restricted physiological ranges of movement. These accessory movements will also be restricted in their range *in this position of the physiological range*.

It is the first group of this section to which other manipulators take exception, yet it is a primary element which this book embraces.

As an example, if a patient is unable to reach above his head because of restricted flexion of the glenohumeral joint (which is a relatively pain-free movement), although stretching accessory movements may gain an initial improvement, full restoration is impossible without also stretching the restricted physiological movement.

3. Stretching

Mobilizing techniques to stretch have three other roles:

1. Slow passive movement to retain range.
2. Stretching to increase an otherwise normal range to make it more mobile (perhaps some would call it making the range hypermobile).
3. Stretching to lengthen contracted or fibrosed muscle tissue.

Stretching to retain range

The thought behind this statement is really using the word 'stretch' wrongly. When a patient is in an active phase of any of the arthritides, there is value in endeavouring to prevent losing range of joint movement. However, this should not be done at the expense of exacerbating the pain. The treatment movement therefore, should be neither oscillatory nor repetitive. The movement should be a single movement in the functional directions that are important for the patient's daily needs. Obviously the treatment movement would not be forceful. Similarly the movement should be performed very slowly and well within the patient's comfort.

Stretching to increase the normal range

There are many fields of endeavour (sport and dance for example) where it is necessary, for the participants who have special potential, to have a greater range of movement than is normal for the average person. For a ballet dancer to achieve recognition as a good dancer, good 'turn-out' is essential. Some young dancers have this either naturally or gain it by their exercise and training programmes. Others may have good range for other aspects of dance, such as 'point', yet be lacking in 'turn-out' despite persistent training. When such a person has very good potential in the other requirements of a professional dancer, passive movement by a physiotherapist can be utilized to gain range in the 'turn-out'. When this is applied, the dancer's active training and warm-up periods must be coupled with the stretching treatment.

Such a use of passive movement techniques is not detrimental to the person provided common sense is exercised by the physiotherapist. The dancer must not experience any latent pain reaction from the treatment and must be able to keep good muscular control of the increased range. A good example of such a treatment is given on page 238.

Stretching fibrosed muscle tissue

In these stated circumstances, the movement used is the one that stretches the contracted fibres. This, then, will be a physiological movement. There is no place at all for 'accessory movements at the limit of the range'.

Other forms of manual physiotherapy treatment should also be used, to both assist in the lengthening of the contracted tissue, and to strengthen the antagonist(s).

4. Relieving pain by using special techniques

A patient may have considerable joint pain which limits his active movement, although there is no loss of passive range. In other words, if the examiner were prepared to ignore the patient's pain, and press on regardless, he would find the range of movement full in all directions though obviously they would be extremely painful. Mobilization has a definite part to play in the treatment of these painful joints.

With these joint disorders there is usually a degree of inflammation, the cause of which is not always evident. There may be an outside factor causing it, for example rheumatoid arthritis or its variants, or there may be a mechanical irritating origin. The latter group can be successfully treated by special passive movement techniques. If the mechanical treatment eliminates the mechanical irritating cause, the patient loses his pain.

A patient may have more than one cause for an inflammatory reaction in a joint. For example, it is common for a patient to have osteoarthritis producing an inflammatory reaction, superimposed upon a mechanical factor provoking further inflammatory reaction. When this is so, passive movement treatment can effect a degree of improvement commensurate with the extent of the mechanical cause.

Frequently at a first consultation it is impossible to determine whether a combination of factors is causing the painful reaction. However, if a short trial of controlled passive movement is administered, the extent of the mechanical cause may be determined in retrospect by assessment. If the treatment lessens the patient's pain and improves range then at least part of the patient's pain must have been mechanical in origin. However, if there is no improvement there is no mechanical factor.

If a patient has an *active* osteoarthritis in a joint, mobilization will not improve the pain but anti-inflammatory medication or intra-articular injection may. However, if the diagnosis is osteoarthritis, passive movement treatment should be a foremost consideration because symptoms may well be mechanical, being superimposed on previously imposed joint changes.

It is in this area of determining what is the best thing to do to help a patient with distressing, yet not disabling symptoms, that the physiotherapist has an important role to play in conjunction with the referring medical practitioner. The patient with post-traumatic arthritis and an exacerbation of symptoms without signs of inflammation is an example.

Most of the patients referred by doctors to physiotherapists for treatment of musculo-skeletal problems seek help because of pain rather than stiffness. The joints should be tested for range and pain, and the muscles should be tested for strength and pain. If the examination is carried out correctly it will be found that most musculo-skeletal problems have two components, a pain component and a stiffness component. Spasm may also be present and this may cloud the assessment, particularly if it prevents movement early in the range.

These components, or 'joint signs', in musculo-skeletal disorders must be recognized and assessed independently. All physiotherapists will have treated patients who have a painless stiff joint. They will also have treated patients who have pain associated with the stiffness. However, it is surprising how few physiotherapists recognize the group of patients who have painful joints that are not limited by any stiffness. It is important to be aware (a) that such patients *do* exist, and (b) that they can be treated by special passive movement techniques. When the concept of treating the pain component is understood, accepted and used, then treatment by manipulation can be utilized to its fullest extent.

5. Sports injuries and trauma

Sports injuries can be considered in two categories. Firstly, there are those people who have their cause in the 'over-use', 'mis-use' or 'abuse' category. They form a special group because people competing in any sport subject their bodies to the maximum level they can achieve. By continuous training and competing, they may place a greater stress on some structures than those structures are able to stand. This extra stress superimposed on an 'over-use' situation will result in symptoms. The treatment of the symptoms requires many forms of physiotherapy of which manipulative physiotherapy is one – it is not necessarily the main one, but it is an aspect of overall management which is neither adequately recognized nor used. However, it does play a major role in prophylaxis.

The second category of sports injury is the same as the trauma group referred to earlier, which relates to the injuries caused by blows and falls, particularly in the heavy contact sports.

Other trauma included under this heading includes the results of car accidents, machinery related injuries, and even post-surgical trauma. All comprise damage to what may have been otherwise healthy tissue. As with the first group of sports injuries many forms of physiotherapy, including manipulative physiotherapy, have a role to play in treatment. What many people do not seem to realize is that passive movement treatment can achieve desired changes which other forms of physiotherapy cannot achieve – two examples are achieving maximum attainable range of joint movement and muscle length, and achieving best results from the effects of pain-inhibition. Also it may be the only way of clearing a protective muscle spasm.

3

Communication and the person

The patient is a person,
a person needing our skills.
Our duty is to the person.

Our goal is to promote mutual confidence and gain
respect and trust.

One of the most important contributions we can make in the successful management of a patient's symptoms (the 'problem' being both his disorder and the effects it has on him as a person) lies in our being able to understand him, even to the extent of actually feeling, within ourselves, what he feels. This effectively means that we can interpret his expressions and nuances in the way HE hopes they will be interpreted. Perhaps the statement, 'being able to "read" the person', is an expression that covers the situation. This is not always easy because each of us develops from different genes and within different environments. We all, also, have different experiences in our lives which affect us and influence us in different ways. A person's genetic make-up, the environment he grows up in during his formative years, and the experiences during his life-time are referred to as his 'frame of reference'. We all, patient or therapist, have a personal and different 'frame of reference' which must be understood as being different and affecting us differently.

Therapists must be able to accept people for what they are without placing judgements or interpretations on them just because they are different. From the very first eye contact with a patient at the very first consultation (and, of course, thereafter), it is the therapist's responsibility to gain the patient's confidence and trust by showing belief and concern

– even 'understanding' when understanding is not initially possible. To start making inflexible judgements from the very first eye-contact is to be unjust to the patient, and is certainly not in his best interests. And it is the patient's best interests that should be the therapist's primary concern. The best judgements are those that are made in retrospect – the first contacts with the patient should be ones that draw the therapist and patient together in an atmosphere of understanding and trust.

'Beware how you pass judgement at least until you know how to put yourself in their place and see from their view'[1].

For some therapists, understanding other people comes easily because they have a natural talent, or flair, for it. For others, though it is difficult, much can be learned. There are two ways of learning:

1. The least important of the two methods is to 'read, mark, learn and inwardly digest' from all manner of texts. These may be in terms of lectures, the reading of related books, even sitting-in on interviews between a professional and a client. This latter infers that the professional (for example a skilled social worker, lawyer, doctor etc.) is discussing a subject of a personal nature with the client on a one-to-one basis. There is, however, a real basis for danger in theoretical learning, and this is borne out in the following quotation:

'It is those who get involved in caring for other people who run the risk of getting depersonalised by the psychological and sociological tools of the trade. There are social workers who are so busy analysing their relationships with their clients

1. Peters, E. *Monks Hood,* Future Publications, London, p. 18 (1984)

that their clients' needs go unregarded. You can see them assessing the situation according to the text books as they talk to you'[2].

2. The second method, which is to teach oneself, relies upon believing and having genuine concern for the patient. It is not difficult to teach oneself, and, in fact, it is the most important method of learning because of its continuing nature. To learn by experience requires certain qualities to be used consciously, uncluttered and not hindered by one's own dogmatic opinions or attitudes.

Teaching oneself is a very humbling experience. While talking with patients we often find out that what we had thought and judged to be 'so-and-so' turns out to be entirely wrong, and that we find out gradually that it was, instead, 'such-and-such'. To be able to see and accept the error is to learn by it: we are not all-knowing nor always right, and to realize this can make future judgements more pliable and open ended. The more open minded and less judgemental a person is, the more likely the person being judged will be understood more accurately.

Prior to initial consultation

There are many things that should be appreciated about people in relation to how their disorder affects them and how they may present their symptoms to the interviewing physiotherapist.

Acceptance

People accept their problems in many different ways. For example, quite incongruously a patient may laugh when telling about what he is unable to do because of his disorder when the disability is not a laughing matter. As concerned therapists, we should realize that while this does seem quite odd, it is not so uncommon as to be pathognomonic, but rather it is to be recognized as being part of the person's make-up to be recognized and not criticized or judged unfavourably. Another patient may burst into tears over something that seems trivial. However there may be many reasons for the bursting into tears. There may be frustration at the lack of understanding of the patient by other members of the family. There may be sadnesses in the patient's life and the present disorder is just 'the last straw'. The tears may come forth because at last someone is listening to their 'tale of woe'. The therapist's responsibility is to accept the tears, show

understanding and concern even if the reason can't be understood initially. Yet another patient may be quite aggressive or even arrogant – accept it, don't fight it and don't bite back. By talking with him, learn to understand why he reacts in this way and so mould the necessary questions in such a way as to soften the responses, or at least, to avoid aggravating the aggression.

Ethnic background

Patients' acceptance is often moulded by their ethnic background or their particular family's handling of the person. This, again, should be taken into account, accepted and appreciated so that the patient can be helped in the best possible ways. The patient must be able to feel and see the therapist's concern, and to be able to believe that they are in caring and understanding hands.

Threshold

People clearly have different thresholds of pain, but what is sometimes not understood is that there are both physiological and psychological reasons for these differences. Professor Keele showed that 60% of the people he tested had what he classed as a normal average threshold of pain, and that while 23% had a lower threshold of pain 17% had a high threshold of pain.[3]

The point to be made here is that because a patient may be judged to be complaining about pain more than seems to fit the disorder, he should not be judged, initially at least, to be grizzling unwarrantedly. Rather the judgement should be in his favour, based on the reason that there is something about the disorder that the therapist is not finding. Later in treatment it may be reasonable to reconsider the verdict – the rule 'the witness is innocent until PROVEN guilty' is the one to use, despite the fact that the opposite is the one more commonly used. It is disheartening to see so many patients who have been cast into the mould of having psychological problems resulting in the physical disorder just because the patient hasn't been adequately understood, examined or treated.

Demonstration

If the patient's mother tongue is not the same as that in which he is having his treatment, and he is not confident talking in this different language, he may

2. Dalrymple, J. *Costing Not Less Than Everything,* London, Darton Longman & Todd, p. 93 (1975)
3. Keele, K. E. Discussion on research into pain. *Practitioner,* **198**, 287 (1967)

feel he has to exaggerate his non-verbal communication to express his complaint. It is easy to see, therefore, that the judgements made must be tempered with reasoning, not dogma.

Some people speak with their arms or their facial expressions – they would be unable to express themselves adequately if they wore a mask or had their hands tied behind their back. Such methods of expression should not give the patient the label of being unacceptable if we, the therapists, have not seen much of this in our experience. The expressions should be accepted for what they are – a means of describing the story. Such over-expressions, if indeed they can be called this, are for some a national characteristic of an ethnic group, or it may be characteristic of some professional groups such as actors or artists.

Worries

There is another aspect which the investigating therapist should bear in mind. The patient may have apprehensions or fears relating to this experience of physiotherapy. The experience may be totally new to him or he may have had other people tell him of their unhappy experiences. The patient may be very worried and apprehensive because the referring doctor may have used the dreaded word ARTHRITIS in his diagnosis, conjuring up thoughts in the patient's mind of wheelchairs and being bedridden. Another area of concern can be that the insurance company's referees may have said, 'There's nothing wrong with you physically, it's all psychological and you should go back to work'. The patient, while he knows or believes it is not psychological, then expects the encounter with the physiotherapist to be yet another distasteful experience.

Financial problems, loss of status, lack of understanding within the family situation, fear of the future because of the disability, are all things that can be factors of the patient's problem – 'the problem', as was stated earlier, 'being the effect the "disorder" has on him as a person'.

The above headings have presented but a few of the situations in which a patient may find himself, and which therapists should be sufficiently open minded about, and understanding of, throughout treatment, but especially from the first moment of a first consultation. I well realize that almost every therapist considers she does care for her patients in this way, but I'm afraid that the depth of her skill in caring is often ineffective in what it achieves in the relationship, and therefore the treatment.

Communication

Verbal and non-verbal communication is the means we have to 'get an idea as exactly as possible out of one mind and into another'[4].

On the verbal side of communication, besides the choice of words used there is the way they are said, the tone, the questioning etc. which adds quality to what is being said: 'He did load the tone of his voice with something of dignity which Mr Crawley might perhaps be excused for regarding as arrogance'[5].

On the non-verbal side of communication there is so much that can be said that a whole book, rather than part of a chapter in a book, could be given to it. Even quite minute nuances can be enormously informative. Yet not everyone has facial expressions that can be 'read', and these are difficult circumstances under which to work: 'Grace, who was still in front of him, could see the working of his face as he read it but even she could not tell whether he was gratified, or offended or dismayed'[6].

At this stage of discussion of the subject, it is important to say that although communication with a patient is a two-way affair, the main responsibilities for its effectiveness lies with the therapist rather than the patient. From the therapist's point of view she should be thinking of three things:

1. I should make every effort to be as sure as is possible that I understand what the patient is trying to tell me.
2. I should be ready to recognize, from the patient's communication, any gaps he leaves which I should endeavour to fill by asking appropriate questions.
3. I should make use of every possible opportunity to utilize my own non-verbal expressions to show my understanding and concern for him in his plight.

The patient, on the other hand, does not have these responsibilities, though many judgemental authorities would have it otherwise. It is the therapist's responsibility to be doing the work, not the patient's, and in the long term if there has been any misunderstanding between patient and therapist it is almost always the fault of the therapist, not the patient.

There are aspects of communication that have a general application in manipulative physiotherapy treatment, and there are aspects that particularly relate to certain areas of the management such as the history taking, the assessment of the effect of treatment the site and behaviour of the patient's symptoms and so on. The general aspects will be

4. Gowers, E. *The Complete Plain Words,* 3rd edn (revised by S. Greenbaum and J. Whitcut), Harmondsworth, Penguin Books (1987)
5. Trollope, A. *The Last Chronicle of Barset,* Pan Books, London, p. 139 (1967)
6. Trollope, A. *The Last Chronicle of Barset,* Pan Books, London, p. 839 (1967)

discussed in this chapter, and the skills associated with the different areas of management will be discussed in their separate chapters.

Communication – General
Verbal communication

The first thing to remember is that the therapist should pronounce and use words in the same way as the patient uses them. When this is not possible because the pronunciation is so wrong, the word should be avoided, certainly it should not be pronounced in a way that would make the patient feel he is being shown up as being ignorant.

Probably the primary requirement of all communication, but particularly for the patient and physiotherapist, is that the listener should correctly interpret what the speaker is saying – correctly, that is, in knowing what the speaker is trying to portray. The difficulties in this process are many and they can nearly all be overcome if the therapist keeps one thought in mind – ASSUME NOTHING.

However, to 'assume nothing' really means that once the therapist *thinks* she has understood the patient, she needs to confirm it by asking him, using her own words, if what she says is what he meant. However, to carry this out with every little issue is ridiculous, and will irritate the patient, even if it doesn't irritate and frustrate the therapist. However, as therapists learn from their experience, it will become obvious that there are many particular times when this verification must be made so as to avoid misunderstanding important issues.

Therapists should realize that it is not easy for a patient to put into words what it is he is trying to describe. In fact, it is the difficulty of this process that is the first area among many in which errors of communication occur (see Table 3.2).

Although Table 3.1 was used in the fifth edition of *Vertebral Manipulation*, its humour emphasizes its truth. ('Many a serious word is said in jest!') In reproducing it here I would ask the reader the question, 'What is the most important part of the jingle . . . and why?'

Table 3.1 Communication problems

> I know that you
> believe you
> understand what
> you think I said,
> **BUT,**
> I am not sure
> you realize that
> what you heard
> is not
> what I meant

The answer to 'what is the most important part of the jingle' lies in the last three lines, and especially the part 'is not what I meant'. The reason why it is the most important part has already been referred to – each of us at times attempts to describe something, such as an emotion or an experience, yet fail because of the difficulty in finding the right words to express it. Therefore when such an error does occur, we should not blame the patient: instead, think of the number of times we have failed in this one area of 'not being able to say what we mean'.

The next area of folly is the therapist not listening to what the patient has said. This tends to occur later, rather than earlier in a consultation because as time goes on, the therapist may have made up her mind about certain things relating to the patient. Thus she may well hear what she expects to hear rather than listen to the words the patient uses (see Table 3.2). The following quotation is worthy of repetition:

> 'Listening is itself, of course, an art: that is where it differs from merely hearing. Hearing is passive; listening is active. Hearing is involuntary; listening demands attention. Hearing is natural; listening is an acquired discipline'. (*The Age*, August, 1982)

Having heard and listened to what the patient has had to say, the therapist's interpretation of what was said may not be the same as the patient meant, as quoted in the jingle above. If the issue being talked about is important then the rule for the therapist

Table 3.2 Sequential errors in communication

> *The patient:*
>   Difficulty expressing in words what he is attempting to describe
>
> *The therapist:*
>   (a) Being influenced by previous judgements, although hearing what he says, misinterprets because she does not *listen* to what he says
>   (b) Her interpretation of what he said may be incorrect
>
>   ASSUME NOTHING – CONFIRM
>
>   (c) Her wording of the question may not express what it is she is wanting to know
>
> *The patient:*
>   (a) Being influenced by previous experiences he mishears therapist's words
>   (b) Even if he has listened, his interpretation of what she has said may be incorrect
>
>   PATIENTS DO ASSUME – AND THEY DO NOT USUALLY CONFIRM
>
>   (c) His wording of his reply may not express what it is he is attempting to express

'assume nothing', should be invoked and the interpretation should be 'confirmed'. During the interview, if the interpretation of the patient's comment has been correct the comment will probably lead the therapist to ask a related question. In doing so, she has to work out in her own mind how to express the question in words that the patient will be able to understand. The question should be expressed as *simply* as possible and it should be as *short* as possible.

Avoid asking two questions in one sentence and although the question should be as short as possible it should not be curt or spoken bluntly.

An error that can occur in this process is that the words and phrasing of the therapist's question may not exactly express what it is she is wanting to know (Table 3.2). If however the thoughts are expressed accurately, the next problem, as listed in Table 3.2, is does the patient 'listen' with an open mind and does he interpret the question properly? If he does, he then has to go through the same processes of thinking about his answer and thinking about how to express it so that it will be understood.

This then brings us back to the beginning of Table 3.2. It is easy to see that in the process of asking just one question and getting a meaningful reply, there are many areas where misunderstandings can take place.

The fault is ours

In relation to the concept that this book endeavours to portray, there is a very important approach, or attitude, to the situation when the patient has not answered the question for any one of the reasons discussed. The error becomes evident when the patient's answer does not relate to the question asked by the therapist. The concept rules that the therapist should accept that the error has occurred because of the way she has asked the question and that the misinterpretation is her mistake and *not* the patient's. If, then, the therapist merely repeats the question using the *same* words, she is insulting the patient. She should:

1. Apologize for giving the wrong impression of what the question was about.
2. Rephrase the question after saying 'I'm sorry – what I really meant was . . . ?'

Pausing

A general rule that is worth cultivating is either to speak slowly, or, better still, to allow pauses of sufficient duration so that the patient has enough time to think about what is being said. There is a natural time-span between hearing something being said, listening to its precision, and interpreting its meaning. If there are other factors that bring stress or worry into the patient's situation, the time required for the transposition is longer. When waiting for the answer to a question, time should be allowed for the patient to relate the question to his own 'frame of reference' and to his 'disorder' before thinking out his answer. He then has to think how best to say it so as to give the relative answer to the question he thinks he is being asked.

He may even be allowed time for considering the reasons why he thinks the therapist is asking the question she is – does it have a hidden purpose or a double meaning?

Quality of voice

In non-verbal communication, there are nuances of behaviour and elements of body language which speak for themselves. So, too, in the spoken word, the quality of voice can give indications of how strongly the patient feels about answers to certain questions. His tone may be harsh, the answer blunt and curt, or he may carry on quite a tirade which shows the therapist exactly how he feels.

The patient may put stress on certain parts of his description of his symptoms to inform the therapist of his feelings about their importance.

The therapist can also make use of tone, etc. For example, 'How important is it TO YOU (louder for emphasis) . . . pause (for the emphasis to be further emphasized) . . . that you be able to sit for longer periods without pain in your hip?'

In other words, it is not only *what* is said, but *how* it is said.

Non-verbal communication

Non-verbal communication does not refer to the tone and quality of the sounds being produced when using words to communicate, but rather to the nuances of behaviour that accompany (or replace) the words; the raised eyebrows, the tilt of the head, the scowl or frown. Not only are these nuances expressive of the emotion that lies behind the accompanying words, but generally, especially if they are quick reflexive responses, they can be trusted more than can the accompanying words. The following quotations are interesting examples of non-verbal messages taken from novels:

'Her mouth was set in grooves of dull belligerence'[7].

'His face went through the motions of remembering'[7].

7. MacDonald, R. *Black Money,* Collins Fontana Books, London, pp. 107, 105 respectively (1970)

'The question took him by surprise. For a moment his face was trying on attitudes. It settled on a kind of false boredom behind which his intelligence sat and watched me'[8].

Conflict

Non-verbal nuances do not always fit with the verbal discourse, and when this is so, some plan should be implemented to attempt either to make them agree or to find reasons why they do not agree. The speed of the non-verbal response has been referred to already in relation to its reliability, but sometimes people deliberately use nuances to their own advantage. This possibility should not be discounted, especially if they affect treatment decisions or influence the forming of judgements.

The therapist can also use her own non-verbal communication to good effect. At the outset of this chapter, the importance of gaining the patient's confidence and making him aware of the therapist's honesty and concern for his welfare during the first moments of an initial consultation was emphasized. It could be said that for the first 15 minutes of that initial consultation, the therapist should consciously use non-verbal communication and verbal expression to demonstrate that honesty and concern. Obviously it should be expressive throughout every stage of treatment, and it would hopefully be natural, instinctive and not requiring any conscious effort. After all, there is only one thing worse than treating an unemotional, unexpressive 'dead-pan' patient, and that is being treated by an unemotional, unexpressive, 'dead-pan' therapist. Nevertheless it is necessary to be sure that the right messages are read by the patient, and this may require conscious effort and even over-expression by the therapist. The same applies during a retrospective-assessment session when the reasons for treatment reaching a stage when symptoms have plateaued during treatment are being sought.

A very good text for learning more about non-verbal communication is *Bodily Communication*[9]. The book also contains a very useful bibliography.

As in verbal communication, a person's non-verbal communication is influenced by environmental factors as well as genetic factors. This applies equally to patients and therapists. So, once again, differences in 'frames-of-reference' have to be appreciated and an attempt made by the therapist to understand the patient as a person and so understand the basis of his non-verbal expressions. Where favourable she should use nuances that are compatible with the patient's.

Questions

There are other important aspects of communication which have a general application. Each relates to gaining the maximum in depth and quality from an interview other than that which can be gained by the simple process of questions and answers. They are:

1. Paralleling.
2. Keying.
3. Biasing.
4. Immediate response.

Paralleling

When the patient is answering a question, his mind goes through a process of sorting through his relevant information, and in doing so establishes a line of thought, and highlights information in a sequence of importance. It is important, therefore, to make use of this process by following his line of thought with related follow-up questions. By doing this, points that may seem minor, and perhaps even irrelevant, will be expressed which may otherwise be lost: certainly the degree of importance they bear to the patient will never be known by the therapist. To interrupt his train of thought in mid-flight, so to speak, and ask a different question quite unrelated to his current state of thinking will lose an important advantage.

Paralleling is not an easy skill for the beginner to use because it requires experience of many interviews:

1. To know what the questions are that she wants answers to by the end of the interview.
2. To be able to retain the answers to the questions in the paralleling process without losing the other questions she wants answers to which are not parallel with the patient's current line of thought.

It is vital that the therapist should not lose control of finding out what she wants to know, and so initially she may need to sacrifice the invaluable gains from paralleling to keep that control. Nevertheless the gains in knowing the importance of things as they appear to the patient are so great that at times the 'control' should be sacrificed in preference for the 'gains' from paralleling.

Keying or key words and phrases

Frequently, during a patient's discourse he will make a statement or use a word that could have great significance – *he* may not realize it, but the

8. Ludlum, R. *The Aquitaine Progression,* Granada Publishing, London, pp. 106, 47 (1984)
9. Argyle, M. *Bodily Communication,* Methuen, London (1975)

therapist must latch onto it while the patient's thoughts are moving along his chosen path. She should use it immediately either by waiting until he has finished his sentence or by interjecting. For example, she might say:

Q 'You just mentioned your mother's birthday – what does that relate to?'
A 'Well, I can remember that it was on my mother's birthday that I first realized I was aware of discomfort in my shoulder when I reached across the table to pick up her birthday cake.'

By instantly making use of his train of thought (paralleling) the development of the progressive history of that patient's shoulder pain is easier to determine for both the therapist and the patient, because, in fact, his mind is clearly back at the birthday party.

Biasing

It is very easy to fall into the trap of asking a question in such a way that the patient is influenced to answer in a particular way. For example, the therapist may wish to know whether the last two treatments have caused any change in the patient's symptoms. The question can be asked in three ways:

Q1 'Do you feel that the last two treatments have helped you?'
Q2 'Has there been any change in your symptoms as a result of the last two treatments?'
Q3 'Have the last two treatments made you any worse in any way?'

The second or third questions are acceptable because if the therapist is hoping there has been some favourable change, the patient's answer, if he has improved, will be reliable. Question 2 has no bias and question 3 biases the patient away from a favourable answer. Question 1 on the other hand influences him towards his replying 'Yes'.

Immediate-response questions

This section relates to responding to statements that are made by the patient. During treatment sessions when the patient is being asked questions he may word his reply in a way that is either not complete, or is ambiguous. For example, he may say he is 'better'. Statements such as this call for an immediate-response question – 'Better than when?' or 'Better than what?' The patient's statement of 'better' can be misinterpreted unless it is qualified. He may have been worse from the treatment, but he is 'better' than that now, or he may be 'better' than when he first started treatment.

There are many times when immediate-response is called for, but mostly they arise during the assessment of changes that may take place as a result of treatment.

Examples will be given in the relevant chapter in dialogue form with explanations as to why the 'immediate-response' question is called for.

In summary

The importance of the relationship between patient and therapist cannot be over-emphasized, nor can the importance of the role that communication has, in establishing the most favourable relationship, be over-emphasized. Probably if the therapist learns to communicate, and believe in the patient, and shows this belief by skilful use of non-verbal communication with the verbal communication, she will achieve much.

Although there are many important areas that work together to make up successful manipulative physiotherapy, communication has not, in the past, been given adequate attention. This must change.

4

Examination

When a patient with skeletal pain consults his doctor, the examination includes many tests which do not concern us here. However, if this patient is then referred for physiotherapy the minute details of joint examination immediately become the physiotherapist's concern.

Although physical examination of posture, deformity and muscle length, strength and assessment of other joints are important, the detail of their examination will be omitted from the following discussion so that emphasis can be placed on the examination directly concerned with treatment by passive movement.

The examination can be divided into subjective examination (that part of the examination related to learning what the patient's problems are) and objective examination (the physical findings). In subjective examination the information being sought is what *the patient* feels his problems are and in what structures the therapist feels the causes of these problems might be. During the subjective questions and answers, there are two parts.

The first is making sure that the points made by the patient are understood and that there is no misinterpretation of what he feels his problems are. If there is a mixture of complaints, the relationship between them needs to be established and appreciated by both patient and therapist. The aspect that must be stressed here is that the therapist should see the problem *in the patient's terms*.

The second part of the subjective examination is orientated around asking the patient specific questions which are going to assist in determining:

1. The functions that are at fault in anatomical and pathological terms.
2. Determining the diagnosis in terms of its stage of progression and its stability.

Once this stage has been reached the therapist can plan what she feels needs to be examined physically.

Subjective examination

It may seem impertinent and childish to state specific dialogues to be used under certain circumstances. However, experience teaches how to ask questions in such a way that ambiguities and misunderstandings are avoided. With this in mind, the specific wording of some questions will be given (represented by the letter 'Q') together with the thoughts related to them (represented by the letters 'ET', examiner's thoughts). Any pertinent answers by the patient in the dialogue will be prefixed by the letter 'A', and 'S' for statement.

The patient's problem

At a first consultation it is the therapist's responsibility to establish a pleasant relationship with the patient so that he may feel at ease and feel an early confidence in the therapist. Once the initial introductions (learning how to pronounce the patient's name the way he pronounces it) and pleasantries have been completed the more serious and searching questions can begin.

Q 'As far as YOU are concerned . . . [pause] . . . what do YOU feel . . . [pause] . . . is YOUR MAIN PROBLEM?'

ET It is essential to establish that the patient should feel free to complain and be listened to. By emphasizing this first question in the way suggested, there can be no doubt in his mind that the therapist wants to know what *he* sees as his problem rather than what the doctor(s) has said about his problem.

The first part of the subjective examination aims at establishing the KIND of disorder from which the patient is suffering. Some suggestions of varieties of problems that might fall within the physiotherapist's field of expertise are as follows:

1. Establish the 'kind' of disorder.
2. Why has the patient sought treatment, or been referred for treatment:
   (a) Pain.
   (b) Stiffness.
   (c) Giving way.
   (d) Instability.
   (e) Weakness.
   (f) Loss of function.
   (g) After:
      (i)   trauma;
      (ii) surgery;
      (iii) manipulation under anaesthesia; or
      (iv) hospitalized traction;
      (v)   plaster following fracture;
      (vi) dislocation.
   (h) Differential diagnosis.

Having asked the question quoted above, the patient's answer may establish the KIND of disorder, or it may give information that guides the therapist's line of questioning needed to establish the KIND of disorder.

A 'My knee frequently lets me down.'
ET This could be an instability situation or a pain inhibition. To avoid influencing his answer by asking 'is it painful when it lets you down?' the unbiased question is:
Q 'Do you know why it lets you down?' Or 'In what way does it let you down?' Then:
Q 'Do you in fact drop to the ground?'

Once the patient has expressed his disorder as he sees it, and the therapist has established in her mind the KIND of disorder she is likely to be dealing with, she can follow one of three paths of thought:

1. The history of the disorder.
2. The behaviour of the disorder.
3. The diagnosis.

The choice is best guided by the patient, with the therapist using her skill and ability to parallel his line of thought (see page 18).

Most patients referred to physiotherapists have pain as their main problem and so it becomes necessary to establish the area, nature and behaviour of the patient's pain.

Components

Pain presents in many different manners as well as sites. A patient may have a dull but constant ache in a certain area as well as having a sharp stabbing pain in the same area on certain movements. This becomes easy to accept when it is realized that a fall, for example, injures more than one structure associated with a joint. Each structure may respond to the injury with different kinds of pain.

Therefore, when questioning the patient regarding his symptoms, the possibilities of different components in the disorder must always be kept uppermost in mind.

Area

In the search for the area of pain the findings should be as precise as possible because they form the foundation on which the examination is built. If the area overlies a joint, the patient should be asked specifically if his pain is 'within' the joint, if necessary grasping the joint firmly, surrounding it while asking if the pain is 'deep inside'.

There may be more than one site of pain. For example, a patient may have a painful foot which causes pain and makes him limp. Though he may say in answer to the initial question that this pain is in his foot, more detailed interrogation may reveal that he has three sites of pain; one along the medial side of his foot, a second area along the lateral border of the foot, and a third site which he describes as being through and inside his ankle.

Failure to ascertain such details will lessen the effectiveness of examination, assessment and treatment.

If a patient has sustained an injury, or if the history of the disorder has indicated that structures elsewhere than his main complaint may be affected, he should be questioned about related sites (see Table 4.4, part A3, page 30). If they are symptom free they should be designated as such by a tick ($\sqrt{}$) on the body chart (Figure 4.1).

Any area of paraesthesia or anaesthesia should be marked on the body chart used to outline the areas of pain (Figure 4.1).

Behaviour

In relation to the 'behaviour' of the pain the patient should be asked to describe his pain (sharp, dull, throbbing, constant, variable or intermittent) and whether all areas of the pain occur simultaneously or whether different actions or positions reproduce different pains (Table 4.1).

It is essential to know which is the main area of pain and what particular movements provoke it; whether the joint is painful while at rest, whether the resting pain is caused by some mechanical

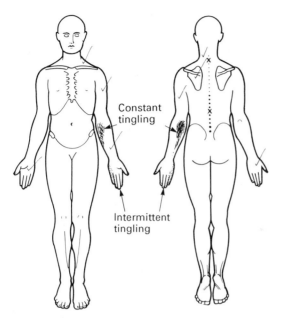

Constant
tingling

Intermittent
tingling

Figure 4.1 Body chart

whether it is pain or stiffness that is of greater concern to the patient.

Pain can behave in so many different ways. However, there are two aspects that are commonly not appreciated. The first is that the patient may be able to carry out a day's activity with minimal inconvenience, but finds that his pain develops *after* he stops these activities. A second variation can be that the pain only develops after a particular position has been adopted and maintained for some considerable period. It may develop following the sustaining of only one particular position or it may follow several different positions. A further example is evinced where a joint has been comfortably kept in a particular position for a length of time, then on moving from this position sudden sharp pain occurs. It may subside immediately, possibly leaving the patient pain free.

If the pain varies in any way (for example in area or intensity) an attempt should be made to find out what particular activities provoke the pain and how long the increased symptoms take to subside. If the patient's pain is only intermittent, its frequency and duration should also be determined.

'Behaviour' of the symptoms is important because the physiotherapist must know how and why the pain varies throughout a 24-hour period.

These differences of pain pattern must have some significance in relation to diagnosis but it is doubtful whether anyone as yet knows the reasons for the different patterns, and unfortunately there are physiotherapists who are unaware that pain can

degree of stretch or compression affecting the joint, or whether by an active inflammatory process. If the joint is painful only when moved or exercised, the offending movements must be determined and the differences in the various directions of movement appreciated. Furthermore, it must be determined

Table 4.1 Initial questions to ask before asking the more direct questions

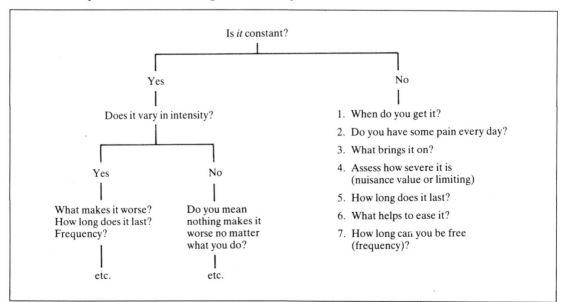

behave in so many ways. This leads to incomplete examination followed in turn by an incomplete understanding of the patient's problem.

When the pain is aggravated by movements the patient should be asked to demonstrate the way in which he is restricted by the pain. Analysis of the movement then forms a primary part of the objective examination. It is also useful to know whether there are any positions he can adopt that aggravate or relieve the symptoms. Analysis can be left until the objective examination is begun if it breaks the examiner's train of thought to do it at the time of the demonstration.

Irritability

This term has a very specific definition, and purpose, in this book; the word is not used lightly or loosely. Irritability relates to a particular aspect of the behaviour of the patient's symptoms and it should be determined for every patient at the initial consultation. Its importance lies in the fact that if it is not determined as a separate entity, the physiotherapist may negligently carry out too extensive a consultation, resulting in an exacerbation.

'Irritability' is determined by relating the vigour of an activity that causes pain, firstly to the degree of pain that ensues, and then to the length of time taken for this increased pain to subside to its prior level (see Table 4.4, part B2, page 30).

Two examples may provide useful comparisons. Firstly, a schoolteacher with shoulder pain is unable to write more than a few lines on the lower part of the blackboard without experiencing moderate pain which continues for more than an hour. This joint condition is irritable; it takes very little activity to cause considerable pain which takes a long time to subside. For this reason the patient should not be subjected to prolonged examination of painful movements because of the inevitable exacerbation. Treatment by passive movement in this instance must be gentle and the amplitude of movements used should be small. A second example is a patient who notices sharp momentary shoulder pain only if he mis-hits a drive at golf, or sustains similar jarring. This condition is not irritable, and to determine the joint signs by which treatment can be guided examination of his passive movements would probably need to be taken to the limit of the range and the various movements tested in finer detail and with greater strengths than with the first-mentioned patient. Also, treatment would probably require more vigour than the first patient's shoulder could tolerate.

The purpose of assessing irritability is to try to discern just how much movement the patient's disorder can be subjected to without causing an exacerbation.

At the first consultation, in relation to the three elements of irritability, it should be realized that this estimate is related by the patient *to his activities*. However, the patient's activities and the therapist's examination and treatment are not always easy to relate to each other because passive movements are not protected so much as are his activities.

At the second consultation the irritability can be re-evaluated in relation to the first consultation's examination and treatment. By the third consultation the irritability can be directly associated with the passive movement treatment – and it is this evaluation that is the information that the therapist is striving to assess from the first consultation:

1. *Irritability at first consultation*: Related to patient's activities.
2. *Irritability at second consultation*: Related to examination and treatment at first consultation.
3. *Irritability at third consultation*: The sought-after irritability, related to passive movement treatment only.

When referring to the irritability component of the patient's disorder (or discussing it in front of the patient) it is important to make it clear that it is the irritability of the disorder that is being discussed, not the irritability of the patient. It may seem a facetious comment to make; however, when using the word in front of the patient, make it quite clear that it is the irritability of the disorder being stated otherwise the patient is almost certain to think that the therapist believes that it is he who is irritable; he will not like that inference.

'Irritability' has two other valuable uses. Firstly, assessment of joint irritability provides details by which progress can be assessed from treatment to treatment. During the treatment, discussion of the progress of the irritability being made can benefit both physiotherapist and patient. Assessment, which forms a vital role in treatment, will be discussed later.

The other reason for assessing joint irritability lies in its relation to treatment. This will be considered later, as it has an important bearing on the type of movement chosen for a technique.

Nature

Table 4.4 (part B3, see page 30) refers to situations which, by virtue of their 'nature', may limit how such objective examination and treatment can be carried out. The word 'nature', in the context of this text, needs a degree of explanation:

1. Each patient has his own personality and character which must be recognized. Some people are stoics, others may tend to complain excessively. The patient of the latter kind cannot be treated vigorously. The stoic, on the other hand, is difficult to treat most effectively

because he does not complain soon enough (if at all). It is so easy to over-treat him because he does not talk about what he feels during treatment. Similarly, treatment can be too gentle and thus be ineffective because of this lack of feedback.

2. Pain threshold, and pain acceptance, can be high or low. The person with a low pain threshold has to be treated with the greatest of care. The firmness of the technique that may be required may be more than the patient can accept, so the progress towards this firmness will be slow.

3. Some patients are hostile towards the medical system – and here again the communication and the treatment technique have to be modified to suit the patient first, and then suit the disorder.

This next group of 'nature' considerations relates to the family unit:

4. Different ethnic groups and different social groups have different ways of expressing and handling their symptoms.

5. There may well be a familial or genetic component in his disorder. This applies more to the 'spontaneous-onset' group than to the 'traumatic-onset' group. Nevertheless a patient may have an injury superimposed on familial factors.

6. A patient may be a 'slow-healer' and this possibility should be considered.

7. Occasionally a patient is a member of a family which has a tendency towards exotic disorders rather than the predictable complaints.

The last groups relate more to the 'kind of disorder' or the diagnosis. Such things as:

8. Stability of the disorder.

9. Episodic disorder (its present stage in progression).

10. Active inflammatory disorder.

History

History taking is a skill that one develops with experience based on the knowledge required to relate the behaviour of a patient's complaint to theoretical neuro/musculo/skeletal knowledge and an understanding of pathology. At what stage the taking of the history fits into the subjective examination should be quite flexible. It will depend partly on the therapist's experience, partly upon the patient's statements and answers concerning his main problem, and upon whether the problem has had an insidious or traumatic onset. In the 'spontaneous' group it is necessary to determine how long it took to develop and the manner in which it developed. In the trauma group, where possible,

the manner and extent of the trauma should be ascertained, thus enabling an idea of which structures have been damaged and how extensively they have been damaged.

The therapist's experience – The therapist must not lose track of the discussion with the patient. The more experience the therapist has had, the freer her mind is to mix questions relating to the presentations of the disorder with those of the history.

Patient's comments – While asking the patient the opening questions he may immediately start talking about an incident that occurred 6 months ago. This gives the therapist the opportunity of paralleling (see page 18) his line of thought and thus gaining the advantage of learning subtle facts about the onset which she may miss if she does not start the consultation with the history.

Insidious onset – It is frequently necessary to know something, or everything, about the behaviour of the patient's symptoms so as to know what questions to ask which relate to the history. This is particularly so with the chronic disorders of insidious onset. Obviously this means leaving the history aspect until near the end of the subjective examination.

To save time, the present history should be sought before any previous history, but this is not an inflexible rule.

Acceptability

The obvious goal of history taking is both to make a diagnosis and to understand the extent the disorder has on the patient. Five determinations need to be made:

1. What is the extent of the disability in the patient's terms?

2. What does the disorder prevent the patient from doing? Or

3. What 'price' does the patient have to 'pay' (in terms of pain or disability) *after* performing any particular activities or adopting any particular sustained positions?

4. What is the present stage and the present stability of the disorder?

5. (a) Is it pain, or stiffness or a combination of both (or weakness, or instability) that prevents the patient from being normal? (b) If both pain and stiffness are present which is dominant?

Within these goals, the patient's story of the history has to make sense. For example, if he relates a trivial incident as being the cause of what seems to be a gross disability, then there has to be something else (which the therapist should seek out) to make the trivial incident acceptable. The trivial incident may be just 'the last straw which broke the camel's back'; the 'something else' may be the strain or overuse situation, or it may have underlying pathology:

1. Sprain.
2. Strain.
3. Overuse.
4. Misuse.
5. New Use.
6. Abuse.
7. Disuse.
8. Joint locking.
9. Sub-clinical disorders.

The questioning skill comes from knowing to what extent strain and overuse etc. can predispose to breakdown and symptoms, and also to know the effects of pathological disorders. There may be other predisposing factors in the history of a patient's disorder such as having a genetic or familial predisposition, or he may be a person who always takes longer to 'get over' any sickness he has had. There may be a vital involvement; his general health may be poor or he may be excessively tired. There is the possibility of a previous injury (many years previously) which predisposes him to the present disorder. No stone should be left unturned to make the history match the disability. The predisposing factors are as follows:

1. Familial.
2. Genetic.
3. Unusual or new activity.
4. Sustained posture.
5. Virus.
6. Slow healer.
7. Fatigue.
8. General health.
9. The possibility of an injury many years ago causing the current symptoms.

Questions should be asked to determine which structures might be involved in the disorder as outlined below:

1. Intra-articular.
2. Capsular.
3. Ligamentous.
4. Tendon of attachment to bone or ligament.
5. Tendon of attachment to muscle.

Above all else the following rule should be kept in mind:

> ## MAKE FEATURES FIT

The history has to be acceptable in relation to what is determined about the behaviour of the symptoms. After the subjective examination, the history also has to match what is found during the physical examination. Similarly the history has to match any medical tests such as X-rays, blood tests, internal examinations, etc. All of these elements must fit with what the patient feels is his problem.

The history of patients who are referred for treatment by physiotherapy can be very loosely grouped into two categories:

1. There are those whose symptoms are chronic or have developed spontaneously without the patient really knowing why or how. The therapist may uncover a trivial incident that had occurred, whereas the patient had forgotten about it because it *was* so trivial. Another alternative is that predisposing elements may exist, and that it is on this predisposing situation that the current disorder has developed.
2. The second category is quite different in that the presenting disorder is the direct result of trauma.

1. The chronic and spontaneous onset group

The progression of the disorders in this group should be sought in depth if the state and stage of the disorder can be reasonably understood. The depth of questioning is given in an example which follows. The dialogue form is used to reinforce the information contained in Chapter 3.

This true story that follows concerns a 74-year-old lady who asked her medical specialist to refer her for physiotherapy. She had considerable shoulder pain which was preventing her sleeping. X-rays of her shoulder showed gross osteoarthritic changes with a complete loss of joint space. She could only lift her arm to shoulder level. The specialist felt that excision of the head of the humerus was the required treatment, but as physiotherapy was unlikely to do her any harm he acceded to her request.

There were faults in her medical examination which would not have occurred if the following concepts taught in this text were applied.

(i) Present history

She had only had her present degree of pain for a period of 6 weeks:

Q1 'Mrs Smith, as far as YOU are concerned, what do YOU feel, at this stage, is YOUR MAIN problem?'

ET I want to know what *she* is seeking treatment for; what does *she* want to get better from?

A 'It's this pain in my shoulder. I get it mainly at night, I can't get comfortable and it stops me from sleeping normally.'

ET At this point there are two paths to take. Shall I find out where precisely the pain is or shall I seek 'history'? To seek the site of pain will be paralleling her thinking so it would probably be more valuable to sort this out first.

Q   'Can you show me where you feel this pain?'

And so the questioning goes on until we find out that she feels it within her glenohumeral joint.

ET   Having found the site of pain, the history can be sought.

Q   'How did IT start Mrs Smith?'

ET   By using the word 'IT', Mrs Smith is given a free rein to let her mind wander to what she spontaneously feels about the onset. That is she can think about time, she can think about incidents that may have started it off. She may drift into talking about 'previous history' if *she* feels it is more relevant.

A   'I suppose I've had it for about 6 weeks now.'

ET   This tends to indicate that there was not any specific incident on any specific day that triggered it off; however, I should endeavour to confirm this line of assumption.

Q   'Did it come on suddenly one day or did it take a week or so to develop?'

A   'No, it came on fairly quickly.'

ET   'Fairly quickly' is not precise enough and so demands an 'immediate response question'.

Q   'By fairly quickly, do you mean you didn't have it one day but did have it the next day?'

A   'Yes, that's right, it came on one day.'

ET   Now, does this mean she probably had an incident which caused it on that one day or may she have done something the day before without really noticing anything, but wakened with the pain that night or on first getting out of bed in the morning. In other words, was it an AFTER-effect or was it a painful incident?

Q   'Can you remember what day it was when you first felt it?'

A   'Yes I can because it was my son's birthday, it was on a Friday, August the twenty seventh, that's his birthday.'

Q   'Do you remember whether the pain came on when you first got up or was it later in the day?'

A   'Aw now you're asking me something: I don't really remember as far back as that . . . wait a minute . . . I remember . . . it was when I was taking a chocolate cake out of the oven that I first felt it.'

Q   'Did you drop the cake?'

ET   I hope she didn't, not a *chocolate* cake.

A   'No, it just hurt in my shoulder a bit.'

Q   'What was IT like for the rest of the day?'

ET   Using 'IT', again leaves the opening for emphasis in Mrs Smith's thoughts.

A   'No, I didn't feel much for the rest of the day, but of course, having the party for my son

kept my mind occupied – no, I noticed it more when I went to bed.'

ET   Now I want to know the progress of the symptom-history . . . how quickly and how severely did the symptoms develop?

Q   'Was it when you first went to bed or did it waken you later in the night?'

A   'Yes.'

ET   'Yes' what. Being elderly it is likely to be the latter so I'll confirm by asking the opposite; that is, I'll bias it opposite to my supposition.

Q   'You mean you noticed it when you first went to bed?'

A   'No I was all right when I first went to bed.'

Q   'So when did you first feel it?'

A   'It wakened me after I had been in bed for a while. I had been asleep and it wakened me when I turned over in bed.'

ET   This is a good example of 'confirming' what turned out to be a wrong assumption. Really though, does it matter when and how it starts? Yes it does. The more a therapist can understand about the development of the symptoms the more chance she has to learn about the choice of treatment and its predictability. A short cut to finding out the progression of the symptoms would be to say the following.

Q   'What are the night-time symptoms like now compared with the first night?'

A   'I think they're very much the same.'

ET   Confirm.

Q   'So do you mean that over the intervening 6 weeks it hasn't become any worse?'

A   'No – I mean yes; sorry – it hasn't got any worse.'

(ii) Previous history

Q   'Have you had trouble like this with your shoulder before?'

ET   By saying 'like this' her line of thought can be manoeuvred which may save time. If it doesn't, then other questions will have to be asked.

A   'No, not like this; I've always had 'the arthritis' in it, but not pain like this. I can't remember when I could ever get my arm above my head – my mother had 'the arthritis' too, but hers was in her leg.'

ET   Interesting information (familial component?), definitely useful and didn't have to be sought.

Confirm and clarify the range of movement.

Q   'So the fact that you can't lift your arm up high is not new?' OR
'Could you lift it ANY higher than now than, let's say, 3 months ago?'

A 'Oh, yes, I could get it a fraction higher but not much.'

Q 'How much – can you show me with your other arm?'

It turns out to be a matter of about five degrees difference.

ET Very interesting in that it seems as though her present problem can almost be isolated from her longstanding osteoarthritic disorder. The aim of the physical examination will be to determine the relationship of the behaviour of the pain during movement to the available range of movement – is it an 'end-of-range pain' or a 'through-range pain'?

Question: Is the reader able to see that, by delving into the history at depth, the radiological changes are put into a different context to the referring doctor's context and that probably surgical excision of the head of the humerus is not the first treatment of choice? In fact the goal of treatment changes from (a) providing her with a greater range, (but this is not what she wants), to (b) getting rid of her pain (irrespective of whether the range changes) so she can sleep normally again.

2. The trauma group

The history of disorders caused by trauma can be considered in two very loose groups. The first group is one that results from major trauma such as falling from a ladder or being in a vehicular accident. The second, usually related to competitive sport, has a history of a stronger effort added to an accustomed repetitive action, such as the throwing action of a baseball pitcher.

(i) Major trauma

The history to be sought under these circumstances includes:

1. How extensive was the injuring force?
2. How much bruising resulted?
3. Where was the bruising?
4. Was there any swelling?
5. What colour was the swelling?
6. How quickly did it swell?

When injuries occur during competitive sport, information regarding the direction of the injuring force and the immediate resulting disability should be sought in detail.

(ii) Minor trauma

The history of these usually has, what may seem at first, to be a comparatively minor incident, when related to the severity of the disability. The injuring incident is usually superimposed on a predisposition. This predisposition may have a familial/genetic base. However, it is more common for it to have an excessive repetitive action as its base. The example of the baseball pitcher was given above. Here there is an 'over-use' situation (repetitive pitching during training and competitions) as a base, onto which the pitcher tries to pitch harder, resulting in sudden pain from the extra effort. This harder pitch is an extra over-use, or abuse, superimposed on a pre-existing over-use state. The human body has an enormous potential to adapt to demands, but it still has its limits.

The depth of detail of the history under the above circumstances needs to be such that the therapist can have an understanding of the possible degree of 'wear and tear' which existed before the injuring effort exceeded the human body's limit. This knowledge gives many clues as to how speedily the existing complaint can be relieved and how much relief can be expected. It also provides the details related to likely recurrences and prognosis.

Although the foregoing has been related to injuries from sport, it applies equally to the manual labourer or home gardener.

It should be ascertained whether the patient considers his symptoms are improving, worsening or static. As 'assessment' is the fulcrum about which the whole treatment programme is conducted, the importance of minute details regarding the patient's symptoms and their variations can be appreciated.

Routinely, a patient should be questioned regarding his general health and whether any particular tablets are being taken so that their possible effect may be appreciated and any dangers to treatment revealed (Table 4.2).

Table 4.3 summarizes what needs to be known and the sequence used by novices during the subjective examination.

Planning the objective examination

From the point of view of teaching, it is helpful if the student completes a planning sheet (Table.4.4) before commencing the objective examination. By committing her thoughts and plans regarding the objective examination to paper, the novice helps the supervisor to follow her deliberations and thus to guide, correct and assist her.

Reference to the planning sheet shows four sections. Section A refers to the structures that need to be examined as the cause of the disorder. Section B provides facts relating to the patient's symptoms which should guide the therapist in knowing how these symptoms are likely to behave as a reaction to the first day's examination test movements and treatment. Section C requires the student to decide the strength with which test movements need to be performed and to show how easy or difficult the important test signs will be to find. In other words, if a patient has a mild ache generally in his foot following a 10-mile walk then all the answers to the questions in section B will lead the physiotherapist to the conclusion that her examination techniques will need to be 'moderately vigorous', thus avoiding a too-gentle examination routine which ends by revealing nothing. Similarly it also avoids doing too-vigorous examination techniques on a patient who has considerable pain and who would thus be subjected to exacerbation.

Table 4.2 History

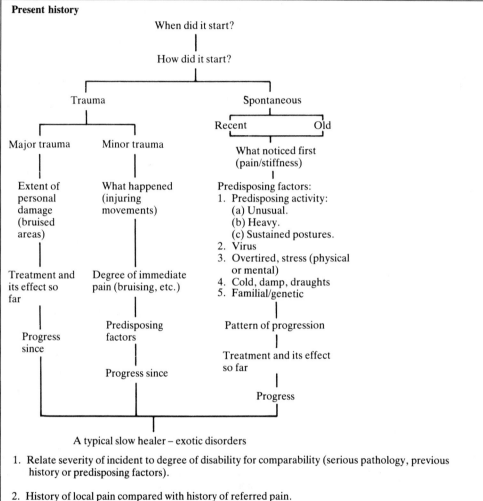

Present history

When did it start?

How did it start?

Trauma — Spontaneous

Recent — Old

Major trauma — Minor trauma

What noticed first (pain/stiffness)

Extent of personal damage (bruised areas)

What happened (injuring movements)

Predisposing factors:
1. Predisposing activity:
   (a) Unusual.
   (b) Heavy.
   (c) Sustained postures.
2. Virus
3. Overtired, stress (physical or mental)
4. Cold, damp, draughts
5. Familial/genetic

Treatment and its effect so far

Degree of immediate pain (bruising, etc.)

Pattern of progression

Progress since

Predisposing factors

Treatment and its effect so far

Progress since

Progress

A typical slow healer – exotic disorders

1. Relate severity of incident to degree of disability for comparability (serious pathology, previous history or predisposing factors).

2. History of local pain compared with history of referred pain.

3. Progress over initial period until 'levelling off' of symptoms.

Previous history

1. Related to this joint.

2. Related to relevant joints:
   (a) Other peripheral joints.
   (b) Vertebral column.

3. Related to other symptoms.

4. Medical history.

Table 4.3 Subjective examination

Beginning with the mandatory question

Kind of disorder
1. The patient's disorder in his terms.
2. The patient's demonstration.
3. Is the disorder one of pain, stiffness or both?

Kind of structures involved

Kind of changes in the structures

History or area
Record on the 'body chart':
1. Area and depth of pain, indicating areas of greatest intensity and stating type of symptoms.
2. Paraesthesia and anaesthesia.
3. Check associated areas, i.e.:
    (a) Of vertebral column.
    (b) Of joints 'above and below' the lesion.
    (c) Other relevant joints.

History or behaviour and symptoms
1. When are they present or when do they fluctuate? Constant, intermittent-frequency?
2. Any pain at night? Need to get up because of it? Able to lie on it? (Is the night pain for mechanical reasons or inflammatory?)
3. On first rising, c.f. end of day?
4. What aggravates, what eases?
5. Functional limitations (dominance of pain or stiffness).
6. Irritability.

History or Special questions
1. General health, relevant weight loss.
2. What tablets are being taken for this and other conditions? (Steroids, pain-killers, anti-inflammatory drugs.)

History
1. Of this attack.
2. Previous history.
3. Are the symptoms worsening or improving?
4. Any previous treatment? Effect?
5. Any contraindications?

HIGHLIGHT MAIN FINDINGS WITH ASTERISKS

Planning the examination

Section D is self-explanatory. It is a second aspect of examination, directed towards preventing recurrences rather than determining the painful structures. Its goals and intentions therefore are totally different from the previous sections and must be seen to be so. It is seeking the cause of the cause (or the cause that caused the *source* of the symptoms to become symptomatic). For example, a patient may have sprained his ankle badly. Sections A–C on the planning sheet will relate directly to treating the damaged structure, restoring range and thereby eliminating the pain. A separate and important aspect to the examination is directed towards preventing recurrences. Here section D of the planning comes into force. In the example above it relates directly to determining muscle weakness around the ankle from the point of view of its power and its speed of stabilizing action and to determining any other abnormalities that may lead to, or precipitate, a recurrence.

Objective examination

Before any movements are tested actively, the physiotherapist should have a clear appreciation of the disorder to know whether to limit tests movements and so avoid exacerbation. If the irritability of the disorder is high, it is far wiser to spread the examination over more than one visit, leaving the less important details of examination until later.

Treatment by passive movement is based on the examination findings of the movements of joints with all of their inert associated structures, and the neural structures, together with the knowledge of any pathology that may be present. An assessment of the patient's active movements should be made to ascertain his willingness and ability to move, and to gain measurements on which future assessments can be made.

Comparable sign/appropriate joint

When examining joint movement the primary aim is to find a 'comparable sign' at an 'appropriate joint'.

A joint sign refers to any aspect of movement of a joint that is abnormal. When dealing with musculo-skeletal problems these abnormal findings will be stiffness, pain, or muscle spasm. A 'comparable' joint or neural sign refers to a combination of pain, stiffness and spasm which the examiner finds on examination and considers to be comparable with the patient's symptoms. The comparability is most commonly linked with pain or protective muscle spasm.

Reproduce or produce?

In relation to pain being linked to comparability, the pain can be one of the following:

1. Reproducing the patient's pain with movement of the structures.
2. Producing a degree or kind of pain that is not the normal kind of discomfort that could be considered as an acceptable normal. However, this 'degree or kind of pain' must be at an appropriate joint for the patient's symptoms.

When pain is 'reproduced' by the test movements,

Table 4.4 Planning the objective examination

'Planning the objective examination' is part of the total examination procedure as a teaching medium to encourage clear, methodical and purposeful thinking.

PART ONE

A. The sources of the symptoms
1. Name as the *possible* sources of *any part* of the patient's symptoms *every* joint, muscle and neural interface which must be examined.

Joints that lie under the symptomatic area	*Joints* that refer symptoms into the area	*Muscles* that lie under the symptomatic area	Related *neural* sites

2. List points 'above and below' the lesion which should be checked, (when appropriate) ....

3. Are there any special tests indicated?
   (a) Neurological examination
   (b) Other – specify ....

B. Influence of symptoms and pathology on examination and first treatment
1. Is the pain 'severe'? *Yes/No* or 'latent'? *Yes/No*
2. Does the subjective examination suggest an easily irritable disorder?
   Local symptoms Yes/No, Referred/other symptoms Yes/No
   Give the example on which the answers are based.
   (a) *Local symptoms*
       Part (i)   Repeated MOVEMENT causing pain...
       Part (ii) Severity of pain so caused ....
       Part (iii) Duration before pain subsides...
   (b) *Referred/other symptoms*
       Part (i)   Repeated MOVEMENT causing pain...
       Part (ii) Severity of pain so caused ....
       Part (iii) Duration before pain subsides...
3. Does the 'Nature' of the disorder indicate caution   *Yes/No*
   (i) pathology/injury – specify..
   (ii) easy to provoke exacerbation or acute episode.
4. Are there any contraindications? *Yes/No* Specify...

C. The kind of examination
1. Do you think you will need to be gentle or moderately firm with your examination of movements?

2. Do you expect a 'comparable' sign $\left\{ \begin{array}{c} \text{to be easy} \\ \text{or} \\ \text{to be hard} \end{array} \right\}$ to find? – why?

3. What movements do you anticipate to be 'comparable'?

*   *   *   *   *   *   *

PART TWO

D. Associated examination
1. Provocative 'neuro/musculo/skeletal/medical' factors leading to the cause of the symptoms.
   What associated factors must be examined
   (a) as reasons why the joint, muscle or other structure has become symptomatic
   and/or
   (b) Why the disorder may recur? (e.g. posture, muscle imbalance, muscle power, obesity, stiffness, hypermobility, instability, deformity in proximal or distal joint, etc.)...
2. The effect of the disorder on joint stability ....

E. Treatment
1. In planning the TREATMENT (after the examination), what advice should be included and/or measures would you use to prevent or lessen recurrences?
2. Do you expect to be treating pain, resistance, weakness or instability?

AN ALTERNATIVE TO SECTION 'C'

The following text is a useful substitute for part 'C'. It helps both teacher and novice.

C. THE KIND OF EXAMINATION

1. At which point(s) under each of the following headings will you *limit* your objective examination? Circle the relevant description.

Symptoms

Local Pain	Referred Pain	Paraesthesia Anaesthesia	Dizziness	Extent of Objective Tests
–	Short of P_1	Short of symptom $prod^n$	Short of D_1	Active movement short of limit
point of onset or point of increase of resting symptoms	point of onset or point of increase of resting sysmptoms	point of onset or point of increase of resting symptoms	point of onset or point of increase of dizziness	active limit of movement
partial reproduction	partial reproduction	partial reproduction of symptoms	partial reproduction of dizziness	active limit plus over-pressure
total reproduction	total reproduction	–	–	'when applicable tests'

2. Do you expect a comparable sign to be easy/hard to find? Why?
3. **DOES THE SUBJECTIVE EXAMINATION SUGGEST THAT:**
   (a) The symptoms (nature/severity) are comparable with the history?
   (b) Functional activities (when possible) need to be included in the objective examination.
   (c) One or more of the following factors may be causative in symptom production (posture, stiffness, instability, loss of muscle strength/endurance, leg length discrepancy, tension, deformity in a proximal or distal joint, virus, fatigue, etc.)
   (d) The symptoms could be arising from 'T4–6 area', thoracic outlet syndrome, 'juvenile disc syndrome', apophyseal joint, nerve root.
   (e) Do you think you will be treating pain, resistance but respecting pain, resistance, or into resistance to provoke 'bite'?

   (Compare your decision now with your finding on objective examination).

Reproduced in part by kind permission of the South Australian School of Physiotherapy.

their significance is obvious. However, 'producing' local pain at a significant joint but without 'reproducing' (when a patient has referred pain) is less definitive. Nevertheless, it is frequently just as significant, and sometimes it is only appreciated in retrospect.

Movement signs are relevant only if they are 'comparable' with the disorder. It is quite common to find minor joint signs at an appropriate joint but which are not comparable with the patient's disability. Such examination findings would reveal only mild pain and any stiffness present would be minimal.

Not only must the joint signs be comparable with the patient's disability they must also be in an 'appropriate joint'. In other words, there may be stiffness and pain on passive flexion of the metatarso-phalangeal joint of the big toe yet the patient's complaint may be pain felt anterior to the ankle joint. Obviously, the joint signs found at the big toe are not in an 'appropriate joint'.

The aim of examining movements is to find one or more **comparable** 'signs' of an **appropriate** structure or structures.

Finding a comparable sign is not always easy, and signs that may seem comparable at the first treatments, may prove to be otherwise later. This may be so when the patient does not improve with treatment. Under these circumstances, re-examination should be carried out with careful stronger test movements in an endeavour to find different signs that prove more comparable. Having found such a sign and made use of it in treatment, the patient's symptoms and signs should improve. As improvement occurs, comparable signs may change and a new comparable sign may become evident. These changes of comparable signs will require changes in treatment techniques.

Active movements
'MOVE to PAIN or MOVE to LIMIT'

Following the subjective examination and the planning, a decision needs to be made as to whether the test movements of the objective examination should be either:

1. Taken to the limit of the available range.
   OR
2. Taken to that point in the range when pain commences, or commences to increase.

In the latter circumstances some assessment of the behaviour of the pain should be made *just beyond* that point in the range where the pain commences (or where the constant pain commences to increase).

When PAIN is the dominant factor in the patient's disorder test movements are taken only to the point in the range where pain commences (and just beyond). When stiffness is more important than pain, the test movements should be taken to the LIMIT of the available range.

1. 'Move to limit'

This means that over-pressure may be applied to all test movements in order to determine:

1. End-of-range 'feel'.
2. Symptom response to the over-pressure.

2. 'Move to pain'

1. This means that when the patient has the severest of pains, the accessory movement tests should be assessed in neutral physiological positions which are:
   (a) fully supported.
   (b) as free of discomfort as possible; and
   (c) avoiding compression of joint surfaces.
2. It also means that the accessory movement should only be taken to the point in the range when the pain is first felt (or where it is first felt to increase). When this assessment has been made the movement should be taken fractionally beyond this point to assess how quickly the pain increases or how quickly it spreads and to where.
3. Physiological movements, if tested, should also only be taken to the point in the range where pain is first felt.

Functional demonstration/tests
(See Table 4.5)

The first movement to be sought is the one(s) that the patient can demonstrate as being associated with his disorder. To begin the objective examination, a question could well be:

Table 4.5 Objective examination

Observation

Watch for patient's willingness to move the structures

Functional demonstration/tests

1. **Their** demonstration of **their** functional movements affected by **their** disorder.
2. Differentiation of their demonstrated functional movement(s).

Brief appraisal

Watch for:
1. Abnormal patterns of movement.
2. Willingness to move.
3. Deformity.
4. Swelling.
5. Wasting.
6. Inflammation, etc.

Active movements

Physiological movements (repeated faster).
Specific movements which the patient can demonstrate as being painful (analyse).
The injuring movement.
Movements under load (antigravity or resisted).

Resisted full range if tendon sheaths affected.

Isometric tests

Test muscles under the painful area for cause of pain and weakness (pain inhibition).

Other structures in 'plan'

Joints above and below.
Relevant spinal area.
Relevant intra-, extra-neural tests.

Passive movements

Special tests. (These will be discussed in detail with each joint.)
Physiological movements (may need over-pressure).
Accessory movements with joint in a neutral position.
Accessory movements in other positions between 'neutral' and at the limit of the physiological range.
Relevant intra-, extra-, neural tests.

Palpation

Temperature, swelling, wasting, sensation, relevant tenderness and position of structures.

Check case records and radiographs

HIGHLIGHT MAIN FINDINGS WITH ASTERISKS

After treatment

Instruction regarding activities, rest, exercises, pain and recording

Q 'Is there anything you can show me, here and now, which causes (provokes or reproduces) your problem?'

Having been shown the movement, and let us consider that he demonstrates his golf swing, it needs to be analysed.

Q 'At what stage of your swing do you feel it?'

This analysing should start with:

Q 'And does the pain go immediately when you've completed your swing?'
ET There are three basic aspects of the golf swing pain that need to be clarified:

1. The pain may disappear immediately the swing is completed. However, with repeated swinging, the degree of pain may:
   (a) Remain the same with each swing.
   (b) Become more painful as he continues provoking the pain with each swing.
   (c) Lessen with each swing until it becomes painless.

   (a)–(c) indicate end-of-range pains which will be treated with small-amplitude techniques that reproduce the symptoms, but in varying degrees for each of the three.)

2. Repeated swinging may produce an ache after two or three swings, and increase in intensity as he continues swinging (this indicates a through-range-pain which will require techniques being performed smoothly and slowly with a large amplitude).

3. At what part of the golf swing does the pain occur – at the end of the backswing? Before striking the golf ball? At end of the follow through, or during the swing?

Once this is determined, the patient should adopt the painful position and the therapist analyses the movement by differentiation tests to determine the main components movements effecting the patient's pain.

Differentiation

As part of objective examination procedures (and treatment techniques) it is often necessary to carry out 'differentiation tests', to determine *accurately* the source of the patient's symptoms. By the very title, 'differentiation tests', the tests differentiate between two or *more* possible joints or structures.

The tests are performed so as to determine *which* painful movement of *which* structure is the precise source of the person's symptoms.

There are five kinds of differentiation:

1. If a patient's buttock pain is reproduced in standing, by fully rotating his body without moving his feet, is it because of the rotation including (a) the hip; (b) the sacro-iliac joint; (c) the lumbar spine? Differentiation tests will tell you.

When a movement provokes pain which can be directly related to a patient's disorder, and which includes simultaneous movement of more than one structure, these special tests are carried out to determine which of the joints and structures is the main culprit or the sole culprit. If more than one of the joint–movement complexes is at fault, the test is then used to define which is the primary source of the disorder, or what percentage of the source of the disorder can be put down to each structure. A good example of this is pain as shown in Figure 4.2, which is reproduced by full supination of the patient's *forearm*, *wrist*, and *hand*. Figure 4.3 describes the test.

2. An example of the second kind of differentiation arises when it is difficult to know whether a patient's symptoms, in say the deltoid area, are arising from a cervical spine disorder or a shoulder disorder.

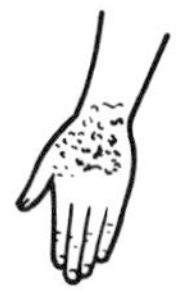

Figure 4.2 Site of symptoms requiring differentiation tests to determine the source(s)

3. The third kind of differentiation relates to deciding what part of a patient's shoulder and arm symptoms are caused by a shoulder disorder and what part is from a neurogenic or dural disorder.

4. Then there is the time when the site of the patient's symptoms are very closely located at a joint. Here there is the need to differentiate between intra-articular sources and periarticular sources.

5. When a patient has referred pain, it is necessary to differentiate between (a) referred pain from a joint, (b) referred pain from viscera, (c) pain from traction or compression on peripheral nerves, and (d) radicular pain.

First group

It is essential to know very precisely the exact spot where the symptom emanates. Sometimes the patient is unable to identify an exact spot, yet can identify an area.

In this example, the pain is reproduced when passive supination is produced by the therapist supinating the patient's forearm and hand with the grasp being applied at the patient's hand.

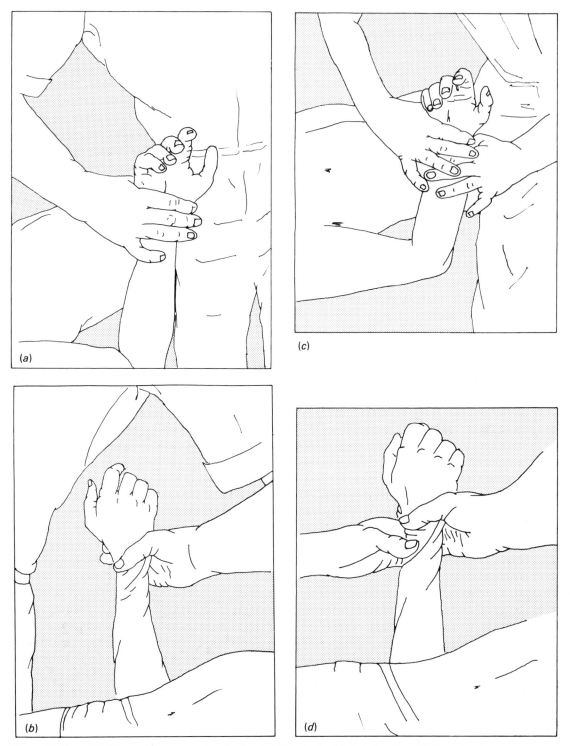

Figure 4.3 (*a*) and (*b*) Views of the grasp and supination to 'bite' of pain. (*a*) Anterior view. (*b*) Posterior view.
(*c*) and (*d*) Further supination of radio-ulnar joint (and a resultant lessening of the wrist supination). (*c*) Anterior view.
(*d*) Posterior view. (*e*) and (*f*) Increasing supination of the wrist, hand and creating a resultant lessening of it at the inferior
radio-ulnar joint.

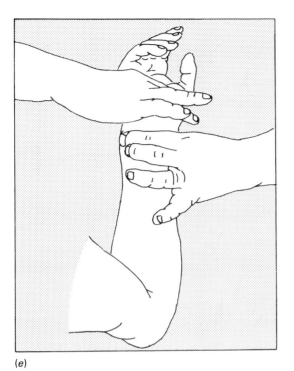

(e)

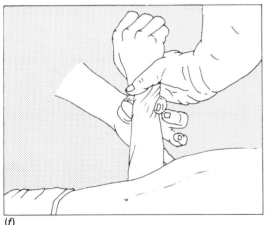

(f)

Figure 4.3 continued.
(*e*) Anterior view. (*f*) Posterior view

The first example to be described will be one whose disorder is chronic with pain being of nuisance value rather than being very painful. This is described in a step-by-step sequence because its principles apply to all such differentiations.

1. The therapist supinates through the right hand up to that point near the limit of the range that not only reproduces the patient's pain but she cautiously further supinates to provoke a sharp 'bite' of pain. She must be able to control this position/'bite' with one hand with the minimum

area of contact on the patient's hand (Figure 4.3 (a) and (b)).
2. The therapist should slacken off the pressure fractionally when she has full control of the supination so as to decrease the intensity of the 'bite' of pain for the patient's sake.
3. While retaining the grasp for supination with the right hand, position the index finger and the thumb of the left hand against the radius and the ulna respectively in such a position as to be able to supinate them further. (Figure 4.3 (c) and (d)).

   When in this position, reimpose with the right hand, the 'bite' position of the supination. Use non-verbal (flinching) and verbal messages to know the 'bite' position is accurate.
4. Maintain the supination 'bite' position with the right hand, and with the left hand, delicately pronate the inferior radio-ulnar joint (Figure 4.3 (e) and (f)).

Although the movement of the patient's inferior radio-ulnar joint is PRONATION, there are distinct advantages in using the terms 'de-rotate' (or de-supinate). Using 'de-rotate' takes away the confusion about what is taking place at the different joints – it makes, most clearly, the point that rotation is taking place at the joints: the radio-ulnar joint is having its supination lessened and therefore the wrist/hand's supination increased.

When the de-rotation is performed, the patient's symptoms will either increase or decrease. In fact, what has happened is that the supination stress has lessened at the inferior radio-ulnar joint while at the same time increased the supination stress at the wrist/hand. So, if the reproduced pain ('bite') *decreases* the symptoms must be coming from supination of the inferior radio-ulnar movement. If the symptoms *increase* the culprit must be the wrist/hand supination.

When *pain* is the patient's complaint, the technique requires different handling:

1. Supination, using the right hand, is only taken to that point of supination where pain starts to increase (P1) (Figure 4.4 (a)).
2. While maintaining the precise P1 supination position, the left hand gently and slowly further supinates the inferior radio-ulnar joint. This is de-rotating (or de-supinating or pronating) of the wrist/hand supination (Figure 4.4(b)). *The position of the patient's hand and the therapist's right hand must remain unaltered in relation to the patient's body.*

   If pain increases with this technique, that increased pain must be from the further increase of supination of the inferior radio-ulnar joint. If the pain decreases then that decrease must be as a result of the decreased supination of the wrist/hand.

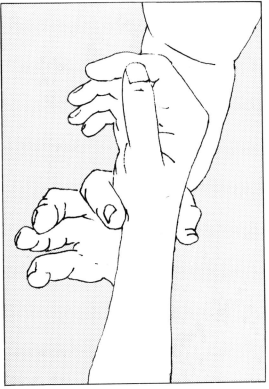

(a)

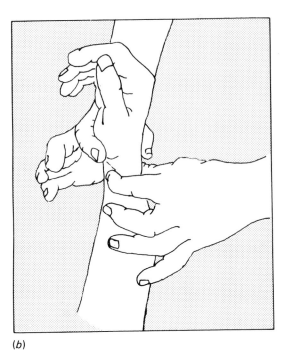

(b)

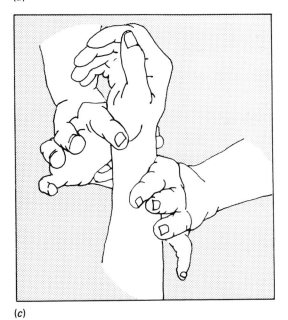

(c)

Figure 4.4 (*a*) Hand and forearm supination to the point when reproduced pain starts to increase (P1). (*b*) Supination of radio-ulnar joint is increased and at the wrist it is decreased. (*c*) Supination of wrist/hand is increased and inferior radio-ulnar pain is decreased

The reverse direction can be performed to confirm the findings of test above.

3. Returning to the same starting supination position (P1) as shown in Figure 4.4 (a), the rotating described for Figure 4.4 (b) is reversed. That is, the radio-ulnar supination is decreased and thus the wrist/hand supination is increased (Figure 4.4 (c)).

If pain increases on performing the test (Figure 4.4 (c)) it means that the wrist/hand is at fault, while if pain decreases it is the inferior radio-ulnar joint that is at fault.

Confirmation tests

With the differentiation tests of this kind there are, in fact, four ways of confirming each of the findings. The tests are described for the onset of, or the beginning of increase of, the reproduced pain to demonstrate the delicacy of the testing movements:

1. *The test finding* – The first confirmation is that if further supination of the radio-ulnar joint increases the pain, the radio-ulnar joint is the culprit.

2. *Second confirmation* – If the further supination of the radio-ulnar joint increases the pain, the desupination of the same inferior radio-ulnar joint should decrease the pain because the wrist/hand supination has decreased. If this does happen, the first test is confirmed, i.e. the above two findings agree with each other.

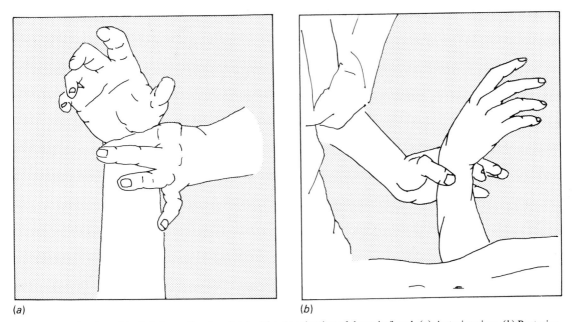

Figure 4.5 Supination of the inferior radio-ulnar joint without supination of the wrist/hand. (*a*) Anterior view. (*b*) Posterior view

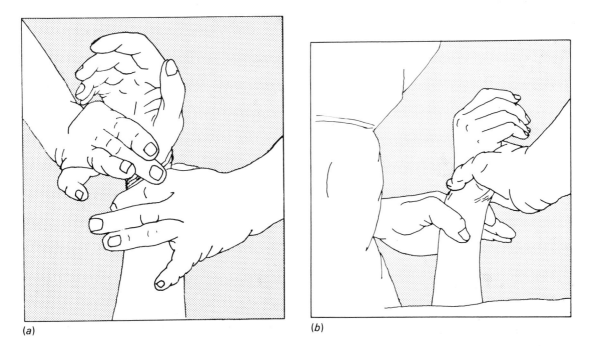

Figure 4.6 Supination of the wrist/hand without any supination of the inferior radio-ulnar joint. (*a*) Anterior view. (*b*) Posterior view

3. *Third confirmation* – If the radio-ulnar is the culprit, supination of the inferior radio-ulnar joint on its own (i.e. no wrist/hand movement) should increase the pain, thus confirming the first finding (Figure 4.5).
4. *Fourth confirmation* – Supination of the wrist/hand without any movement of the inferior radio-ulnar joint should be pain free (Figure 4.6).

This is the moment to say that whatever movement (of the multiple joint complex) reproduces the patient's symptoms, it is fundamental and obligatory to carry out *that exact movement* for the differentiation test(s).

It is not necessary to carry out all of the four test movements on every occasion. However, they are the four ways that can clarify the examination findings. To know them and use them puts the therapist in a position where there can be no mistake.

Second group

An example describing this group has symptoms in the deltoid area which require differentiation procedures to determine whether they are caused by a cervical spine disorder or a glenohumeral disorder.

It is not uncommon for a person to seek relief of pain in the area suggested above. The patient may never have had neck or shoulder symptoms before. On examination of the physiological movements, the shoulder may be painful at the end of range(s); and the cervical spine's physiological movements may be symptom free. Two other examination movements of the cervical spine must be tested before it can be said that the cervical spine is NOT affected:

1. Compression of the cervical spine should be assessed by the therapist gradually increasing compression through the crown of the patient's head endeavouring to compress structures on each side alternately, positioning the patient's head and cervical spine in some extension, together with lateral flexion and rotation towards the side of the pain. If the cervical spine is implicated, performing the procedure towards the side of the pain will probably be more uncomfortable than when performed on the side opposite to the site of the pain.
2. The second test is the primary test. This uses careful palpation of the appropriate vertebrae. The inter-vertebral spaces are assessed to determine whether there is any abnormal position or thickening of related intervertebral levels. If there is a difference, such as thickened in-

tervertebral tissue or prominence of relevant zygapophyseal joints, pain will probably be felt deeply when oscillatory unilateral pressure is applied in a postero-anterior direction through the zygapophyseal joint. This is classed as an abnormal examination finding.

Confirmation of no cervical structure contributing to the patient's deltoid area symptoms will be evident if the cervical spine is treated at two consecutive sessions without producing any change in the symptoms. Conversely, successful treatment of the spine with palpatory techniques will produce favourable changes in:

1. The test movements of the shoulder.
2. The symptoms felt by the patient.
3. The palpation signs of the cervical spine.

Other examples requiring this kind of differentiation are:

1. Chest and abdominal symptoms from the thoracic spine.
2. Hip from the lumbar spine.
3. To a lesser degree, pain in the elbow and knee being referred from the cervical and lumbar vertebrae.

Third group

This group is different from the second group in that it is differentiating the cause of shoulder (and arm) symptoms being from a shoulder disorder, a neurogenic or dural disorder.

Tests for the glenohumeral joint are well documented and do not require description here. Neurogenic signs are determined by 'upper limb tension tests' first described by Elvey[1] and they have been described in *Vertebral Manipulation*[2]. The arm positions, if they are tested and found to be positive, probably implicate the peripheral nervous symptom, whereas if cervical movements cause an increase in the symptoms while the arm is kept in a moderately pain free, upper limb tension test (ULTT) position, then the structures implicated are far more likely to be at fault within the spinal canals.

Fourth group

The differentiating here is between intra-articular and periarticular disorders. There are three distinctions:

1. The therapist grasps the patient's humeral head with the thumb posteriorly and the fingers anteriorly with one of her hands. With the other hand she stabilizes the acromio-clavicular area.

1. Elvey, R. L. Brachial plexus tension-tests and the pathogenic origin of arm pain. In *Proceedings of Multidisciplinary International Conference on Manipulative Therapy,* Melbourne, Australia, pp. 105–111 (1979)
2. Maitland, G. D. *Vertebral Manipulation,* 5th edn. Butterworths, London, pp. 185–189 (1968)

Then, while asking the patient if he feels his symptoms 'in here' she rocks the head of the humerus back and forth in the glenoid cavity. The patient quickly and easily understands where 'in' is, and those who have an intra-articular disorder are quick to reply 'yes'.

2. Patients having intra-articular pain always have symptoms (pain or aching) at the particular joint. They may have a spread of symptoms but this is relatively uncommon. The periarticular disorders often have referred symptoms which can be indiscriminate. An exception is the hip, which very occasionally can cause knee pain without any hip pain.

3. Mid-range oscillatory movements of a normal synovial joint are symptom free, and mid-range oscillatory movements of a symptomatic synovial joint *may* also be pain free. However, if the same oscillatory movements are performed while compression of the joint surfaces is added during the oscillatory mid-range movements, pain will be provoked. If the intra-articular disorder is a long-standing chronic disorder (and is of nuisance quality rather than constant pain) the compression component may need to be both sustained and performed strongly before the symptoms are reproduced. This technique will provoke any discomfort (remembering of course that the oscillations are performed in mid-range and not at the end of the available range).

Fifth group

This group relates to patients who have referred pain.

1. There are those who have referred pain from a synovial joint yet without any local pain at the faulty joint. Two common examples are:
   (a) The patient having pain felt in the knee yet having its only source in the hip.
   (b) The patient having pain at the deltoid insertion, with its source being at the shoulder.

2. The non-contractile tissues of a joint can be responsible for referred pain covering a whole limb. A reasonably common example is again the hip but this time causing pain in the whole length of the leg and into the foot (dorsum of the foot usually, or lateral ankle).

3. There is the example of visceral structures causing referred pain. Two examples: the gall-bladder causing right shoulder pain, and the heart causing left arm pain.

4. Peripheral nerves when damaged by traction or compression will refer symptoms, and may do this without pain at the local site of damage. Fortunately, neurological signs are often present, and these signs are directly related to a peripheral nerve and not to a nerve root compression. Traction or pulling of the nerve reproduces the symptoms; and pressure on the area where the peripheral nerve is at fault will be unusually sensitive and will provoke the referred pain.

5. Radicular pain is produced by pressure on the nerve root within the vertebral canals. It is usually easily recognized, especially if neurological changes and signs are present. The neurological changes accompanying referred pain from a peripheral nerve (the elbow may cause pain in the medial one and a half fingers) differs from that of a nerve root (it cannot affect half a finger). Many other obvious tests can help in the differentiation of peripheral nerve disorders from nerve root disorders.

While the joint is at rest and before carrying out any test movements of the joint the patient should be asked if he has any pain, discomfort or awareness. The joint should then be moved in a particular direction until pain is first felt or, if the joint has some degree of pain while at rest, the patient should be asked to move to the point where pain starts to increase. This range should then be noted and recorded by the physiotherapist.

If the irritability of the disorder assessed during the subjective examination indicates that exacerbation is unlikely to occur, the patient should then be asked to continue the movement into the painful range as far as possible. Changes in the severity, or area, of the pain with the further movement should be noted and recorded together with the range at which pain started and the range that proved to be the limit of the patient's active movement.

If the subjective irritability of the disorder and the severity of the pain permit, the patient should repeat the movement from the starting position to the limit of the range while the physiotherapist watches for abnormalities in the normal rhythm to determine in which individual joint the fault lies. It is obvious that such a test of the knee or elbow will reveal less than a test of the foot or shoulder where many joints work in harmony.

Countering abnormal rhythms

The method used to look at rhythms of movement can be likened to a camera which has a 'wide-angle' lens and a 'telephoto' lens. If, for example, gait is being examined, the therapist should at first use her vision as though using a wide-angle lens to observe the whole. If, on doing this, the therapist notices something that is not normal she should then view the area using her eyes as a telephoto lens, to hone in on where she believes the main fault lies. It may mean that while the patient continues to repeat the movement, she has to see-saw her vision from wide angle to telephoto until she can see the abnormality so understandably that she can, in fact, perform the abnormal rhythm herself.

Abnormalities of normal rhythm of movement can occur in any movement of any joint. Everyone is familiar with the abnormal scapulo-thoracic movement during flexion of the upper limb when the glenohumeral joint is very limited – the scapula begins rotating, protracting and elevating very early in the range. Many people have minor abnormal rhythms of movement. It is because people can have abnormal rhythms that are normal and pain free for them, that it becomes necessary to assess a patient's abnormal rhythm to determine whether it is related to his disorder. The only way to do this is to counter the abnormality when it occurs, and compare the pain response during the uncountered movement with the countered movement. If pain is reproduced when the abnormal movement is countered (and successfully prevented from occurring) yet when not countered it is either pain free or much diminished, then the abnormal rhythm is directly associated with the disorder.

There are however two factors that can influence the interpretation of the above pain response. The first is that some part of the abnormal rhythm may be old, in terms of years, having occurred during an earlier episode of the same disorder. In such circumstances some of the current abnormal rhythm may be old and some may be new owing to the current disorder. The second factor is related to protective muscle spasm. This spasm occurs at the moment when the normal rhythm would be painful but the protective muscle spasm comes into play to prevent the pain occurring thereby producing an abnormal rhythm: but sometimes this spasm is so protective, or so strong, that the abnormal movement cannot be countered no matter how hard the countering is attempted.

Because of these difficulties related to the interpretation of the effect of the countering, it is necessary for the therapist:

1. To know how successful she is being in countering or preventing the abnormal movement.
2. To compare the pain response during the countering with that from which the patient is suffering.

This determination, at times, can only be made reliable when considered in retrospect assuming of course that treatment produced favourable changes.

SEEK ABNORMAL RHYTHMS AND
COUNTER THEM

Speed

Sometimes it is necessary to introduce speed into the test movement to find abnormalities in the rhythm when none are evident if the joint is moved at a normal speed. The speed of the test movement may then reveal abnormal rhythm and may also provoke and reproduce pain that otherwise would be missed.

Over-Pressure

All movements of a joint are assessed, and if it is felt that a movement is full range and painless a moderate degree of pressure is then applied at the limit of the range to assess whether the movement is in fact both full range and painless. The pressure should not be excessive but applied with full appreciation of the age and general condition of the patient. Of equal importance, the over-pressure must not be too light. This is an essential test because a patient often considers his movements are normal when in fact there is some pain or restriction if over-pressure is applied. If the physiotherapist does not apply the required degree of over-pressure, the information she records is likely to be incorrect.

A joint's movements can never be classed as normal unless *firm* over-pressure can be applied painlessly.

When movement causes pain, measurement of the range should be based on that given in the booklet *Joint Motion. Method of Measuring and Recording*[3]. The method of examining these active movements will not be discussed here as reference to the booklet, which has been widely accepted for the benefit of universal standards, can be made separately. It is important to point out, however, that with some joints, if the movement is assessed first in the standing position and then in the supine position, different measurements will be recorded. This is more obvious in weight-bearing joints but it also applies to the shoulder joint where gravity assists flexion in the supine position but resists it in standing.

Range/pain

It is important that the person examining the patient's joint movements should take into account simultaneously both pain and range. When recording examination findings the physiotherapist should not record the range of movement that a joint may

---

3. *Joint Motion. Method of Measuring and Recording* American Academy of Orthopaedic Surgeons (1976)

lack without also recording the site, type and degree of the patient's pain felt with that test movement. Similarly, she should not record any findings in relation to the patient's pain with movement unless it is also related to the range at which or through which the pain is felt.

During examination and assessment **pain** should **never** be considered without relation to **range** nor **range** without relation to **pain**.

Combining movements

There are times when a patient has a relatively good range/pain-response of, say, shoulder flexion such that it cannot be classified as being 'comparable' with his disorder. If the patient is then asked to perform the same flexion movement but with the arms medially rotated, then laterally rotated, it may be found that flexion/medial rotation is most restricted, the restriction including a comparable pain response felt in his shoulder.

The physiotherapist should be sufficiently flexible to introduce combinations of movements and changes in the sequence of the movements in an endeavour to find the most comparable signs.

Recording

When *recording* range of movement and the symptomatic response to that movement, one should develop a pattern of recording and stick to it. By doing so, more facts can be remembered, while at the same time leaving the therapist's mental processes more time to take in other details. In the following text the following example is used:

Sup √√

This example means supination (Sup) has a full range of movement (the first tick, √) and has no abnormal pain response when over-pressure is applied (the second tick, √).

Compression and movements under load

The effect of compression on weight-bearing joints while in the standing position can be important and indicate the need to introduce compression into the examination of active movement to elicit joint pain. A common example is a patient with minor knee symptoms who may have a full painless range of active knee movements when tested in a supine position but when asked to stand and squat fully, finds flexion is very painful.

Movements under load

When other test movements are not productive in terms of 'comparable findings' the patient should be asked to perform movements against gravity. If this is also non-productive, the physiotherapist should increase the loading to the movement being tested. This may require innovation, but where there's a will, there's a way.

During examination, if a joint sign comparable with the patient's symptoms cannot be found, the patient may be able to recall the exact movement that caused his injury. Gentle repetition of this movement, *simulating the condition under which the injury occurred*, should be used as a test. However, not all joint pain has a traumatic origin and details of trauma cannot always be recalled.

If the physiological movements are tested and no positive signs are found, the joint affected should be subjected to strongly resisted active movements under load. Performing the movements against gravity may be sufficient load to provide joint signs but if this is not so then increased resistance must be included in the test movement.

Neural movement tests

When joint tissues are abnormal, peripheral nerves in the area could be also. Nerves are easily damaged, either directly during a joint injury, and/or indirectly because of exposure to blood, oedema or scar. There are two likely sources of symptoms – mechanical or ischaemic damage to nerve fibres, or irritated connective tissue sheaths.

A peripheral nerve must glide alongside adjacent tissues and also stretch as it adapts to body movement. The study of the movement mechanics of the peripheral nerves and the mechanical and physiological consequences of altered mechanics is complex. One main reason is that the nervous system is a continuum, and an abnormality in one part will have repercussions elsewhere along the trunk, including the neuraxis (central nervous system).

In line with the principles of this book, the examination and treatment of the nervous system is detailed in a text by Butler[4].

ISOMETRIC TESTS

Muscles that lie under the area of the patient's pain should be tested strongly isometrically to see if the pain can be thus reproduced. At the same time, notice should be taken of muscle power and a determination made as to whether the weakness is neurological, rupture or pain inhibition. Muscle length should be assessed.

---

4. Butler, D. S. *Mobilization of the Nervous System*. Churchill Livingstone, London (1990)

OTHER JOINTS IN 'PLAN'

Routine examination should include quick tests of the joints above and below the painful one so that, hopefully, they can be excluded from the clinical examination; if found to be limited or painful then they will have to be examined in detail. The relevant area of the spine should also be examined.

Passive movements

One of the main functions of examination by passive movement is to find a movement or movements with signs (pain, resistance or spasm) that can be compared with the patient's symptoms. If more than one such movement is found, their respective signs are compared. For example, during the examination of a man who has pain encompassing the right shoulder region, all movements of the glenohumeral and acromio-clavicular joints are tested passively to determine the extent and nature (range, stiffness, pain, spasm) of limitation of movements and the pain which may be present in each direction. The important examination findings are those movements that reproduce pain comparable with the symptoms, while the movements that produce a small amount of pain become less important. The movements are recorded in order of severity, and any loss of range in each of these directions is also noted.

Passive movements can be broadly divided into two groups. The first is the group of passive movements that can also be performed actively, i.e. passive physiological movements. In the second group the movements cannot be performed actively, they can only be produced passively: i.e. passive accessory movements. For example, shoulder flexion is a physiological movement whereas movement of the head of the humerus up and down in the glenoid cavity is an accessory movement.

Although the gross range of both passive and active physiological movements is similar, the joint–surface relationships during their movements are not necessarily so. For example, as soon as muscles contract to produce active movements the joint surfaces are compressed. During passive movements there is no compression unless the examiner deliberately applies it.

Another difference relates to the gliding of the joint surfaces which occurs during movement. This is best seen in the glenohumeral joint. The glenoid fossa is shaped to allow an upward and downward movement of the head of the humerus. While the arm hangs by the side of the body, the head of the humerus occupies the upper part of the glenoid cavity, but as the arms are raised above the head the muscular action moves the head of the humerus downwards in the glenoid cavity. This means that when the arm is raised actively, the head of the humerus, at any one position in the range, always occupies a constant position in the glenoid cavity. If, however, the same position in the range is maintained passively, the head of the humerus can be moved into various positions in the glenoid cavity. Thus, passive accessory movements may be performed during the passive physiological movements.

The need to use compression to elicit joint signs was discussed in relation to testing active movements. When passive movement tests do not elicit pain they should be repeated while compression is applied. The test is particularly appropriate if the disorder is thought to have an intra-articular component.

Physiological movement tests

The first movements to be tested passively should be those physiological movements that have been tested actively. These tests are repetitions of the active movements given in the booklet *Joint Motion. Method of Measuring and Recording*[5] performed as passive movements, and as such will not be described here. However, there are other test movements not included in the above booklet that form an important part of examination when the routine test movements do not give conclusive answers. These will be described in detail in the chapter relating to each joint.

As relaxation is essential for effective testing of passive movements the tests should be performed with the patient in a reclining position. It is the position of choice even when a joint such as the wrist or even an interphalangeal joint is being examined.

Firstly the patient should be asked if he feels any pain, and if he does, its site should be determined. The joint should then be moved through the range to the position where pain is first felt and this position should be noted. Then the joint should be moved further, the physiotherapist watching the patient carefully to endeavour to assess the degree of pain being experienced. Unless the pain becomes excessive, the joint should be moved to the limit of the range. The available range together with any change in the site or degree of pain should be recorded. The nature of the limitation, whether muscle spasm or stiffness, should also be noted. This assessment should be made for each direction of movement that has been performed actively so that a comparison between the active and passive movements can be made. A marked discrepancy between a range of movements performed passively and actively may be due to loss of muscle power or

---

5. *Joint Motion: Method of Measuring and Recording* American Academy of Orthopaedic Surgeons (1976)

an inability to move further because of pain. This text is concerned solely with joint-pain problems and excludes those disturbances of movement that are due to loss of muscle power or function, having a neurological origin.

Accessory movements

Measurement of passive physiological movements is generally accepted as routine examination but it should be realized that the range of passive accessory movements can and must also be assessed; these latter, performed in different directions, are very small and their assessment is therefore more difficult. However, if the joint is to be treated by passive movement their assessment is most important. If the accessory movements are limited and painful, the active movements cannot be normal. A loss of range in one accessory movement can explain why a particular physiological movement is restricted.

The meanings of the words 'move to pain' and 'move to limit' have been discussed in relation to active movements (see page 32). They also relate to passive movement tests just as much as, and in the same way as, they apply to the active movement tests. However, there are two qualifications. When the passive accessory movement tests are applied to the 'move to pain' group, they are tested with the joint positioned in its *loose-packed, mid-range, least painful, position.* Conversely, when they are applied to the 'move to limit' group, they are assessed at the limit of the physiological range or in a position just short of that limit.

Single joints

Accessory movement tests of single joints need to be considered differently from multiple joints such as is found in the hand and foot. The first relates to joints such as the glenohumeral joint and the knee joint where large movements are easy to assess. In these instances, the accessory movements, produced by thumb or hand pressure against the head of the humerus or tibia respectively, can also readily be assessed for range and pain response. In joints such as the sternoclavicular joint or acromio-clavicular joint these accessory movement tests may be the only tests to give positive findings. For example, if the sternoclavicular joint is the source of minor symptoms the active and passive shoulder girdle tests of flexion, depression, protraction, retraction and rotation may be painless, whereas accessory movements of the joint performed with thumb pressures, reproduce the deep pain. The temporomandibular joint is another familiar example.

Multiple joints

This relates to a movement comprising the movement of many joints working in harmony, as in the hand. When both active and passive wrist flexion are painful, it is often only by the accessory movement tests that the painful lesion can be localized to a particular joint.

It was pointed out earlier that passive accessory movements are possible at any stage of flexion of the arm (see page 42). This principle applies for every joint, even when many joints work together, as in the hand. To examine accessory movements in different positions of the joint range may be the only method of finding joint signs comparable with the patient's symptoms. As finding such a movement is sometimes missed because of difficulty in testing and lack of perseverance, treatment by passive movement may not be successful. For example, a patient who intermittently experiences sharp pain somewhere deep in the radial side of his hand while pouring tea from a teapot may have active and passive physiological movements which reveal very little. However, careful examination may reveal that the sharp pain can be reproduced by a postero-anterior gliding of the first metacarpal on the trapezium if the joint is put under compression. The important point is that pain with this test movement is comparable with the patient's symptoms. Testing accessory movements in different physiological joint positions is often essential to determine the most painful or most limited part of movement.

Gliding tests

Many anomalies occur clinically that do not entirely agree with what is thought to be known anatomically and physiologically. Description of movement between the capitate and hamate provides a useful example of the comparison between the theoretical considerations of a joint movement and the clinical assessments.

Under normal pain-free circumstances the capitate may be held anteriorly and posteriorly around the lateral border of one hand with the middle finger and thumb, while at the same time holding the hamate between the fingers and thumb of the other hand around the medial border of the hand. With this grasp it is quite easy to slide both bones back and forth against each other to produce and feel movement at the joint. If the movement is stretched at each extreme, and the joint is normal, then the movement and stretching will be painless.

If the patient has pain in his hand which is felt during various functional movements, accurate examination of the intercarpal area may indicate, for example, that the pain is arising from the joint between the capitate and hamate because some of the movements occurring at the joint, when performed passively, reproduce the pain. Figure 4.7 represents diagrammatically the normal relationship of the capitate–hamate joint.

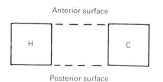

Figure 4.7 Neutral position of the left hand under normal circumstances. View of the proximal surfaces of the hamate and capitate

Circumstances may exist where if the capitate is stabilized so that it does not move and the physiotherapist pushes the hamate anteriorly with her free hand, the patient's pain may be reproduced (Figure 4.8(a)). In theory the pain should also be reproduced if the same movement is stretched in the same direction but this time the hamate is stabilized with one hand while the capitate is moved posteriorly with the other hand (Figure 4.8(b)). Clinically this is not always so even though theoretically the same movement is being produced by both methods. Importantly, the movement that reproduces the patient's pain should be the movement used in treatment. The movements may be further investigated by comparing the movement described above firstly with the capitate and hamate distracted and secondly with them compressed.

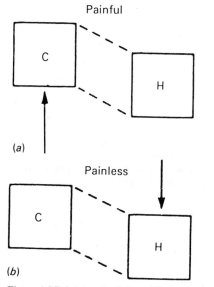

Figure 4.8 Painful and painless. (*a*) Capitate stabilized. Hamate moved anteriorly. (*b*) Hamate stabilized. Theoretically if one method of performing the movement is painful it is reasonable to expect that both ways of performing the movement should be painful. However, clinically one can be painful (*a*) and the other painless (*b*)

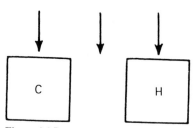

Figure 4.9 Postero-anterior pressures on the capitate, the hamate, and the joint line

Thumb pressure movement tests

The above description is related to only one movement of the joint between the capitate and hamate. Further examination of this joint is performed by producing posteroanterior pressures on the capitate, then on the hamate, and then on the joint line between the capitate and hamate (Figure 4.9). Each of these three posteroanteriorly directed pressures produces a different movement in the capitate–hamate joint and any one of them may reproduce the patient's pain, and one may be more dominant than the others.

The joint movements produced by the posteroanterior pressures can be further varied by inclining them medially and laterally (Figures 4.10(a) and (b)), or cephalad and caudad (Figures 4.11(a) and (b)).

All of these directions can be combined to test the various movements. For example, Figure 4.12 shows one combination. It depicts movement between the capitate and hamate produced by a posteroanterior pressure on the joint line combined with a medial

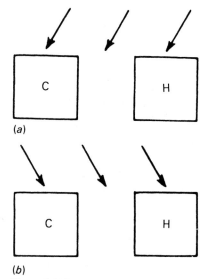

Figure 4.10 Postero-anterior pressures directed (*a*) medially; (*b*) laterally

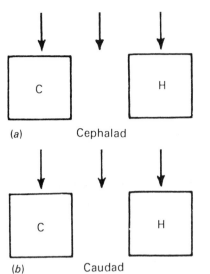

(a)　　　　　Cephalad

(b)　　　　　Caudad

Figure 4.11 Postero-anterior pressures directed cephalad and caudad

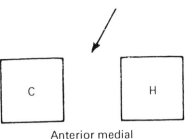

Anterior medial
and cephalad
on the joint line

Figure 4.12 Postero-anterior pressure on the joint line directed medially and cephalad

inclination and a cephalad inclination. This pressure is applied at the joint line. The same direction of pressure could have been applied on the capitate or hamate.

Figures 4.9–4.12 all depict the left hand.

When testing these fine movements with thumb pressures, the angles of the pressures should be explored extensively because there may be as little as one or two degrees between (a) the right direction and (b) being off-centre. The same applies to being on the precise spot to apply the pressure or being a pin's head away from it.

To test the joint still further, variations of pressure against each bone and the joint line should be done in the anteroposterior direction. Particular note should be taken of:

1. The position of bones in relation to each other (normal or abnormal).
2. The limitation of joint movement in any direction found by the examining palpation techniques.
3. The site and degree of pain produced by each of the movements; is it comparable with the patient's disorder?

The examination findings guide which technique should be used for treatment because the pressure techniques of examination can give such clearly defined detail.

Lastly, the clinical examination findings, bearing in mind the discussion above, will give information in relation to position, range of movement, and pain with movement. The therapist is then able to decide whether treatment is going to be directed towards:

1. Restoring to normal the relationship between the capitate and hamate.

2. Increasing the range of movement between the capitate and hamate.
3. Making the available range pain free.

Thus the therapist is in a position to relate her knowledge of the state of the movements and their symptomatic responses with the disorder and give her a clear indication of the intention of the treatment technique that can be used.

As the passive tests used in examination are the same as those used in treatment, their description will be left until the joints are discussed individually. A general plan of the objective examination is given in Table 4.5.

With each test movement, assessment is made of the range of movement relative to the symptoms felt in each direction. From this information comparisons can be made between each direction of the joint's movements. However, range and pain alone do not give sufficient information to guide the manner in which the joint will be moved passively in treatment. Adequate detail is required to appreciate the relative position in the range of the onset of the pain and the onset of resistance, the type of resistance, the rate of increase in strength of each of these factors (that is, their behaviour during movement) and the relationships all of these elements bear to each other.

Some readers may consider the extent of this detail unnecessary, but it should be realized that all experienced skilled manipulators have this appreciation of joint signs whether it is conscious or unconscious and they modify their handling of a joint in accordance with small changes in the signs that occur during treatment. The finer the therapist's appreciation of the details, the better will be the handling of the joint.

Teaching this perception in clinical terms to newcomers is exceedingly difficult. Not every patient is suitable demonstration material, and even when a suitable patient is available it is not possible, in the best interests of the patient, for all students to handle the joint. In addition, and importantly, a teacher cannot be sure that newcomers have, in fact, felt what they should have felt. Nevertheless, there will never be first-class handling and assessment of joint conditions unless the physiotherapist acquires a high degree of sensitivity to symptoms and signs in movements of the abnormal joint. New concepts of teaching this aspect of manual skill are needed, having, at least in part, a theoretical basis. If a theoretically based method can be used, students will come to handle joints more perceptively and learn far more from each experience which comes their way. Those students with little natural aptitude will be helped by having a theoretical basis for their work and a means of insight into what they should be able to feel.

'Geography would be incomprehensible without maps. They've reduced a tremendous muddle of facts into something you can read at a glance. Now I suspect economics is fundamentally no more difficult than geography except that it's about things in motion. If only somebody would invent a dynamic map'[6].

The Movement Diagram is the *dynamic map for 'passive movement' which can be likened to such a map for economics*. It 'reduces a tremendous muddle of facts into something you can read at a glance.' The theory of the movement diagram is described in detail in Appendix 1, as is its practical compilation. It is the detail of the latter that the good manipulator must have, especially when related to palpation techniques of examination, as described on pages 307–313, and their use in treatment.

The complexity and subjectivity of the aspects of examination discussed here make them extremely difficult to learn, but unless they are learned, the handling of joints does not reach a high standard. Movement diagrams provide a method of gaining insight into the way these factors control, and are controlled by, the skilled use of passive movement both in examination and treatment.

Joint chapters

Within each chapter for peripheral joints, two objective examination 'tables' are given which list:

1. The tests that should be performed to test all of the individual joints that combine in the movement of a joint unit, such as the shoulder girdle. This table is titled 'composite joint', and it is used *only* for *chronic disorders of minor disability*. Its purpose is to list each of the passive test movements which MUST be performed either to exclude the area as being a source of the symptoms, or to provide a basis of test movement findings from which 'differentiation tests' would be made.

   Each of the test movements should be commenced gently (IV) but progressing to strong over-pressure, while comparing any pain response with that which can be produced on the sound limb, before the movement can be declared 'clear'.

2. The tests that should be performed, with over-pressure, to prove that the joint is normal, titled 'proving unaffected'.

6. Snow, C. P. *Strangers and Brothers* Penguin Books, Harmondsworth, p. 67 (1965)

5

Principles of technique

To apply any technique of passive movement treatment the position adopted is governed by the following factors:

1. The patient must be completely relaxed if treatment is to be effective without placing unwarranted strain on the structures supporting the joint.
    Even treatment of the thumb should be performed with the patient lying supine.
2. The patient must be comfortable and have complete confidence in the operator's grasp. The grip should not be tighter than that required to perform the movement, and the position should make full use of the mechanical advantage of levers.
3. Wherever possible, the operator should embrace the parts to be moved or stabilized. In accompaniment with this the operator should hold around the joint so as to feel the joint movement as the technique is performed.
4. The patient must feel confident that the joint will not be hurt by being moved further than he expects. The physiotherapist, therefore, must position herself carefully so that she prevents the movement going beyond an established point.
5. The operator's position must be comfortable, easy to maintain and the most economical in which to carry out the treatment with minimum effort.
6. The operator's position must afford her complete control of the movement.

Before carrying out a technique, the direction and type of movement to be used is determined from the movement signs and the starting position adopted. The patient must be in a comfortable, fully supported position so that complete relaxation is possible and the physiotherapist must have complete control of the part to be moved. Whenever possible, part of the grasp must be around the joint so that the movement can be felt. During treatment minor changes may be needed, depending upon the 'feel' of the movement; smaller or larger amplitudes might be used and the rhythm made slower or staccato, or the movement performed earlier or later in the range than originally planned. These minor changes, which are made during small exploratory movements, also help to give the patient confidence in the physiotherapist's control of a painful area. The technique is then performed for a planned period with a planned discomfort response, and the patient's signs are then reassessed.

Grades of movement

As will be evident from the previous chapter, any part of a range of movement may be used in treatment, and widely varying amplitudes and speeds may be chosen. It is both tedious and time consuming to refer to a treatment movement as 'a large-amplitude movement performed in the early part of the range' or 'a small-amplitude movement performed firmly at the limit of the range'. To overcome this exigency, and to make the recording of treatment quicker and simpler, a system of grading movement is suggested. Although recording treatment will be discussed in detail later, it is necessary to introduce these grades of movement (the seeds for which were proposed by Miss Jeanne-Marie Ganne in 1965) here, because of their application to the treatment techniques in following chapters.
    Grades from I to IV are used to describe the treatment movements but like all similar gradings (for example rating 1 to 5 for muscle power) the

values overlap; that is there is also a place for plus and minus values. The grades of movement which are described below can be depicted in relation to a straight line representing a full average range of passive movement (Figure 5.1).

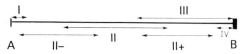

Figure 5.1 Grades of movement. A = Beginning of range of movement; B = end of normal average range of passive movement

Grade I: Small-amplitude movement performed at the beginning of the range.

Grade II: Large-amplitude movement performed within a ***resistance-free*** part of the range. If the movement is performed near the beginning of the range it is expressed as 'II−', and if it is taken deeply into the range, yet still not reaching resistance or the limit of the range, it is expressed as 'II+' (Figure 5.1).

Grade III: Large-amplitude movement performed into resistance or up to the limit of the range. This movement can also be expressed with plus and minus values. If the movement is pushed firmly towards the limit of the range it is expressed as 'III+' but if it nudges gently into the resistance, yet short of the limit of the range, it is expressed as 'III−'.

Grade IV: Small-amplitude movement performed well into resistance. This too can be expressed as 'IV+' or 'IV−', depending on its vigour as described for grade III.

In relating 'IV−' and 'IV+' to the 'limit of the range', it is easy to become confused. So, where is grade 'IV' if it is not at the limit of the range? And likewise, what is a grade 'IV+'? The position of a grade IV relative to 'IV+' is a subjective assessment which depends on how strongly a therapist is prepared to push. Grade IV is strong pressure into the resistance, so obviously a grade 'IV+++' must be very strong indeed. In this edition of *Peripheral Manipulation*, the point 'B', representing the limit of the range, is now much thickened. This has come about because position 'B' (end of range) for a timid therapist may be well short of the skilled therapist's passive end of range. This subjectiveness helps the novice to learn from seeing and comparing her diagrams with those of a skilled therapist.

If the normal range of joint movement is limited by the joint disorder, grades III and IV are restricted to the new limit of the range, and grade II movements are restricted to smaller amplitudes (Figure 5.2).

Similarly, pain may arise from a hypermobile joint that is slightly stiffened. Such a situation alters the positions of grade III and IV movements as shown in Figure 5.3.

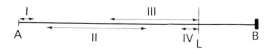

Figure 5.2 Restricted grades of movement. A = Beginning of range of movement; B = average anatomical limit; L = pathological limit of range

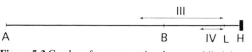

Figure 5.3 Grades of movement in a hypermobile joint. A = Beginning of range of movement; B = average anatomical limit; L = pathological limit of range; H = patient's limit of normal hypermobile range

Rhythms of movement

Joints can be moved in many different ways from a stationary holding, through slow smooth movements, to a staccato type rhythm and manipulation performed at speed. For example, a joint that has much pain will be best treated with grades performed slowly and evenly; a stiff small joint, in say the hand, would be treated with sharp staccato movements.

Of the many techniques described in the following text some are used commonly, others less commonly, and some only on a few occasions. Not all techniques must be taught in detail. If the principles and application of the important ones are understood, this will be enough to ensure that the least important ones can be done when the need arises. Their presence in the text shows how techniques can be modified to suit unusual circumstances. The most commonly used techniques are marked with three asterisks (***), the less commonly used with two asterisks (**), and the techniques that are used least and need not to be taught in detail at the undergraduate level with one asterisk (*).

Where applicable, techniques will be applied to the joints on the right side of the body. The patient will be referred to as 'him' and the physiotherapist as 'her' although the operator is depicted as male in the figures. The physiotherapist is called 'her' in order to emphasize the fact that brute strength is not essential to the use of manipulative treatment − rather, what is required are perceptive hands and an agile, methodical mind. Unless otherwise stated the patient will be lying supine for all techniques. Each joint will be described separately and more than one starting position may be given for one direction of movement.

Many techniques are performed in positions similar to those used for examination; others have different positions for the operator. The physiotherapist tests many directions of passive movement during examination, each being performed only once or twice. This may indicate the use of one position. In treatment the movement is repeated many times in only one direction although the position in the range may alter.

The gentler grades of movement sometimes require different starting positions from the stronger grades. The positions described are suitable for learning the various techniques but they may not suit all physiotherapists. Therefore, as the skill is learned and the feel of joint movement becomes instinctive, each physiotherapist should modify her positions to suit her own circumstances.

When the treatment movement is carried into the painful range and the patient finds it difficult to relax, the treatment movement must be regular, it must be performed slower than usual and the rhythm must be even. The patient will then know exactly how his joint is being moved and will find it easier to relax.

Direction of movement

When an oscillatory movement is used in treatment, the treating direction of that movement is most commonly performed at a speed that is faster than the retreating movement. For example if a general wrist *extension* is the movement to be made painless, and it is extended from the fully flexed position, these rules apply:

1. It would be quite pointless to perform a flexion – extension oscillation at the limit of the flexion.
2. It would be equally pointless if the speed of the flexion part of the oscillation equalled that of the extension.
3. The requirement of the technique was determined by the examination: extension *from* full flexion reproduced the patient's symptoms most clearly, and the technique was planned to provoke a degree of pain. The treatment movement is performed thus: the patient's wrist is slowly taken to the limit of its range of flexion, from which it is then immediately extended through the range, and at a quicker speed, so that the symptoms are reproduced. The slower flexion is then repeated, and so on.

This can be thought of as a *release technique* and it has a place in mobilization that most practitioners appreciate.

Broken rhythm

Some patients have difficulty in relaxing completely, even when pain is minimal. They periodically tense their muscles without realizing they do so. If large-amplitude treatment movements are hindered by this tensing, treatment movements of **broken**

rhythm and changing amplitude should be employed in an attempt to trick the muscles. Sometimes these movements need to be performed almost as a flick.

Examination

When a technique is initially used in treatment, it is commonly employed in an exploratory manner to determine the response of the joint. Hence the treatment movement is continually modified to meet the demands of the condition. The movements used may vary in depth, gradually moving in deeper and receding according to what is felt at different depths. This exploratory technique is an extension of passive movement examination.

Stationary holding

When attempting to increase the range of movement by stretching a stiff joint which is painful at its limit, the movement should be applied slowly within the available range up to the point when pain becomes a limiting factor (Figure 5.4). This new position

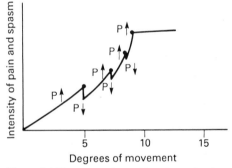

Figure 5.4 Slow steps of stretching. P = pain; ↑ = increase of pain; ↓ = decrease of pain

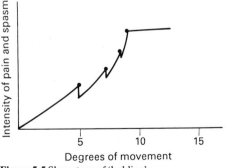

Figure 5.5 Slow steps of 'holding'

should be held stationary until the pain subsides after which a further slow stretch is added (perhaps only 1 or 2 degrees) until the pain increases again.

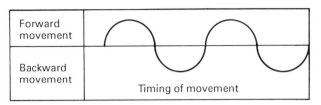

Figure 5.6 Smooth change of direction of movement

When the tolerable limit is reached, the movement is again held until the pain decreases. The procedure is continued in these small steps until the pain does not decrease (Figure 5.5). Small slow oscillatory movements are then performed just short of this limit.

Slow smooth oscillations

The *change* of direction of the movement from backward to forward should be imperceptible (Figure 5.6). This particular rhythm (probably grade II) is used when the disorder is causing a lot of pain.

Distraction and compression

There is a place in treatment when joint surfaces should be kept apart (to avoid contact) while still being able to treat by passive movement yet avoiding the aggravating element. Equally, and more commonly, there is a place in treatment for moving a joint while compressing (and rubbing) the adjacent joint surfaces together.

When the patient has much pain, or if the disorder is very irritable, the joint surfaces must be kept apart. This distraction is only a very small movement (less than 1 mm) and does not resemble traction forces.

Compression is another matter. The circumstances under which this is used apply to chronic disorders, chronic in terms of symptoms, not necessarily 'long term'. Two common examples are hip pain and shoulder pain. These are examples of pain being provoked by lying on the affected joint. The longer the person is able to lie on the offending joint before pain begins, the stronger the compression needs to be while performing the treatment chosen and the longer the treatment technique needs to be applied. Lowther refers to these movements as 'stirring movements'[1], and 'cyclical loading'[2].

There is one aspect about performing the techniques which, in my view, is probably the most important part of applying any manual technique – it is a very personal thing and sometimes it cannot be achieved.

Question: Have you been to an orchestral concert for piano or flute (and I suppose this applies to other solo artists playing with an orchestra)? If you have, have you seen the extent to which the soloist involves himself with the meaning of the work – with the composer's emotions when he wrote the music?

You may feel that what I am trying to say is nonsense and has no place in this book. However, it is absolutely essential to involve ourselves with our patients and their problems in the same sort of manner. I suppose what I'm trying to do is reply to a statement often made, 'you can't learn manipulation from books', that is quite false. But you can't learn from books unless you commit your whole self, your whole being, to trying to *feel* what is going on with the technique while you are performing it.

Please bear with me as I quote from the conductor André Previn.

"A musical concept of learning from writing and doing."

'As a conductor your responsibility first and last is to those notes (techniques) as written, wiping from your memory all preconceived notions. What I mean is that you must forget the day to day circumstances of a composer's life [author's life] and how such circumstances might or might not have found expression in the music [text]. A lot of the time it's difficult, but that is what you must at least *try* to do.

More importantly is, how accurate are those written notes, those dots and dashes.

Musical notation [manipulative texts] can at times be really hopelessly vague even when dealing with absolutely fundamental ingredients of music [treatment]. Let's look at those four notes [grades and rhythms] as they appear in the score [text].

The fourth note is marked with a pause over it. Well how long should that pause be?

1. Lowther, D. A. The effect of compression and tension on the behaviour of connective tissues. *Aspects of Manipulative Therapy*, 2nd edn., pp. 16–22 (1985)
2. Lowther, D. A. The effect of mechanical stress on the behaviour of connective tissue. *Australian Journal of Physiotherapy*, **29**, 181 (1983)

Is it like this? . . . or is it like this? . . . .

And it's marked with two F's (ff) – Fortissimo – very loud.

Well, wait a minute.

How loud is loud? How soft is soft?

And when a composer like Stravinsky [Therapist A] specifies loud, is it the *same* degree of loudness – or even more importantly, the same quality of attack – as when you play Mozart [Therapist B]? Of course not.

So how do you, as a conductor or instrumentalist [physiotherapist] decide that *your* interpretation of the notes is the only possible correct one? After all, no two conductors are alike; no two performances are identical, and much more to the point –

Every time you play a piece you discover new details you haven't noticed before.

The truth is that there's never any single or definitive interpretation. Indeed I would go so far as to say that the greater the composition, the more your understanding of it is likely to develop over the years.

Think about it for a moment. You can write a letter putting words to paper and while you're writing those letters you understand those words mentally without having to hear them out loud. It's the same with composers who have learnt to put musical notes on a manuscript paper as easily as words of a letter, but everybody works differently, and while Beethoven's habit was to jot down his ideas in sketchbooks, Mozart, apparently, resolved every detail in his head before he committed the entire works onto paper, he hardly ever changed so much as a note.'

What I am trying to say is that when you are trying to improve the quality of a sick joint's movement by a passive movement technique it is necessary to put yourself or your mind inside the person, or, more accurately, inside the joint area, and to involve yourself emotionally with what the joint is trying to tell you about how it wants to be moved. I believe that this commitment is the difference between the good physiotherapists and the bad physiotherapists.

When – Which – Why

Having talked about grades and rhythms, what does one choose? There are many factors that influence the choices:

1. There is a choice of accessory movements or physiological movements.
2. A choice of minimal distraction or compression.
3. A choice of sagittal plane, coronal plane, horizontal plane or longitudinal direction (in any of the planes just mentioned).

4. A choice of combining techniques in varying sequences.
5. A choice that is directed by pathology and other such factors (recent injury, chronic disorder).
6. A choice that is dependent on the therapist's experience and skill.

The following text relates the manner of performance of the chosen technique rather than choosing the technique.

Pain and irritability

If the patient has a very irritable disorder and the degree of the pain is both constant and severe, the technique must obviously be gentle. It then avoids the circumstances when the technique causes pain during treatment and also aims to avoid any latent reaction or exacerbation. Under such circumstances the grade used would need to be painless, with as large an amplitude as painless range will permit. The rhythm would be very smooth in its changes of direction of the oscillation, and it would be performed slowly. Again, the speed should be as fast as the disorder will permit while still maintaining painless oscillations.

This is probably a good stage to state one of the rules associated with passive movement treatment. If the disorder presents its pain as a through-range-pain, it should be treated by a through-range-technique – in other words, a large amplitude. This rule may be dictated by the disorder being an intra-articular disorder. If may also be used to treat (maintenance treatment perhaps) a joint that has pathological changes within the joint as seen in osteo-arthritis.

In the first stages of treatment, the prudent choice is to use accessory movements rather than physiological movements, as it is easier to produce a larger amplitude painlessly and more smoothly. As the symptoms decrease, so the amplitude and the combination of different accessory movements can be used.

Chronic aching

Under this heading the patients do not have severe pain but have an ache which they feel is greater than they class as acceptable. The range of movement may not be markedly restricted, but if the movement is stretched the pain will increase. This is an *'end-of-range-pain'* without a *'through-range-pain'* component. Under these circumstances there is no need for large-amplitude movement. The choice lies in the end-of-range technique, that is the grade IV type technique in both accessory movements and physiological movements. For the grade IV accessory movement techniques it may be necessary to place the structures on stretch in a physiological position to make the accessory movement technique effective.

If the range gained is highly satisfactory, but the end-of-range-pain has increased; or if the painful range now occupies a larger extent, a *'treatment-soreness'* technique should be used. This technique uses a much larger amplitude and it must be in the same direction and range as the grade IV but performed as a grade III−; slowly and smoothly gradually trying to reach a stage of being able to perform a grade III painlessly. If this can be achieved there will be no soreness resulting from the treatment.

If the patients' circumstances are such that restriction of range is far more important than pain, the technique of greatest value is the same small-amplitude end-of-range technique but the rhythm would be staccato.

Muscle spasm

When strong spasm is present to protect the area from painful movements or positions, there is only one technique to use. The structure has to be moved to the point in the range when the spasm comes in to play. At this point the stretch is sustained without movement. When the pain level lowers, as it will, the stretch can be increased and held again. The range of movement will gradually increase until a certain stage is reached when the spasm will not let go. At this point the position should be sustained but interspersed by tiny slow smooth movements. *It*

is at this stage, and only at this stage, when the technique is reaching and attacking the disorder.

Techniques such as 'slow reversal', 'reciprocal relaxation' or 'contract–relax' can be used. These techniques can achieve the same initial result as the stepped passive stretch. However, when the plateau has been reached, the neuromuscular techniques will not attack the disorder. Passive movement is the only technique that may achieve that small extra range so vital to improving the range that the disorder will allow.

In conclusion

There are hundreds upon hundreds of techniques. Preferences vary from therapist to therapist, but the important thing to remember is that the speed, amplitude, pain response during performance, pathology and diagnosis all have an influence on HOW the technique is performed (Table 5.1). Essentially we must endeavour to be guided by what is happening during the performing of the chosen grade and rhythm and also what the patient feels as a response.

Table 5.1 Grades of movement in various conditions

Condition	Grades used
Through-range pain	II− to III+
Intra-articular pathology	II− to III or III−
End-of-range pain	IV to IV+ or IV++
Technique soreness	II or III− to III or III+ painlessly

6

Disorders

It is not the purpose of this chapter to provide a comprehensive discussion on all orthopaedic and rheumatological disorders, but rather to categorize the most common of the disorders treated by the physiotherapist. For a further description of each disorder and a wider cover of disorders, the reader is referred to Apley[1] and Corrigan and Maitland[2].

The word 'disorders' is used in this text to cover any complaint from which any patient may suffer and be referred for physiotherapy. The title then includes those disorders that can be given an accurate titled diagnosis as well as those that, though perhaps being recognized as a syndrome, cannot be precisely titled. It should also be remembered that there are occasions when a patient is referred to a physiotherapist to assist in the diagnosis ('differential diagnosis'). This occurs most commonly when abdominal or chest pain is present and its source uncertain. Even limb pain (e.g. hip/knee pain) occurring in conjunction with an active disease process such as a malignancy, may have a mechanical component unrelated to the malignancy itself. This can be differentiated and in turn treated.

Musculo-skeletal disorders

Musculo-skeletal disorders may be loosely grouped into those whose symptoms have developed gradually, and those whose symptoms have a notable traumatic origin (Table 6.1).

Within the insidious or spontaneous onset group, by far the greatest majority will have a story and presenting symptoms and signs that fit into a regular and readily recognized pattern. Cyriax's 'capsular patterns' are perfect examples of typical (regular) patterns. When irregular symptoms and signs are present, there is probably an underlying 'misuse' or 'overuse' basis, or a structural, functional, or disease reason that will account for the irregular pattern.

Table 6.1 Classification of musculo-skeletal disorders

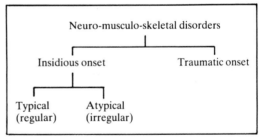

Disorders and their histories

Developing the background history of these groups is an interesting exercise. It is one that helps the physiotherapist to develop a skill in prognosis – not only a prognosis related to treatment expectation, but also related to the likelihood of recurrences and to the development of preventative measures. It is the history of the patient's known onset of symptoms that provides part of the background to the disorders – BUT, it is only part of the background (and it is the easiest part to develop in the history taking skill). The therapist's skill in seeking what basis preceded the onset of the

1. Apley, A. G. and Solomon, L. *Apley's System of Orthopaedics and Fractures,* 6th edn., Butterworths, London (1982)
2. Corrigan, B. and Maitland, G. D. *Practical Orthopaedic Medicine,* Butterworths, London (1983)

symptoms is the main part. To be able to ask the right questions to extract this important part of the history requires knowledge about the possibilities for the different groups.

Understanding the cause of the insidious onset is essential to understanding the patient's presenting signs and symptoms and assessing the prognosis for recovery (Table 6.2). Some patients have a familial or genetic predisposition to develop certain disorders when other factors are present. Other disorders develop as a result of predisposing activities. Then there are those who have had an unrecognized trivial incident. In all three situations the patient is often unaware of the reason for the onset of symptoms. Skilled questioning is essential to establish the relationship of any predisposing factor to the presenting symptoms.

Table 6.2 Causes of insidious onset

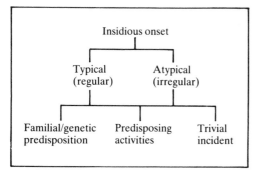

Familial/genetic predisposition

An example of this is those patients who might loosely be called 'jointy people', often referred to as having 'acute joint awareness' or 'genetic sensitivity'. They have symptoms in different joint areas from time to time. The symptoms may 'come-and-go' for no obvious reason and they rarely seek treatment unless the symptoms persist or restrict their normal activities. Tracing familial components to the disorder often reveals somewhat similar symptoms in another sibling or in one of the parents.

The actual onset of symptoms for patients in this category is never straight forward, yet it does have a general pattern. The current symptoms for which they seek treatment do have a reasonably standard onset. The onset is either (a) that the patient has noticed developing symptoms during and after performing an activity with which he would normally have no difficulties, or (b) that he has noticed aching in different joint-areas for short periods (2 or 3 days) over the preceding few months (2–3 months or more). This commonly begins when the patient is in his early thirties. He knows of no reason why they should have developed.

The delving into the background of the disorder's earlier history might have a dialogue similar to the following:

ET There has to be some reason why the symptoms should have begun and somehow we should be able to 'make the features fit'.

Q 'Can you recall when you FIRST had ANY symptoms, however mild they may have been?'

ET If he seems to be taking an inordinate length of time trying to answer, I'll help him by giving two extremes for him to choose from.

Q 'Are you thinking in terms of weeks or years?'

A 'The recent trouble has been about 3 months, but I was trying to think about the months, and even 2 or 3 years you mentioned because as a child I was supposed to have had what they called "growing pains".'

Q 'Well, if we say your present problem started 4 months ago, are you saying that 5, 6, or 7 months ago you were totally symptom free?'

A 'No, not totally free. I have had the occasional awareness of an ache in my shoulder or hip, even my elbow and knee, for a day or two at a time, but otherwise I would say I have been without symptoms.'

Q 'Can you relate those 1 or 2 days of aching to anything?'

A 'No, I don't think so.'

Q 'Could you have been doing anything different at the time?'

A 'No, not that I can think of.'

Q 'Might you have been unwell or overtired?'

A 'I could have been overtired. I am under pressure at work from time to time.'

Q 'And have these been at times when you had symptoms?'

A 'They could well have been.'

ET This isn't getting me far, but there is one useful avenue I could follow up.

Q 'Do you do different things at the weekends from what you do during the week at work?'

A 'Yes, quite different. I work in the garden most weekends.'

Q 'And does that cause any symptoms?'

A 'Well it does, but I feel that more on Mondays.'

Q 'And what is it like on Tuesdays?'

A 'Much better, nearly all gone – certainly gone by Tuesday evening.'

Q 'And is that pain much the same as your present problem?'

A 'Yes, much the same but it is more general.'

ET I wonder if he has ever had an episode of pain similar to this episode. I feel I have a responsibility to exclude this possibility anyway. If he has had an acute episode it may indicate that he could have a predisposition to a more 'active' disorder.

Q 'Have you at any time had more severe symptoms, perhaps even temporarily preventing you from doing certain activities; may have lasted a few weeks?'

A 'No, not at all.'

ET Well that clarifies those predisposing possibilities.

Q 'Have any other members of your family, parents, brothers, sisters, had any aches and pains like yours?'

A 'Yes, my sister and mother have had problems. My mother's is mainly in her hip but my sister has much the same as I.'

ET That is a big help to me. It seems that (a) there may be a familial or genetic predisposition, (b) his body can't, at the moment, take exercise like gardening without complaint, and (c) if the growing pains are part of the history, his disorder, in one form or another, is very long standing. It influences my treatment goal – I would hope that I can settle his present symptoms to their previous state – I might also be prepared to treat the other symptoms. I know that he can't be made symptom or sign free but I know I have three prophylactic measures that may improve his future:

1. Gravity-assisted, large-range, loose swinging type movements.
2. If his body can accept the gravity assisted exercises I can add isometric and then isotonic exercises.
3. Perhaps the most useful thing would be to teach another member of the family to passive mobilize gently the symptomatic areas using large-range symptomless movements.

This should be explained to him in full so that his expectations are put into their proper perspective. He can then know and understand that his care is an ongoing one for which he can return for treatment if his own home treatment is not sufficiently successful.

Predisposition through use

As a distinctly separate group, there are the people who have predisposing activities as the background to the onset of their symptoms. This is a complex section with many subdivisions and much overlapping. The predisposing components are widely varied and often relate to the office worker who, at the weekend, performs different and physical activities. It also applies to people playing sport, subjecting themselves to ever-increasing levels of their particular activity. This latter group also includes middle aged people who decide that they should endeavour to become fit by doing a regimen of exercises for the first time. They develop symptoms when the exercising exceeds that to which their bodies can adapt.

All of the subdivisions of predisposition through use relate to two factors. The first is the type and vigour of an activity being performed and the second is the state of the structures being used and their ability to accept the use. It is this second factor that is frequently not adequately taken into account. The human body has an enormous capacity to adapt to demands, and if the demands are gradually and progressively increased within the limits of pain, ligaments can thicken and strengthen, muscles can develop and support more strongly, and even bony growths can develop to support around joints and in ligaments/tendons. The different types of predisposition through use that can exist are:

1. New use.
2. Misuse.
3. Overuse.
4. Abuse.
5. Disuse.

'New-use' is self-explanatory. It relates to a person performing some activity that he has either not performed before, or has not performed for a long time. The result from performing this new activity (a) for too long, (b) too strenuously, or (c) beyond the capacities of the structures involved at their present state of health, will be pain.

If each part (a–c above) in the 'new use' activity in unfavourable, the resultant pain will be great, and the recovery time will be long.

The historical questions that need to be asked are:

'How heavy a job was it?'
'How long did you do it for?'
'Have you ever done this before?' (A 'No.')
'Did you stop because the job was completed, or because you couldn't physically go on with it any longer?'
'Did you feel any discomfort or pain while you were doing it or was it after you stopped?'
'Have you had any symptoms (grades of pain or weakness) in this area before?' (This is seeking predisposition by virtue of lowered capacities of the structure involved.)

The answers to these questions, and their relation to the severity and duration of the presenting disorder, provide the information needed to make a treatment–success prognosis.

'Misuse' relates to having had to carry out a function that was awkward or an activity that was performed in an unnecessarily silly manner, either of which, if performed without constraints, would have been done differently. In other words the muscles, ligament and joints have been stressed by the awkwardness of the function.

Under these circumstances, as with 'new use', the awkwardness and the severity of the symptoms need to be related to the severity of the activity, and any predisposition would be determined and interrelated. There is one objective examination test that may need to be carried out and that is to ask the patient to simulate the function that caused the symptoms while the therapist tests the structures in this function.

'Overuse' is another self-explanatory term. All of the structures that together form the human body have a breaking point. Many of these structures in most people can have their breaking point raised by training. However, there is a limit to how far the body can adapt, and this varies enormously from one individual to another. I well remember a man whose talent and training enabled him to be a successful 'weight-lifter' and 'bottom-man' in a balancing and acrobatic team. He had a pain free life until he was 85 years of age when he developed shoulder pain from manually clipping the edges of a lawn while on his hands and knees. The point of interest was that he was fortunate enough to have a body which, during his active life, could adapt to the demands he placed upon it. His vertebrae had bony bridges between them and his tenomuscular and musculotendinous junctions were reinforced by bony components. Yet he had not had pain throughout his life until the short-lived shoulder pain. The human body is extraordinary beyond our comprehension, a point never to be forgotten.

When a patient presents for treatment with symptoms that can be put down to a vigorous 'overuse' situation, the problems are only just beginning. People playing high-grade competitive sports, especially if the sport consists of long durations of the activity at a time, are prone to develop symptoms. This is because they exceed the limit of the body's adaptation to the demand. This does not mean that they will not respond to treatment and appropriate retraining, but the mixture of treatment and retraining requires a very sensible understanding attitude by the patient.

The information needed for the history is:

Q   'Can you demonstrate for me now the action that causes the pain?'
'How long have you been doing it in this particular manner?'
'For how long do you do it at a time?'
'How often do you do it?'
'Did the pain first start as a sudden onset at one particular moment?'

If it had a sudden onset, it could be classed as 'abuse' (see below) superimposed on 'overuse', or as 'overuse' reaching the breaking point of structures beyond the body's ability to adapt to the demands.

If the symptoms develop gradually over a period of 1–3 weeks of daily repetition, then breaking point has not quite been reached, but the warning is there, and it soon will be reached if the same demand is continued.

The gradual onset of symptoms is an 'overuse' situation. It can normally be remedied if the activity is stopped prior to the onset of pain. When pain is the limiting factor, treatment by passive movement should be performed intermittently, slowly, smoothly and gently through as full a RANGE as possible such that no pain is reproduced. Once the pain is relieved, controlled exercises combined with a gradual increase of the overuse-activity can be implemented. Fry[3] provides an excellent paper on this overuse in which he says:

'Overuse syndrome in musicians, a common disorder, is characterized by pain and loss of function in muscles and joint ligaments of the upper limb. In wind players the same process can affect the muscles forming the embouchure, the soft palate and the muscles of the throat. Individuals vary in *susceptibility*, so *the threshold of overuse cannot be known* in advance . . . the condition is typically *brought on by an increase in the duration and intensity* of practice or playing. . . .'

'Abuse', as with the other terms, is self-explanatory. It relates to a person who physically abuses his body (or parts of it) beyond reasonable limits. If the abuse is considered in the 'spontaneous onset' group the history will not contain a once-only abuse resulting in sudden injury or pain, but rather, it will consist of repetitive abuse until pain is felt. The person usually continues the abuse until he becomes disabled. These abusive actions are those that, no matter how fit or well trained the person is who performs them, he would still be classified as abusing his body.

The history is straightforward, but it is necessary to know:

1. How long the abusive activity has been going on for.
2. At what stage it became symptomatic.
3. How long it was continued before he decided that he could not continue any longer.
4. Were there any 'predisposing factors' that may indicate that the degree of abuse: (a)caused the pain sooner than would have been the case otherwise; or (b)is the severity of the disability greater than would otherwise have been the case?
5. Has the abuse-effect been further worsened by its causing an active inflammatory response?

In defence of the person who does perform abusive type activities, it must be realized that he must be

3. Fry, H. J. H. Overuse syndrome in musicians: prevention and management. *Lancet*, **ii**, 728–731 (1986)

getting an enormous gratification from whatever it is he is doing. It is not necessarily right to stop him doing it because of the long-term ill-effect it may have. To stop him may have a longer term ill-effect.

'Disuse' merely puts the body at a disadvantage at a time when the person may be in a position where an active demand is put on him. If the same demand is put on a person who is normally active, symptoms will not develop. In terms of history taking, the requirement is to determine how unfit, in terms of use (disuse), is the part of his body on which the demand is to be put. That is the first approach to the history. The second is to determine the 'disuse' in terms of laziness compared with genetic inability, and to previous injury/disease resulting in forced disuse. The importance of this questioning lies in the information it gives about the prognosis of rehabilitation and preventing recurrence of symptoms.

The longer the body is subjected to any of the above predispositions, (new use, misuse, overuse, abuse, disuse), the greater the likelihood injury will occur. For example, in relation to the underlying overuse: (a) the greater the vigour and frequency of the overuse, and (b) the longer the duration of the overuse (i) per day and (ii) per lifetime, the less the structures being overused can tolerate, and therefore the less the injuring force needs to be to cause disability. Further, when one predisposition through use is superimposed on another, the effects are compounded.

Disadvantaged joints

To repeat, the word joint here is used loosely to cover widely all inert components associated with the moving joint. A disadvantaged joint has some structural anomaly for change which renders it prone to cause symptoms if it is subjected to a stress. The same stress to a 'normal' joint with a normal configuration would not cause symptoms. Examples demonstrate three varieties of 'disadvantaged joints'.

1. Poorly shaped femoral condyles that predispose to recurrent subluxation of the patella. The joint is disadvantaged structurally (genetically).
2. The 'overuse' and 'abuse' situations. Here, repetitive stressful asymptomatic use of a joint, such as to the knee and ankle in people who compete in events such as the springboard/vaulting-horse, disadvantages the joints for their future.
3. A joint sprain that ruptures a ligament such as the medial ligament of the knee, renders the joint disadvantaged.

(2) and (3) have been referred to in the sections on 'newuse, misuse, overuse, and abuse', but they were not characterized as being 'disadvantaged'. However, it is the first one, the genetically structured joint

described above, which is the 'disadvantaged' joint which may be the underlying basis for a disorder.

Trivial incident

It is common for patients to present with the history of an incident that is trivial. One example of the trivial incident group is when a person leans over the back of the front seat of a car to lift a parcel from the back seat. This action causes a sharp pain in the shoulder which lasts no more than a second. This incident is forgotten, but the shoulder develops a moderate ache some weeks later. Such a trivial incident produces lasting symptoms; the therapist should look for a predisposing factor.

Traumatic origin

Sprain and direct injury are included under this main heading, and each has its differences.

As with the 'insidious onset' disorders, 'typical' and 'atypical' also apply. For example, the common type of sprained ankle or torn medial meniscus of the knee are typical in their presentation of history symptoms and signs. In contrast, a pedestrian or cyclist being knocked over by a motor vehicle will not be typical or regular in the presentation of symptoms and signs. Though they may have parts of their symptoms and signs that resemble regular patterns, overall they will be very irregular in their presentation (Table 6.3).

Table 6.3 Presentation of trauma

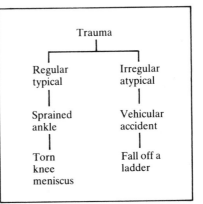

Sprain indicates that the person has had an unexpected unguarded movement forced on the part which becomes injured. A sprained ankle is the one that most readily comes to mind. The history is important.

Q 'What actually happened? How did you "go over" on your ankle?'

A   'I don't really know. I was playing football at the time – I had just got hold of the ball and twisted to get away from the opposition and just went over on my ankle.'

Q   'Did you go over on the ankle on the inside of the direction to which you twisted?'

(Don't go on to say 'or was it the foot on the outside of the direction you twisted?' To understand the reasoning for stating this, just read out each of the ways of asking the question to yourself a few times and assess which is the easiest to formulate the answer for.)

ET   The examiner's question would have been 'What, as far as YOU are concerned . . . is YOUR . . . MAIN problem?'

His answer would have been something like 'pain in my ankle when walking on uneven ground or when running.'

Q   'Show me where you feel this.'

Which he proceeds to do. Then,

Q   'What caused it?'
A   'I sprained my ankle at footy.'

Two thoughts might come to mind: (a) that spraining an ankle at football might not be the same as spraining an ankle when, say, stepping down a gutter; and (b) the areas of pain he has indicated would probably, under these circumstances, be different from the more common sprained ankle. As the pain isn't totally typical, detailed questioning is needed. He stated that it was his ankle on the outside of the direction to which he twisted which he 'went-over' on.

Q   'Did you fall?'
A   'No I just couldn't keep going.'
ET   NEVER ASSUME ANYTHING.
Q   'Why couldn't you keep going?'
A   'The other bloke slammed his foot on top of mine and pinned it to the ground.'
Q   of readers: 'Would you have thought of that?' I wouldn't (and didn't).
ET   The examiner may have found this out by asking him where his bruising was, to which he would have probably indicated the common areas for a sprained ankle, plus a few more, plus two football boot sprig holes on the lateral–proximal dorsum of the foot.

So it becomes obvious that it is necessary to determine just in what directions and how the sprain occurred. This applies to any 'sprain' of any moving part (muscle, ligament, tendon, capsule, nerve). It is then often necessary to ask the patient to demonstrate the spraining movement as well as other movements that reproduce the symptoms.

In fact the above is the story of a real patient, one who had not responded to other physiotherapy which had been applied in a manner to suit the common variety of sprained ankle. It is necessary to be open minded and alert to what might be atypical. When he described his injury, and was then asked to demonstrate how it happened, he stood up, asked that the right foot be held firmly on the ground, then he twisted his whole body towards the left, and with his left foot facing in almost the opposite direction to his fixed right foot he flexed his body forwards (twisted of course) over his flexed left knee and hip, then tried to pull his right foot off the fixed position on the floor. 'His' pain was reproduced by the movement. Treating this with gentle oscillatory stretches in this position, and gradually increasing the strength of the oscillatory stretches as pain decreased, was the primary treatment which relieved him of his disability.

MAKE FEATURES FIT

This statement of 'making-features-fit' cannot be overemphasized. Just suppose that a patient had sprained an ankle a year ago and it had still not recovered (say there was still a 40% degree of disability) despite continued treatment which sounded to have been reasonably sensibly applied, then the 'features don't fit'. So, why? *What is different about this sprained ankle?* One should not just give up and say 'you'll have to live with it' without delving more deeply into the story, previous history, other associable illnesses, pattern of symptoms, immediate responses to physical treatment, what the patient's body (in this example, his foot) can tell him about what it likes and dislikes having done to it – there is almost no end to the probing to be done to make sense out of the story – why isn't it getting better? He can't be just left like this, what can we do? As well as the probing questioning there is the probing physical examination – using combinations of movements, using functional resisted movements at speed, movements with strong compression. There must be something to find, questioning or examining, to make the features fit before deciding that it is an hysterical disorder, and there aren't too many of those.

Unguarded movements, unprotected movements, flicking movements beyond muscular protection, are among the most difficult disorders to restore to normal. They create a degree of damage that is far greater than one would expect. It is important to remember this when endeavouring to 'make features fit' in relation to treatment response and examination findings.

Direct injury is quite different to sprain though sprains may be part of the total injury. Knowing details of the accident provides considerable useful information which may guide treatment, so this forms an important part of the history. Any previous history in the areas injured by the accident often help to 'make the features fit' more exactly. But really, the most important part of the examination (and subsequent direction of treatment) lies in the answers to the question:

Q 'At this stage – what is your main problem?'
Q 'What is it that you can't do at this stage?'

An example of this is a young man who had had his right arm from his hand to his shoulder badly squashed in a car accident. Question: what can't he do at this stage (some 9 months after the injury)? He couldn't lift a motor car tyre off the floor. So what? He was a motor mechanic and if he could only lift a car tyre off the floor he could return to work despite his other arm injuries and disabilities. And so it is obvious where the aim of treatment would lie at that stage.

Differential diagnosis

A patient may have pain which he feels is in his shoulder whereas in fact its source may lie in his cervical spine or its neuromeningeal elements. With pain in the right shoulder, the cause may even be in the gall-bladder (visceral origin). The physiotherapist may be asked to determine the source of the symptoms thus forming one aspect of differential diagnosis. Even when the symptoms do arise from the shoulder complex, the subjective and objective examination needs to differentiate between the different structures that make up the shoulder. However, it is not this aspect that is being considered here under the 'differential' aspect of diagnosis.

A somewhat different aspect related to differential diagnosis which can again be related to the shoulder (though it is not uncommon in other joints) presents itself when the patient has pain in the vicinity of the insertion of the deltoid muscle into the humerus, without any pain being felt in the shoulder. This is an example of referred pain. Another common example of this aspect is pain felt only in the knee yet arising from a painless hip disorder. The mechanism of such referral is not

clearly understood, nevertheless the clinical entity is common, and the site of the cause is regularly able to be proved.

Viscerogenic pain can be referred into areas of the musculo-skeletal system. An example related to the gall-bladder and right shoulder pain was cited above. Similarly, left arm pain associated with cardiac disorders is quite common. There are other examples where the referral is in the opposite direction. That is, pain can be referred to an area which the patient describes as being in one of the viscera. The referral under these circumstances however is usually vertebral column rather than from the peripheral joints. Nevertheless, pain in the testicular region can have its origin in the hip.

Table 6.4 lists the possibilities when the physiotherapist may be called upon to assist in the making of a diagnosis.

Intra-articular/peri-articular

When symptoms are felt in the region of a mobile joint, and it is determined that it *is* the particular joint (including its inert supportive structures) that is the source of the symptoms, it becomes necessary to determine whether it is an intra-articular or a peri-articular disorder (Table 6.5). Although this may seem a simple process, it is not always so.

Within this context, the behaviour of the symptoms, both on movement and at rest, become a primary consideration.

1. On movement

It is indicative here to determine whether the symptoms are felt on movement only at the end of the available range of movement (EOR pain), or that they are felt to be amplified through a large section of the range (through-range pain). These findings are not exactly clear cut when recent severe traumatic injury is the cause of the disorder. Under these circumstances there will probably be through-range pain as well as increased pain at or near the end of the available range. Similarly when moving

Table 6.4 The possibilities for referred symptoms

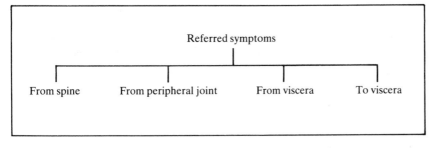

Table 6.5 Differentiation between intra-articular and peri-articular disorders.
EOR = End of range

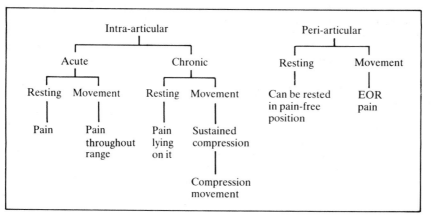

an osteoarthritic (say) hip, when it is an active phase, it will have a through-range pain, but will also have an increased end-of-range pain when being stretched. This can mean, of course, that the disorder has an intra-articular and peri-articular component.

Compression with movement

In the more chronic disorders when pain is not severe, movements through-range and movements to the end-of-range may not provoke or reproduce any discomfort. It is under these circumstances that the through-range movements should be tested as repeated oscillatory movements while at the same time the joint's two articular surfaces are held firmly compressed together. Chronic intra-articular disorders of a joint will be uncomfortable or painful if tested in this way.

2. At rest

Considering the situation when the joint is at rest, peri-articular structures will not be painful provided:

1. That they are neither in a position of stretch or squash.
2. That the structures are neither inflamed nor severely damaged.

On the other hand, when the disorder is a painful intra-articular one, it will ache when at rest, even if it is positioned in an unstressed, well-supported neutral position.

Compression sustained

Another consideration related to resting pain is that a patient with a chronic intra-articular disorder may

have discomfort if he lies on his painful joint. On examination of this joint, it should be possible to reproduce these symptoms by compressing the adjacent articular surfaces together and sustaining the strong compression. Peri-articular disorders will not be painful with this test.

In the subjective part of the examination, the questions are asked:

Q   'How does it feel when you waken in the morning compared with when you go to bed?'
ET   The word 'it' is used to allow for spontaneous responses about anything the patient may feel at that time, rather than to restrict his thinking by asking 'How does the *pain* feel etc.'. Within the confines of (1) and (2) above, peri-articular symptoms will be improved, whereas intra-articular symptoms will be approximately unchanged or they will be worse.
Q   'How does it feel when you first get out of bed?'
ET   Both may feel stiffer than at other times but the length of time they remain stiff is different.
A   'It feels a bit stiff and painful.'
Q   'How long does that stiffness and pain last?'
OR
     'How long does it take for that to subside to its usual level?'
A1   'Only a short time – it's all right by the time I've had my shower.'
ET   This is not an intra-articular or an inflammatory disorder.
A2   'It gradually settles down.'
ET   That is not enough depth of information
Q   'What length of time are you thinking of, (ET Help him) 10 minutes or more than half an hour?'

A   'I suppose it's more like an hour or so.'

ET This is likely to be intra-articular and inflammatory. In fact it is not uncommon for such a disorder to make it impossible for a patient to be unable to stay in bed all night. He may well have to get out of bed, at least once, for half an hour or more before the increased symptoms subside enough to allow him to go back to bed. As a side-issue to this, but worth stating here, he should be taught how to do pendular movements which he should do when he is forced to get out of bed. These pendular movements should be small-range oscillatory painless movements produced by other parts of the body rather than the prime-movers of the joint(s) affected. These movements, if well performed, will reduce the pain and enable him to go back to bed much more quickly.

Sub-clinical arthritis

This is an extremely difficult subject to discuss without disputation and laying oneself open to criticism. Nevertheless, it is extremely important to have some understanding of:

1. What it is, and how it presents with patients.
2. How it relates to the arthritides.
3. What medical test results would indicate its presence.
4. What medical treatment can be used to indicate its presence.
5. What interpretations can be put on it in relation to treatment and prognosis.

Because there *is* a recognizable pattern of both the patient's symptoms on subjective questioning, and his physical signs on the objective examination, and because the varying responses to passive movements are clear and predictable in terms of (a) the value of physical treatment and (b) the indications for specific medical treatment, the subject should be tackled.

Definition of title 'sub-clinical arthritis'

1. Arthritis

This word simply means that there is an inflammatory process within a synovial joint, and as the 'arthritis' is here tied to the word sub-clinical, the inflammation will not necessarily show itself in terms of being 'red, hot, and swollen.' The word is also not saying that it is an osteoarthritis nor any other diagnosable arthritis disorder, such as, for example, rheumatoid arthritis.

The word arthritis should not be used as a synonym for osteoarthritis, and if the word is used to describe to a patient what he has wrong with him, it is essential to explain that he has **not** got osteoarthritis and he will not be confined to a wheelchair in the future. Some people have a fear of being crippled by osteoarthritis and this fear must be allayed.

2. Sub-clinical

This use of the word sub-clinical is meant to emphasize that a diagnosis of 'arthritis' cannot be given on a basis of positive blood tests, of radiological changes in a joint, or any other medical tests. However, it can be determined by the history of the patient's symptoms, the behaviour of the symptoms as the patient describes them, and the behaviour of the symptoms on differential physical examination especially if there are any after-effects following such examination.

Presentation

Symptoms

The symptoms felt by the patient are constant though they will vary in intensity. Too much activity and too much rest lead to increased pain. The pain is always at the site of (often better described as being 'within') the joint. If there is any referral of symptoms, they can spread proximally or distally from the joint and they will decrease in intensity as they spread away from the joint area.

On passive movement of the joint in any direction there will be a 'pain-through-range' response. This pain response is heightened if the passive movement is performed while the joint surfaces are held compressed together.

These patients avoid use of the joint affected and prefer to support it in a mid-range position, yet they also choose to move it about in many directions gently and comfortably in between periods of rest. After more prolonged periods of rest, such as during the night, patients find it more difficult to institute movement, the joint feels to have stiffened. However, this stiffness soon disappears following a little movement.

There is yet another aspect of pain present with this disorder. Following either examination movements, or activities that cause discomfort, there is a latent and lingering exacerbation of symptoms. This 'after-effect' is present with other disorders too but it is *always* present in the 'sub-clinical arthritis'. The exacerbation lasts for a longer period with the more active disorder than with an inactive arthritis.

The pain of this disorder differs from that found with a more mechanical type of inflammatory disorder. The latter pain *can* be relieved in particular positions of rest and the position of comfort can be maintained for much longer periods without the feeling of its needing to be moved. In a likewise manner, when it does feel the need for movement, the initial stiff feeling goes much more quickly: it will probably require only three movements before it is freed. These subtle differences are important to be able to distinguish. Perhaps the experience of treating these patients is the only way to be able to distinguish one from the other on the basis of pain alone. Experience teaches so much.

Movements

As stated above, movements in all directions of the affected synovial joint will be uncomfortable. It will be a 'through-range-pain' response to the movement, irrespective of whether the movement is a physiological one or a passive accessory movement.

The faster the movement is performed, the greater will be the pain. Conversely, it *may* be possible to move through 50% of the range without discomfort, provided the movement is performed:

1. Extremely slowly.
2. Passively (not actively because this involves a degree of joint compression).
3. In a manner that avoids any moderately firm contact of the contiguous joint surfaces.

This is in contrast to the more mechanical (this is an unfortunate term if it is taken literally) variety of arthritis (mentioned above under the 'symptoms' heading), where a moderate degree of speed or joint surface contact is not excessively painful.

Comparing a small passive movement of the affected joint, first with the joint surfaces in their usual normal relationship, and then with compression of the joint surfaces, there is a marked difference in the pain responses. The slow uncompressed movement is far less painful than that felt when compression is added.

Examination of movements of a joint that may be thought to have a sub-clinical arthritic involvement should initially be performed slowly. This avoids exacerbation that occurs from over zealous testing. Having tested some of the movements it is possible to have an idea of the likely reaction to the examination. Armed with this information, the following test procedure of a movement will provide definite information as to how primary the inflammatory component of the disorder is. Circumstances can exist where a patient feels pain or discomfort in rhythm with oscillatory movements performed by a therapist. This is not uncommon when these movements are performed at or near the end of a range. With the sub-clinical arthritic disorder, oscillatory movement within range (grade II−) may be felt as a movement within the joint. However, important though this is, it is not as important as the fact that an ache within the joint will develop and it

will increase in intensity as the oscillations are continued. This build-up of ache is a consistent finding with this disorder. To continue building-up the ache is harmful and should therefore be avoided. However, more information of importance is gained if a minimal ache is first provoked with a known number of oscillations. The movement is stopped, and time taken noted for the ache to subside. When it has subsided, the same number of oscillations is repeated and the ache compared, as well as comparing the time taken for it to subside again. A favourable finding is the case if the ache is less with the second oscillations, or if it subsides more quickly.

One point, which may make it easier to understand and recognize this particular disorder, is that the inflammation is primary not secondary. In this way it is different from the inflammation (the -itis of arthritis) that occurs following a sprain or other similar incident. This is probably the reason why it does not recover to a pain-free stage as readily as does the traumatic inflammation.

Treatment response

This aspect is discussed in Chapter 7 but is mentioned here to show the disorder's distinctive nature. When the disorder is in a very low-grade inflammatory stage, oscillatory movements of large amplitude are used and are taken into a very small degree of discomfort. Initially the movements should not provoke any ache that increases in intensity or does not dissipate quickly when the movement is stopped. In the less low grade stages, movements must not provoke discomfort, or even awareness (to the patient) of a feeling of movement taking place within the joint. There must be no development of ache within the joint. Characteristically there will be a very pleasant feeling of warmth and comfort following the correct treatment. Though this may only last from half an hour up to 2 hours at first, the feeling is one that the patient has not had previously and is not produced by any other form of physiotherapy.

Joint locking

This inability to move a joint normally is caused by such events as 'loose-bodies' within a joint or a torn meniscus. The onset of a meniscus injury is usually one of an unguarded twisting movement: loose bodies may 'come and go' (usually with movement) without the patient being aware of the particular movement(s). The role of the physiotherapist is to free the joint from the obstruction to movement by passive movement techniques. Once freed, exercises for joint support and joint-care education are essential.

Hypermobility

There is considerable confusion surrounding this term, as there is also about how it should and should not be treated. Also, the word hypermobility cannot be discussed without also considering the word instability and its definition. In this text, hypermobility is used to infer an increased range of a joint or joints as compared with the average range of movement in that direction for that joint or joints as seen in the general population.

1. The joint may be hypermobile in one direction while other movements of that joint may be of average range or even hypomobile.
2. The hypermobility may be general in that it affects all or most joints in all or most directions. The essential part of the definition is that there is full muscular control of the hypermobile range. To depict a hypermobile range on the baseline of the movement diagram, or on that same baseline used for depicting grades of movement on a normal joint, the line AB extends beyond point B. This is so because B is defined as the 'end of the normal average range of movement'. The end of range for the hypermobile movement is suitably identified as H (Figure 6.1).

If trauma (or disease) results in loss of a ligament's ability to restrict the range of a movement that it normally restricts, that movement will become excessive (hypermobile). The important implication of these circumstances is that there will not be any muscular control of this new excessive range of movement. Without this muscular control, the joint is unstable. This kind of instability is hypermobility, but hypermobility is not necessarily this kind of instability. (A cat is an animal, but an animal is not necessarily a cat.)

There is another form of hypermobility and another form of instability both of which are associated with pain:

1. The hypermobility is seen with the subluxing patella. In this situation the patella has a hypermobile range of lateral displacement.

When the patello-femoral articulation becomes symptomatic the 'apprehension test' becomes positive. That is, if the patella is passively moved laterally while the tibio-femoral joint is in a relaxed extension position, a point will be reached in the range when the patient suddenly, reflexly contracts the quadriceps group of muscles to prevent further movement of the patella. This occurs at the point when the patella, if moved any further laterally, will sublux.

2. The other kind of instability is a pain response phenomenon. It is commonly seen in a painful tibio-femoral disorder. Usually full knee extension, passively or actively, is limited by pain. This being so, when the patient walks and reaches that part of his gait that requires controlled knee extension, he is unable to control the position and the knee wobbles until the knee extension phase is no longer required. This kind of instability is sometimes referred to as 'stable instability' or 'pain alerted instability' because when knee extension becomes painless the instability seen on walking disappears.

Fractures and non-uniting fractures

This is discussed in Chapter 7.

Arthritis

An active arthritic disease disorder that is causing pain cannot be relieved of the pain by techniques such as are described in this text. However, both post-traumatic arthritis and degenerative osteoarthritis can be helped by skilled manipulative physiotherapy. Also, the long-standing osteoarthritis which is only minimally (or moderately) uncomfortable rather than painful, and which is disabling in terms of function, can be helped to gain further range and thus a better lifestyle. Their treatment is also described in the next chapter.

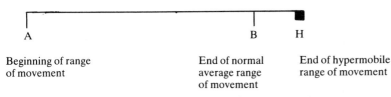

A   B   H

Beginning of range   End of normal   End of hypermobile
of movement   average range   range of movement
                         of movement

Figure 6.1 Movement diagram showing hypermobility

7

Treatment

Reference may be made in this chapter to other forms of physiotherapy and medical treatment, but mainly it relates to treatment by passive movement. Passive movement is not a panacea for all musculo-skeletal disorders. Having said this, passive movement in the assessment, examination and treatment of musculo-skeletal disorders has a much more valuable and important role to play than is generally understood by many therapists. The assessment component is most important no matter what treatment is used, but in this chapter the main emphasis will be placed on the treatment by passive movement as applied to the disorders referred to in the previous chapter.

Passive movements

The two basic movements available for treatment are physiological movements (which are movements actively used in the many functions of the musculo-skeletal system), and accessory movements (Table 7.1).

Table 7.1 Basic movements available for passive movement treatment

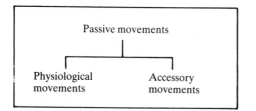

When considering how a physiological movement should be used as a passive treatment movement it is necessary to understand the components of spin roll and slide which take place within the synovial joint during a single direction of a functional movement. This is extremely well discussed in the arthrology section of all latest editions of *Gray's Anatomy*. Rotation within the synovial joint (spin) does *not* produce rotation of the shaft of the bone forming one section of that joint. For example, spin at the glenohumeral joint is a *rotary* intra-articular movement of the head of the humerus in the glenoid cavity. The movement of upper arm, produced by the 'spin' in the joint, is in a flexion extension direction. This is an over-simplification because the spin is not a rotation about one axis, and the flexion extension is not a true sagittal movement, nevertheless the description suffices the purpose. To avoid unnecessary complications, the common terms such as flexion, extension, etc. will be used with the qualification that rotation will often be classified by 'shaft rotation' when thinking of such joints as the hip, knee and shoulder.

Table 7.2 Passive movements at the glenohumeral joint

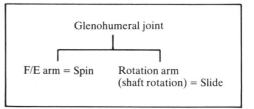

The slide, the spin and the roll if produced separately are accessory movements. They are not the only accessory movements, others being distraction, compression and gliding or translation. The gliding movements (or translations) may be coronal (medially or laterally) or sagittal (anteroposterior or posteroanterior). Obviously they may be angulated, including angulations in cephalad and caudad directions. *Gray's Anatomy*[1] considers rotation at the metacarpophalangeal joints as 'accessory movements first type' and the other accessory movements stated above as 'accessory movements second type', the former being able to be produced actively by grasping a ball. However, this is a fallacy because the hand and fingers may be put into a position of grasping a ball without the ball being there, thus the metacarpophalangeal rotation *is* an active physiological movement not an accessory movement. It may be argued that the passive range of metacarpophalangeal rotation is much greater than its active range, but this is so for all passive ranges compared with active ranges.

Having raised the point of there being or not being two types of accessory movement, passive shaft rotation of a joint is a direction of movement category that fits neatly into the same treatment category as accessory movements of the grade II type. Strange though this may seem, it is a common factor clinically applicable to all synovial joints. Thus Table 7.1 needs to be modified to show this (Table 7.3).

Table 7.3 Modification of basic movements for passive movement treatment

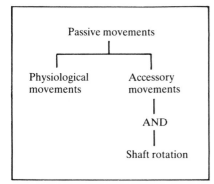

The physiologically functional movements incorporate varying degrees of accessory movements to allow the physiological movement to occur. They also incorporate varying degrees of other directions of physiological movement. For example, a man rarely raises his arm overhead in a pure sagittal plane in daily activities. The relevance of this lies both in examination and in passive movement treatment.

1. In examination

When active movements are assessed, a patient may be asked to perform different movements in unusual combinations so as to determine any anomalies in these movements. As an example, a patient may be asked to abduct or flex his arms, but to do so, not as a normal free functional movement, but with the arms in medial rotation: the symptomatic arm is compared with the normal arm.

2. In passive movement treatment

The same combinations as mentioned above can be used as passive movements in treatment. In addition to these, a physiological movement and an accessory movement can be combined. The combinations can be in the biomechanical direction or even in the reverse direction, for example using, as a treatment, knee extension combined with an anteroposterior pressure applied at the knee.

1. To perform this in the biomechanical direction, the anteroposterior pressure is applied to the femur at the knee.
2. To perform it in the non-biomechanical direction, the anteroposterior pressure is applied to the tibia at the knee. These reverse, or non-biomechanical accessory movements should be used as a routine part of examination by passive movement, as well as during treatment.
3. The accessory movements themselves can be combined and used in examination and treatment. As a typical example, anteroposterior pressure in a laterally directed inclination can be applied to the anteromedial surface of the tibia just distal to the superior margin of the medial condyle of the tibia. This produces a combination of anteroposterior movement with lateral movement and medial shaft rotation of the tibia under the femur. (The knee may be being supported in any physiological position.)

The table is now further expanded to show all the movements available for use as treatment techniques (Table 7.4).

Table 7.4 Movements available for passive movement treatment

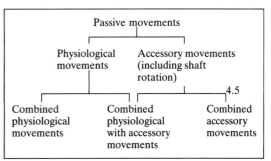

1. Williams, P. L. and Warwick, R. (eds.) *Gray's Anatomy,* 36th edn., Churchill Livingstone, London (1980)

Grades of treatment movements

The available grades with which *any* of the listed movements can be performed has already been tabled (see page 48). Nevertheless it needs to be realized that these grades can be varied very widely. For example, a large-amplitude movement can be used in absolutely any part of the full excursion of a range. As an example, if a person (with a normal shoulder) were to lie supine on a treatment couch, with his shoulder free over the side of the couch a large-amplitude of flexion of the whole shoulder girdle could start from a position of the arm hanging towards the floor and could finish as far beyond the median coronal plane of his head and thorax as is physically available. (Figure 7.1 would be recorded as a maximum range of grade III movement.)

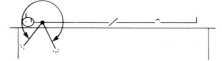

Figure 7.1 Maximum grade III

The same applies, in terms of large-amplitudes, to combined movements, and accessory movements.

On a similar basis, small and tiny amplitudes can be performed *anywhere* in the same full excursion of the range. The only point is that if it is performed at or near the beginning of the range it would be called a grade I, and if it were at the end of the range it would be a grade IV (where some resistance would be felt). Question: what would it be called if it were still a small amplitude but performed in the middle of the resistance-free range (such as might be the case when treating a painful arc)? Suggestion: call it a tiny grade II; or if it is in the first one-third part of the resistance free range, call it 'tiny II−', and in the last third of the resistance free range, why not call it 'tiny II+' – really, it matters not.

Thus the gradings that are available for the movements tabled are enormously variable (Figure 7.2).

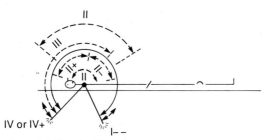

Figure 7.2 Shoulder F, grades I−−; II−, II, II+; III, IV+. III and II = Large-amplitude; III and II = most common amplitude; III and II = small-amplitude. Similarly, I and IV = tiny-amplitude; I and IV = larger-amplitude, but smaller than grade II (IV) or grade II (I)

Rhythms of treatment movement

Many different rhythms are used in passive movement treatment. Movements can be performed at a very low speed, so smoothly that there is no one single point when the direction changes from one direction to the reverse. A movement may be held at one point for as long as 5 seconds waiting for pain or muscle spasm to subside before reversing the direction minimally (sustained). At the other extreme are staccato rhythms which are sharp, more abrupt movements.

The available rhythms can be changed from one to another: i.e. there can be a mixture of rhythms applied as the one treatment technique in the one single direction. This change or mixture of rhythms may include a changing of grades, but this is not necessarily so. For example, a slow smooth rhythm of grade III may be interspersed with one or two staccato movements still in the same grade III range. Conversely, a sustained grade IV stretching movement may be interspersed with smooth grade III− movements to ease the soreness resulting from the stretching. This grade III− movement could hopefully be progressed in a very controlled and assessed way to a grade III movement.

Table 7.5 Rhythms of treatment movement

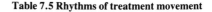
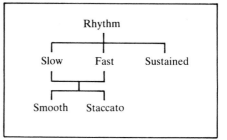

To oversimplify what has been expounded above, the passive movements from which selections can be made consist of:

Physiological movements – Accessory movements – Combinations
Small amplitudes – Large amplitudes – Sustained
Early in range – Late in range – Within range
Smoothly – Staccato
Without compression – With compression

The choice is made with a perfect-effect-goal in mind, but the choice is then modified by (1) the diagnosis, (2) the history and stage/stability of the disorder, (3) the presenting symptoms and signs, and finally (4) by the response to the chosen treatment technique during and after its application.

Table 7.6 Selection of passive movements

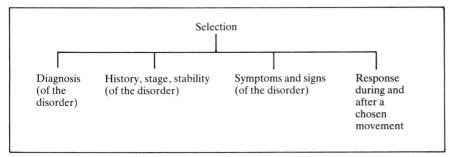

Diagnosis

Where a definitive diagnosis of a patient's disorder can be made, it will influence the choice of passive movement technique used. An example of this is a torn medial meniscus which has resulted in a locked knee. To reduce the locked knee, the therapist must choose a movement or combinations of movements that gap the medial joint space followed by repeated physiological movements of rotation, flexion and extension. How the technique is performed (grade, rhythm) will still depend on information learned regarding the behaviour of symptoms. Similarly the specific movements used to unlock the knee will depend on the history of this and any previous episodes and the presenting signs. Any assessment of the response to the first use(s) of the technique(s) designated by the diagnosis would reveal their role. The 'stage' of the disorder is exemplified by the 'frozen shoulder'. It has three stages, the first being one of severe pain, the second is an association of stiffness without as much pain, and the third is one of stiffness without pain. Each stage requires quite different treatment techniques based on the history, symptoms and signs.

Diagnosis influences the choice of technique in another way. If a patient has had rheumatoid arthritis with obvious changes to the joint and its supportive structures, yet has strained his wrist and is, as a result, unable to lift objects that he could easily lift prior to the strain, any passive movement treatment (any treatment at all, really), must take into account the underlying weaknesses caused by the rheumatoid arthritis. Thus this component of the disorder places restraints on treatment. A reverse situation is the diagnosis of 'frozen shoulder' (an unfortunate term) in its third stage[2]. This stage calls for positive firm treatment techniques with the aim of markedly increasing range. It cannot be omitted to state that the stage at which this treatment is applied is very precise, particularly in its relation to pain at rest.

History, stage/stability

The knowledge related to the onset of the disorder (trauma, spontaneous, peri-articular, intra-articular, sprain, strain) with emphasis also on the stage of progression of the disorder (episodic, pathological development) and the degree of current activity or stability of the disorder itself not only indicate the mode of application of passive movement techniques, but also guide the thinking related to the changes that may be expected to take place with treatment. The latter will be discussed in Chapter 8. The 'mode of application' is relevant here and is described in relation to examples.

An osteoarthritic hip of long-standing duration with episodes of inhibiting pain, and currently being within a painful episode, would require techniques aimed at pain relief. The degree of activity of the inflammation would influence the technique used (painless accessory movements if very active, painless physiological movements if not very active) and its rhythm (slowly and smoothly if very active, quicker if not very active).

An inactive capsular disorder that is stable and late in its stage of progression would require stretching techniques, both physiological movements and end-of-range accessory movements.

A recent sprain (a day or two ago) that has occurred for the first time and that is stable in terms of reaction to the sprain, will require very slowly performed movements in the direction of the sprain and into a very small degree of 'hurt'. At a late stable stage of the reaction to the sprain other physiological movement techniques can be added; and later still, more localized techniques and moderately firm accessory movements are added.

Symptoms and signs

Irrespective of the diagnosis and the history-stage/stability aspects of the disorder, the presenting

2. Corrigan, B. and Maitland, G. D. *Practical Orthopaedic Medicine,* Butterworths, London, p. 52 (1983)

symptoms and signs have the highest of priorities when it comes to the treatment by passive movement techniques. End-of-range symptoms are treated by different techniques (EOR techniques) than are through-range-symptoms (through-range-techniques) or constant pain (accessory movements in neutral physiological positions). Mild aching symptoms felt when lying on the aching joint require special techniques (movement under compression) as do stiff peri-articular structures preventing normal function because of pain as well as the stiffness (stretching techniques into stiffness to the point of provoking the pain i.e. into 'bite').

Response during/after technique

For every aspect of treatment used, the symptomatic response felt by the patient while it is being performed and the effect of treatment over a 24-hour period must be very clearly known by the physiotherapist even to the extent of being able to live them herself. This subjective response is a primary aspect of assessment (see Chapter 8).

The total list of factors from which techniques can be selected are listed below:

1. PHYSIOLOGICAL movements – ACCESSORY movements – COMBINATIONS.
2. SMALL amplitudes – LARGE amplitudes – SUSTAINED.
3. EARLY in range – LATE in range – WITHIN range.
4. SMOOTHLY – STACCATO – SUSTAINED.
5. WITHOUT COMPRESSION – WITH COMPRESSION.
6. SHORT of discomfort – INTO discomfort – INTO pain – INTO 'BITE'.
7. SHORT of resistance – INTO resistance respecting pain – INTO resistance up to 'BITE'.

The treatments that can be applied to disorders that can be precisely diagnosed (this excludes those that have a syndrome title) will be discussed later in this chapter. This allows for a continuity of the reader's thought processes following what has been discussed up to this stage in this chapter.

Phase 1
Treatment of disorders

It is a very complex task indeed to discuss treatment for all of the disorders presented in Chapter 6. In an attempt to make the situation clear, while keeping the complexities of description (and therefore the application of treatment techniques to patients by physiotherapists) at a minimum, the descriptions will be presented in PHASES of skill or PHASES of understanding. The first two phases will be over-

simplifications – it will be easier for the novice to understand and apply. As skills progress and knowledge (clinical knowledge especially) increases, so the phases will be presented as variations on the basic 'first and second phases'.

There are very many times when an exact diagnosis cannot be given other than to state that the disorder is musculo-skeletal and that it should respond to physiotherapy or, more specifically, treatment by passive movement. Many conditions cause joints to be painful, each of which may produce different symptoms and physical signs, and these may alter during different phases of a pathological process. Because of these variations, attempts to relate treatment to pathology can lead to considerable misunderstanding. Instead, it is better to divide the different combinations of symptoms and signs into groups and relate treatment to each group. Although the disorder influences the rate of progress and the prognosis, it does not always influence the type of passive movement used in treatment. Under these circumstances, the techniques used will be guided by the abnormalities of the joint movements.

The three primary physical joint signs found on examination of an abnormal synovial joint and its supportive structures consist of PAIN, at rest or with movement, STIFFNESS, due to contracted structure or adhesions, and MUSCLE SPASM. These can be present separately or in any number of combinations. The following are the main combinations:

1. A painful joint that remains painful even at rest in a neutral position.
2. A painless joint that prevents normal activity because the joint is stiff.
3. A joint that is both stiff and painful.
4. Spasm:
    (a) A joint that is painless during movement because muscle spasm prevents movement.
    (b) Spasm where joint movement becomes painful before spasm appears.
    (c) Spasm in a way that differs from typical, protective spasm.
    (d) Neurological and voluntary spasms.
5. Pain inhibition.
6. Crepitus.

1. Painful joint at rest

The joint may remain painful even when it is rested in a neutral position midway between all of the joint's possible ranges of movement (grade I).

A very important variation is that the patient may say his joint is constantly painful yet if his joint is rested in a neutral position, the pain will go completely. Although it may not require much movement from this neutral position to become painful, the important point is that it *can* be positioned to abolish the pain. The difference is that the pain that can be abolished may be caused by a mechanical focus whereas the example above is more likely to be due to some active inflammatory condition. The inflammation may be chemical in both circumstances (group 1, Table 7.7).

A joint may be painless when at rest and only become painful on movement. There are many variations of the amount and type of pain felt on movement. The joint may give a sudden sharp pain on certain movements but as soon as the movement is released, pain immediately goes. At the opposite end of the scale, the joint may be very painful on movement and when the movement is stopped the pain may continue as an ache of varying intensity lasting varying lengths of time (5 minutes, 1 hour). A patient may have a sudden jab of pain during a trivial action. A common example of this is a jab of pain at the base of the thumb while beginning to lift a kettle (group 4, Table 7.9).

Table 7.7 Readily recognizable patient groupings

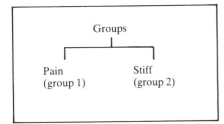

A joint may be painful at rest but if it is moved by the therapist the pain increases rapidly in intensity to the extent where the therapist is not prepared to move the joint further. The amount of limitation of movement due to pain may be very great and this prevents the therapist from knowing whether there is any physical resistance present perhaps beyond this limit. She also cannot know whether there would be any muscle spasm if the joint were moved further. In other words it is not possible, because of the intensity of the pain with movement, to know what other physical factors may be present in the joint movement into the range.

2. Painless, stiff joint

The patient may have a painless joint which prevents normal activities because the joint is stiff. When the joint is stretched it feels tight, and perhaps even a little painful; but the main complaint is one of stiffness, not pain. This patient goes to his doctor because he cannot tuck his shirt into the back of his trousers or comb his hair – he does not go to the doctor because of pain (group 2, Table 7.7).

3. Painful, stiff joint

The largest number of patients with musculo-skeletal problems whom the doctor refers for physiotherapy are those whose joint is found to be both stiff and painful (group 3, Table 7.8). These patients are the most challenging to treat. They require the physiotherapist to be precise in discerning the behaviour of both the pain and the stiffness, and to determine their interrelationships. She must determine whether the behaviours of pain and resistance are associated with each other or not, either in part or in full. In making this interpretation it is necessary for the therapist to know the diagnosis and understand the pathology. With this large group of patients the physiotherapist must build up a concept of the rate of anticipated change which can be affected by manipulative physiotherapy. An essential prerequisite is to know whether the pain is the dominant component (group 3a) or the loss of range due to joint stiffness (group 3b, Table 7.8). These skills can only be developed through precise examination of passive movements combined with continual assessment of changes which can be effected by different techniques.

4. Spasm

(a) Painless spasm

A joint can be painless during movement because of protection afforded by muscle spasm. The protective mechanisms in main are both complex and wonderful. *It is possible for the degree of muscle spasm to be such that it comes into play BEFORE movement becomes painful.*

(b) Pain before spasm

Spasm can also come into play as a more obvious protection for the joint because the joint movement becomes quite painful before the spasm appears.

(c) Atypical spasm

Muscles may contract in a way that differs from the typical protective muscle spasm. It is not voluntary contraction that the patient can release. It is a 'holding' rather than an obvious contraction and it affects more of the muscles surrounding the joint.

(d) Neurological and voluntary spasms

There are two other kinds of muscle spasm which need not concern us in this text but should be mentioned. The first is a neurological muscle spasm caused by an upper motor neurone disorder and the second is the muscle contraction produced voluntarily by the patient to prevent movement.

5. Pain inhibition

'Pain inhibition' is a factor that may be present. It confuses the presentation of the disorder and so confuses treatment decisions. It can be responsible for apparent (not 'actual') muscle weakness, instability, limitation of range of movement. 'Knee extension lag' is a perfect example.

6. Crepitus

Crepitus is another subjective element which is evident as a 'through-range' phenomenon. It may be accompanied by discomfort – it may, or may not, be apparent to the therapist (joint crepitus or tenosynovitis).

Treatment movements

The treatment movements referred to above can be used in one of the following ways.

1. To direct the treatment to relieve the pain.
2. To direct the treatment so as to improve the patients stiff joint which lacks a functional range.
3. To treat the resistance that is present as part of the joint disorder while also being careful to avoid any exacerbation of the pain.

Groupings

Patients with different combinations of symptoms and signs can be divided into four main groups. Two groups of patients' presentations, which are at opposite ends of the spectrum, are readily recognized (Table 7.7): those who are unable to move the joint because of severe pain (group 1) and those who have only a minimal intermittent ache, if any at all (no pain), but who are unable to move the joint because of stiffness (group 2).

There is a third group of patients who have pain related to stiffness, but these patients vary widely in their presentation. Although the pain and stiffness

Table 7.8 Subdivision of patient groupings

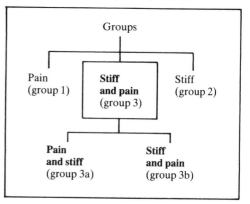

are related, the pain may be severe or it may be moderate and each requires different treatment (groups 3a and 3b, Table 7.8). This group can be subdivided into those where pain is the dominant component (group 3a) and those where the stiffness is the dominant component (group 3b).

Figure 7.3(a) is the diagram of a comparable movement of those with less severe pain. Figure 7.3(b) is the diagram of the comparable movement when stiffness is dominant. If pain is more dominant than stiffness, the initial treatments must be related to pain and can therefore be considered together with the initial treatments of group 1 patients. These patients, unlike those of group 2, cannot be treated with many directions of movement.

A fourth group worthy of separate consideration concerns patients with no obvious loss of joint range but who have 'momentary pain' (intermittent pain associated with particular movements) (Table 7.9).

Table 7.9 Grouping of patients with intermittent pain associated with particular movements

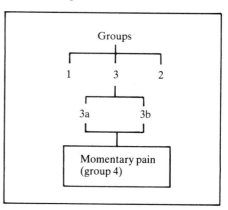

These groups provide a satisfactory basis for describing the application of the different types of passive movement used in treatment. A patient with

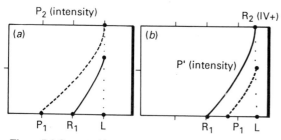

Figure 7.3 Comparable movement; group (*a*), pain more dominant than resistance; (*b*) less severe pain

a painful joint condition therefore fits into one of the following groups:

Group 1: Where pain is the main consideration, the existing limitation of movement is due entirely to pain.

Group 2: Where loss of movement is the main disability and pain is of little consequence.

Group 3a and b: Where pain and joint stiffness are concurrent, the intensity of pain increasing proportionally as the strength of the resistance increases. a = Pain dominant, b = stiffness dominant.

Group 4: Where pain is intermittent and momentary.

Pathology

During the cycle of any pathological process, the joint signs may be as those of one group and gradually alter to those of another. For example, a patient with a 'frozen shoulder' may originally present as group 1 but may gradually change to group 3a, then 3b and may eventually reach a stage that would place him in group 2. If such a shoulder were to be treated by passive movement, the method would need to be adjusted to suit the particular phase of the condition. Similarly, when the treatment of any painful joint lesion alters the signs, the type of passive movement used in treatment must be altered to suit the altered signs.

Scrupulous assessment of symptoms and signs throughout treatment is essential if techniques are to be adapted efficiently. The important signs are checked at the commencement of each treatment session and between techniques during treatment. Only by this method can the effectiveness of each technique be evaluated and suitable changes made. It is assumed, therefore, that with this continual reassessment suitable changes in treatment are made as necessitated by the signs.

Comparable movement

The group into which the patient fits is determined by the examination findings. As was pointed out in the chapter on examination (Chapter 4), the objective examination of every patient must reveal one or more passive movements which are comparable with the symptoms, and a comparable movement diagram for each of the first four groups listed above would be expressed as follows:

1. The diagram of a comparable movement for a patient from group 1 would show that it is pain that limits active movement to less than 60% of normal (Figure 7.4(a)).
2. A patient in group 2 would have movements represented as in Figure 7.4(b) where it can be seen that movement is limited and that pain is minimal.

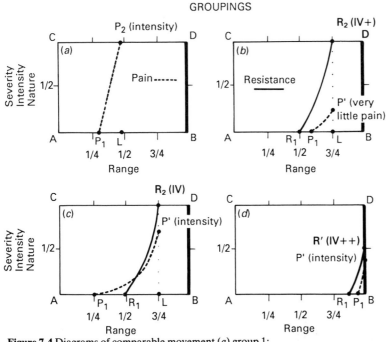

Figure 7.4 Diagrams of comparable movement (*a*) group 1; (*b*) group 2; (*c*) group 3; (*d*) group 4

3. Though patients in group 3 vary widely, the important fact is that, as the severity of the pain increases, the strength of the resistance also increases. An example of a comparable movement is given in Figure 7.4(c).

4. Finding a movement comparable with the symptoms in group 4 is sometimes very difficult. Frequently only one comparable movement can be found. Sometimes physiological movements are normal and it is only when accessory movements are tested in combination with physiological movements can a comparable movement be found. For example, a patient with minor knee symptoms may have a full painless range of all physiological movements. However, when full flexion is combined with medial rotation plus the accessory movement of abduction, pain is elicited and the movement is slightly restricted in range. This then would be the comparable movement. Figure 7.4(d) is an example of such a movement.

To clarify discussion relating the type of movement to the physical findings of that movement, it is necessary to be able to depict the treatment movement; that is, its amplitude and position in range on the movement diagram. The treatment movement is represented by a double-headed arrow directed horizontally as it is on the base line AB used for grades on page 48. The amplitude of the movement is depicted by the length of the arrow, and the position in the range where it is performed is depicted by relating the position of the arrow to the horizontal axis which represents range. For example, if the horizontal axis in Figure 7.5 represents 90° of elbow extension, the double-headed arrow represents a 20° amplitude movement performed 30° short of full extension.

Sufficient detail has now been given to describe how the treatment movements are adapted to the several presentations of pain and physical signs found on passive movement examination. One or all movements of a painful joint may be used in equal or varying degrees. Treatment techniques applied to a painful joint should be considered from two aspects: (1) which movement or movements should be used, and (2) how should the movement be performed with reference to its amplitude, rhythm and position in the range?

The choice depends upon (1) the joint affected; (2) the symptoms and signs; and (3) the pathology.

As treatment progresses, changes in technique are made to match changes in symptoms and signs.

The joint being treated

It is necessary to consider the choice of technique in relation to the joint affected because not all joints respond to the same movement in the same way. For example, longitudinal movement is an important treatment movement for the glenohumeral joint, yet the same movement plays a lesser role in treatment of the superior radioulnar joint. Similarly, small movements produced by thumb pressures on the carpal or tarsal bones are more useful than are similar movements on the hip. Therefore, certain movements are better techniques for certain joints. There are two factors that make one movement a better technique than another. The first is the ease with which the movement can be performed and controlled by the operator. For example, at the glenohumeral joint flexion is a much easier mobilizing technique to perform and control than abduction and, broadly speaking, it is much more useful. The second factor relates to the normal movements of the joint. The glenohumeral joint and superior radioulnar joints are both capable of considerable longitudinal movement passively; but although the head of the humerus moves longitudinally in the glenoid cavity during active movements of the shoulder, the radius does not actively move far in this direction. The treatment technique of longitudinal movement is far more useful in the glenohumeral joint than it is in the radioulnar joint.

Treatment movements that employ the accessory movements are very important in the treatment of both painful and stiff joints. This often influences the physiotherapist to use accessory movements instead of physiological movement. In some joints, for example the hip joint, accessory movements are very small and therefore play a less important part in treatment than they do in others where the accessory movements are large. For example, in the glenohumeral joint, accessory movements play a very important role.

In general, Table 7.10 lists the joints that are frequently more effectively treated by the indicated movements. This list does not mean that other movements should not be used but that, unless there are reasons for deciding otherwise, perhaps the effect of the listed treatment movements should be assessed first.

At the beginning of this chapter patients were divided according to their symptoms and signs into four main groups. The treatment techniques used for group 1 would be quite inadequate for group 2, and those for group 2 would be excessive treatment for group 3. The techniques used for groups 1 and 3 would be completely ineffective for patients in group 4 as may also be those used for group 2 patients.

The value of each technique used in treatment must be assiduously checked throughout the course of treatment and this is done by checking the symptoms and signs before and after the application of the treatment. Sometimes it is necessary to perform the technique twice before an adequate

Table 7.10 Joints commonly treated

Joint	Group of patient's symptoms and signs	Tretament movements
Glenohumeral	1	Posteroanterior movement (arm by side) in neutral pain free Longitudinal movement (arm by side)
Elbow	2 3 4	Flexion or quadrant Extension Extension–adduction
Carpus Digitus	2 and 4 1 and 3 2	Posteroanterior movement Accessory movements Accessory movements at the limit of physiological range or combined with compression
Hip	1 3 and 4	Rotation Flexion–adduction
Knee	1 3 4	Accessory movement particularly anteroposterior movement or rotation Extension Extension–abduction
Tarsus	3 4	Physiological movements Accessory movements
Jaw	1, 3 and 4	Transverse movement

assessment can be made of its value. However, this assessment must be clearly made before the technique is discarded or used in combination with another. The main exception to the rule of assessing techniques singly occurs in the treatment of group 2 patients. These patients do not suffer exacerbation from too much treatment, nor are they examples of any one particular movement being the right one to use; all movements must be used.

Initial treatment

From the outset the physiotherapist must have a plan of treatment in mind and each technique used during treatment must be evaluated. The plan is made following the examination from which the joint irritability and the active and passive movements are assessed. All patients in group 1 have pain which markedly limits movement and the condition is very irritable.

In the past, poorly performed techniques of passive movement have not respected pain adequately. Consequently techniques have been unnecessarily painful and treatment by passive movement has fallen into disrepute. Gentle techniques are guided almost solely by pain, and when stronger techniques are contemplated the effect on pain must be clearly appreciated. Considerable emphasis is therefore placed on pain when discussing the depth and amplitude of passive movement treatment. During treatment, the physiotherapist should at all

times watch the patient, particularly his eyes and hands, for signs that indicate that the movement being performed might be painful. It is essential to use every faculty possible to know how much pain, discomfort or even unusual sensation the patient is experiencing with the movements.

Pain

It was pointed out when describing the first step of the movement diagram (see page 299) that care was required when assessing the onset of pain in the range before treatment could be related to the physical findings of that movement. This is particularly so with patients whose severe pain starts early in the range. However, even the point P1 does not give a complete picture of the patient's pain. During the subjective examination, an assessment must be made of the joint irritability by relating the vigour of an activity that causes pain, to the severity of pain so caused and the length of time taken for this increased pain to return to its usual level. These activities are not, themselves, always painful. Patients in group 1 always have a high degree of joint irritability, and they frequently experience a painful reaction following a comparatively painless activity. Consider this phenomenon in relation to the movement diagram; the joint can be moved back and forth in that part of the range before P1 in Figure 7.4(a) (see page 71) quite painlessly, but if *too much* movement is performed the patient will experience an exacerbation later. The more irritable the joint, the smaller is the amount of movement required to cause this. The fact that oscillatory movements in this painless part of the range can cause an exacerbation at all shows that point P1 in Figure 7.4(a) (see page 71) is incomplete when considering pain, and indicates how carefully the patient's pain needs to be assessed and the possibility of reaction appreciated. If pain starts much later in the range, and particularly if this pain is not severe, there is little likelihood of reaction from painless treatment movement. The point of emphasis is that even though care is exercised to determine where pain begins in the range, movement in the painless part of the range may cause a painful reaction; therefore care in both assessment and treatment is essential.

Joint irritability

When the joint irritability (see page 23 for definition) is an important factor guiding treatment, it must first be assessed by questioning the patient. This information then guides the amount of treatment and the type of treatment movement given. When the patient is seen for the second treatment a clear assessment of the joint irritability can be made, because any exacerbation that has occurred can be directly related to a known amount of joint movement. It is still necessary to bear in mind, however, that at the patient's first visit the joint was moved during examination as well as during treatment. An accurate assessment therefore of joint irritability may not be possible until the third visit though it may prove to have been accurately supposed at the outset.

Treatment in the first instance, with patients whose joints are painful, must be carried out with care. This care refers to the position in the range occupied by the treatment movement in relation to pain, the amplitude of the movement, their rhythm and their speed, and the number of oscillations used in treatment. Although the movement is performed in the painless part of the range, how closely this movement approaches the point where pain is first felt depends on three assessments:

1. Joint irritability ascertained during the subjective examination. If it is high, the treatment movement should be kept further back from P1 than would be necessary if joint-irritability were less.
2. How early in the range pain begins.
3. The intensity of the pain in the early part of the painful range. The earlier it appears and the more rapidly it increases, the further back from where it begins should the treatment movement be performed and the slower and smoother it should be performed. However, if the increase in

pain in the early part of the painful range is moderate, with more severe pain occurring only later in the range, the treatment movement can be brought closer to the point where pain begins.

Grade of treatment movement

The amplitude of the treatment movement is similarly related to how early in the range pain begins and its mode of increase. It is obvious perhaps that when a joint condition is very irritable, a small-amplitude oscillation will cause less exacerbation than will a large-amplitude oscillation in the same part of the painless range. Therefore, the more irritable the joint, or the earlier in the range the pain starts, or the more rapidly the pain increases in intensity early in the painful range, the smaller must be the amplitude of the treatment movement.

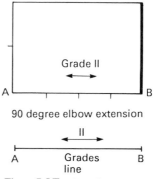

90 degree elbow extension

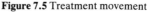

Figure 7.5 Treatment movement

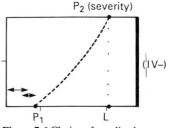

Figure 7.6 Choice of amplitude

Having considered the amplitude of the treatment movement and the position in the range where this movement is performed, there is a relationship between them which should be mentioned. To maintain a constant effect on a joint, having a given set of joint signs, a smaller amplitude must be used as the treatment movement is brought closer to point P1; if the treatment movement is performed back from point P1, a larger amplitude can be used. So a balance can be struck between the amplitude and its position in the range. The two double-headed arrows in Figure 7.6 are comparable

treatment for the particular joint movement depicted. *In practice the larger the amplitude that can be performed when treating pain, the more effective it will be.* In very painful joints, however, judgement must be exercised because if the amplitude is too large it may cause an exacerbation. In Figure 7.6 the technique of choice is demonstrated by the larger arrow which appears earlier in the range.

Oscillation

The number of oscillations given during treatment is the last consideration relevant to care in the initial treatment. When a joint is irritable, a small amount of movement will cause less reaction than a large amount. In other words, if the joint is highly irritable the treatment will need to be not only of small amplitude in an early part of the painless range but the total number of oscillations will need to be small also. The average time spent passively moving joints that are not excessively painful is approximately 4–5 minutes. A highly irritable joint should be moved less and the treatment time varied from a half to 2 minutes.

Direction of treatment movement

The above shows that the initial treatment must be performed in the painless part of the range (Table 7.11). It is important to choose one of the least painful directions for the treatment movement. How far back this treatment movement is performed from the point where pain begins depends upon: the joint irritability, how early in the range pain begins, and how quickly the pain increases in intensity with further movement. If these findings indicate that the treatment movement must be kept well away from pain, it is wiser to treat by using an accessory movement in a pain-free position rather than by using a physiological movement. For example, if active shoulder movements in the standing position are limited to below horizontal by pain, it is wiser to treat by passive accessory movements, such as posteroanterior movement with the patient's arm comfortably supported in a painless position by his side, than it is to use the physiological movements. In this way passive movement of the joint can be administered as a painless movement with less likelihood of exacerbation. Treatment using the technique shown in Figure 10.34 (see page 152) would be performed for 30 seconds or so. Following this, the patient would be asked to stand and raise his arm forward so that a comparison could be made of his range of flexion with that present before treatment. If this movement has improved or is unchanged the treatment should be repeated. If the movement is more painful the same treatment

should be performed in a smaller amplitude further back in the range. Bearing in mind that the patient has had to be examined as well as treated on this first day, the amount of treatment described above would probably be sufficient. It is always advisable, where there is a likelihood of exacerbation, to undertreat than to do too much.

Treatment on the following day would be based on the reassessment of the patient's movements. There should be some improvement to indicate repetition of the same technique. As the joint would not require full examination on this day the amount of treatment could be increased; the amount would be guided by any reaction that might have resulted from the first treatment. It should be anticipated that there would be small but definite signs of improvement in active range in all directions from treatment to treatment. If there is no improvement, a different movement should be used and assessed.

Treatment in the initial stages aims to lessen pain and to allow a greater range of active movement. When pain is severe it is often difficult for the patient to appreciate small improvements, and greater care is therefore necessary on the examiner's part, to discern the changes taking place. Pain may improve in three ways; it may not start until later in the range, it may start at the same point yet not reach maximum intensity until later in the range, or the rate of increase in pain in the early part of the range may not be as great.

As group 1 patients improve, and their active movements become greater than 60% of normal, treatment should be changed from accessory movements to physiological movements. In the previous example of the glenohumeral joint, flexion or the

Table 7.11 Phase 1 treatment

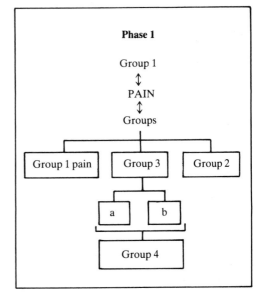

quadrant would be used. However, until the active range is 75% of normal the treatment movement should be kept short of the point in the range where pain beings. As the range nears normal the treatment movement can be taken to the limit of the range and grade III– movements used. The end result of treatment would be a pain-free full range of movement in all directions.

Examination of the patient's joint movements may show that it is pain that is preventing an otherwise full range of joint movement. Special techniques performed in a special sequence can be used to treat this pain.

When pain is to be treated, the following is the routine to be adopted. As the physiotherapist gains experience she may be able to take short cuts hoping for a quicker improvement.

The special type of passive mobilization used to treat pain makes use of the joint's accessory movements and includes 'shaft rotation', while the joint is supported in a pain-free neutral position. At a later stage the physiological movements are performed through a large-amplitude. All of these movements are initially performed short of producing any discomfort or pain in the joint; even any *awareness of movement* felt in the joint by the patient must be avoided initially. As the condition improves they may be used into a controlled degree of discomfort. The accessory movements in a neutral position are chosen for those patients whose active antigravity movements are painful or uncomfortable in approximately the first 60% of the joint's normal range. The change from accessory movements to physiological movements is made when the joint's pain-free range of movement has improved so that pain or discomfort is felt only in the last 40% of its total range.

Assuming that the special passive movement techniques produce the desired improvement in range, progressive stages of the techniques are applied. If we take the example of a patient who has a glenohumeral range of approximately 15–20% of (say) flexion before discomfort is felt then the steps are followed in this order:

1. The joint is placed (if necessary by using pillows, etc.) in a pain-free position in approximately the middle of all the joint's ranges. The technique used is posteroanterior accessory movement. The amplitude should be as large as is possible (painlessly) and it should be slow and smooth. While this is being performed very gently the therapist *should repeatedly ask* the patient if he feels any discomfort. If he does, the oscillatory movement should be performed further back in the range and the questions repeated. If there is still some discomfort during the technique then a much smaller amplitude should be used and it may be necessary to use a very gentle degree of

distraction of the joint surfaces while performing the technique. *The patient must not feel any movement nor anything resembling discomfort during the first treatment.* An example of the technique is shown in Figure 10.34, page 152).

If this accessory movement fails, the second one to try is longitudinal movement (Figures 7.7 and 7.8).

The third choice would be lateral movement (Figure 7.9) or mid-rotation with the patient's arm approximately 25° from his side.

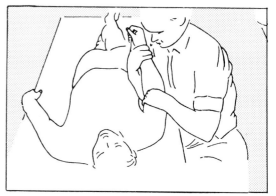

Figure 7.7 Glenohumeral joint; longitudinal movement caudad, arm by side, grade I

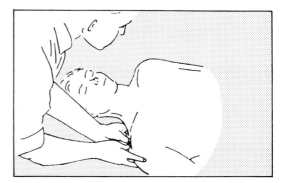

Figure 7.8 Glenohumeral joint; longitudinal movement caudad, arm by side, grades II, III and IV

2. If the careful assessment of the second treatment session shows that there has been some lessening of pain and some small improvement in the pain-free range of movement then the technique described above can be repeated. The physiotherapist must be prepared to proceed slowly; but as soon as it is advisable, as indicated by the improvement shown on assessment, the amplitude of the accessory treatment should be made larger and may also move into part of the range that is painful. On reassessment, if the pain-free

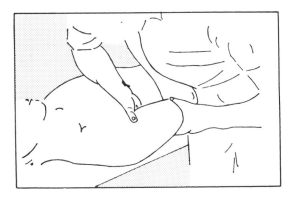

Figure 7.9 Glenohumeral joint; lateral movement arm by side

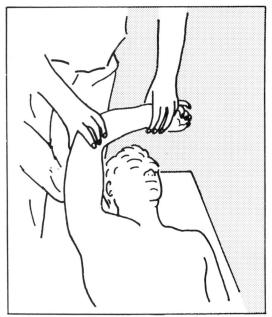

Figure 7.10 Glenohumeral joint, grade II. Flexion

active range improves and pain lessens then the accessory movement can be made larger and larger moving further and further into the range even though it is a little painful, until a stage is reached when full-amplitude grade III movements can be performed.

3. A stage will be reached when grade III+ maximum amplitude staccato accessory movements can be performed with minimal discomfort and at this stage the patient's active pain-free range should have improved in range to 60%.
The treatment movement can now be changed from an accessory movement to a suitable physiological movement performed very gently and carefully as a grade II− slow, smooth movement in such a way as to avoid pain. The amplitude should be as large as possible, but initially it must be a pain-free movement. An example of the technique that may be used is shown in Figure 7.10.

4. As the pain-free range improves still further, the movement can be moved further into the range and may be taken into a controlled degree of discomfort.

5. Gradually, the amplitude and vigour of the movement can be increased until a strong grade III+ movement can be performed without pain Figure 7.11(a) and (b). When this stage is achieved the patient will be symptom free.

6. The method described is a standard routine which may be used for any joint when treating pain. However, it must be pointed out that the change-over from the vigorous accessory movements in a neutral position to the physiological large-amplitude movement short of pain is not a clearly defined point. If the physiotherapist is in doubt as to whether to change over or not, it is usually wise to repeat the accessory movements

for another two sessions and to make them as vigorous as possible. Then the change to physiological movements can be made, but the initial application of these should be performed cautiously. On reassessment, if the joint has become more painful or the active range has worsened, the physiotherapist should revert to the accessory movement for a further two or three treatments. Then if the change to physiological movement is again made, it should be a successful transition.

The above description has been related to joints that have no stiffness or muscle spasm (group 1). However, as has been mentioned earlier, the largest group of patients referred for treatment are patients who have both pain and stiffness (groups 3a and 3b). If the physiotherapist is new to the use of passive movement techniques then it would be wise for her to treat pain first before trying to increase the range of movement limited by the stiffness. If this procedure is followed, the method used for treating pain is exactly the same as that described above. When treating pain, the active range may improve as the pain recedes. However, when the stiffness is quite marked the treatment of pain will only effect a small degree of improvement and will quickly reach a stage when progress, as determined by assessment, ceases. When this occurs, the treatment of pain should be discontinued and treatment of stiffness instituted (Figure 7.12).

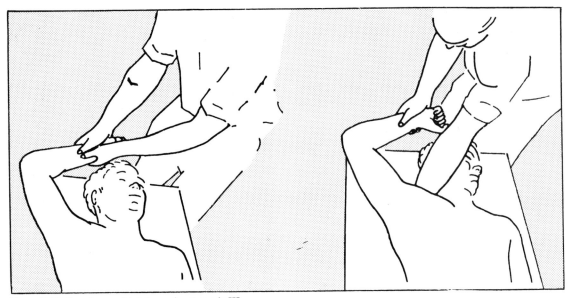

Figure 7.11 Glenohumeral joint; quadrant, grade III

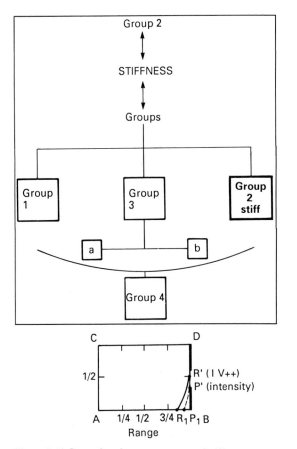

Figure 7.12 Group 2 patients – treatment of stiffness

Group 2 patients have painless stiff joints which require mobilizing at the limit of the existing range in all possible directions. To meet this need all of the physiological movements can be used as treatment movements and, more importantly, all of the accessory movements at the limit of each physiological range are used. For example, if the glenohumeral joint is painlessly stiff, the accessory movements of the head of the humerus in the glenoid cavity posteroanteriorly, anteroposteriorly, laterally and longitudinally may be carried out as stretching procedures while abduction is held at the limit of the range. The same accessory movements may also be performed at the limit of the range of horizontal flexion or flexion. Obviously, if too much treatment is administered, the structures will be made sore but there should not be a painful exacerbation. The relationship between the amount of treatment and joint soreness is watched by careful and repeated assessment. Initially, treatment is carried out daily but as the rate of progress slows or soreness escalates, so treatment is reduced to alternate days, twice weekly and then once weekly, with the patient continuing an exercise routine at home.

When joint soreness is produced by treatment, and this commonly occurs in group 2 patients, large-amplitude movements that approach the limit of range very gently are extremely useful. The large-amplitude movements quickly dispel soreness and because the treatment movement still reaches the limit of the range, treatment of the resistance continues. To intersperse grade III− movements between grade IV movements is an effective technique for these conditions.

When painless stiffness restricts a patient's functional activity, the method of treatment is as follows:

1. One of the stiff, functionally limited physiological movements is chosen and the physiotherapist takes the joint to the limit of this range. At this point small-amplitude oscillatory stretching movements are applied for approximately 2 minutes, attempting to increase the physiological range. Grade IV− movements will be gradually increased to IV+ and even IV++ strength.
2. Then, while holding the joint at the limit of this range the therapist performs the accessory movements that are available at this position. These accessory movements are small-amplitude, strong stretching oscillatory movements (Figure 7.13).
3. The physiotherapist now repeats the movement performed in (1) above and then follows with those described in (2) (Figure 7.14). This alternating between physiological and accessory movements is repeated three or four times at the initial treatment session. Assessment of progress is made during each treatment session and from treatment to treatment.
4. If the technique described above creates any soreness, this can be readily relieved by performing THE PHYSIOLOGICAL MOVEMENT USED FOR STRETCHING, but the movement would now be performed as a large-amplitude movement slightly short of the stretching range, so that little or no pain is felt by the patient. If treatment soreness is minor then this grade III− technique would not need to be performed for very long. The converse also applies.
5. Usually, as the chosen physiological treatment movement improves in range, the other movements of which the joint is capable also improve. When this is so, only one physiological movement needs treating. However, an all-round gain is not always the case and it is sometimes necessary to change to a different physiological movement. The same routine of stretching the physiological movement and the accessory movements at the limit of the physiological range is performed (Figure 7.15).

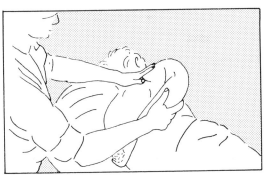

Figure 7.15 Glenohumeral joint; hand behind the back position, adduction

6. When the patient's joint is markedly limited in range, more than one physiological movement and its accompanying accessory movements may be used. When possible, **opposite movments in sequence should be avoided**. Treatment may be more effective if more emphasis is placed on the physiological movements, even to the extent of omitting the accessory movements.
7. The physiotherapist may feel that the joint should be stretched more strongly in an endeavour to separate whatever tight structures are restricting range. However, this should not be done unless the referring doctor agrees that it is necessary, and the patient must be fully informed. The technique is described on pages 83–84.

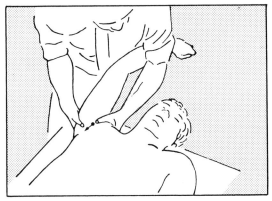

Figure 7.13 Glenohumeral joint; longitudinal movement in full flexion

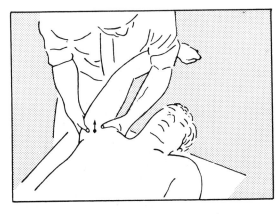

Figure 7.14 Glenohumeral joint; posteroanterior movement in flexion

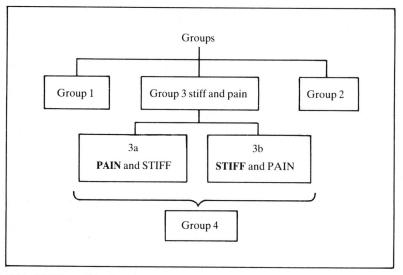

Table 7.12 Group 3 treatment

Not all group 1 patients improve with treatment as described. The examination of joint movement is often necessarily restricted because of pain; under these circumstances not all the physical signs can be determined. As the condition improves, and movement further into the range becomes possible, the presence of physical resistance may become apparent. If resistance is found as pain lessens, the patient's disorder is then considered a group 3 disorder.

When pain is dominant in group 3 patients (group 3a), the initial treatment and the response to treatment are similar to those described for group 1; gentle techniques in the comfortable part of the range lessen the patient's pain and permit a greater active range. As the pain improves, the physical resistance may also show signs of improvement. This occurs commonly in the resistances that have a soft feel, but never occurs in the hard resistances which have a bone-to-bone feel. Obviously the physical resistances in group 3b patients will vary widely in feel, and they may or may not improve with gentle techniques. If the resistance does not improve as the pain lessens, the patient fits into the second category of group 3 patients where pain is less dominant. With less severe pain, treatment will not cause exacerbation, and techniques that aim to improve the range should be used.

Subsequent treatments

When the treatment movements are first directed at the resistance, excessive treatment must be avoided and treatment soreness watched for. Even though every effort should be made to take the treatment movement up to the early part of the resistance, pain felt during treatment must be respected the first time it is carried out. Small-amplitude coaxing movements are performed in one of the less painful directions. Assessment after 24 hours answers the following questions:

1. Is directing treatment at the resistance the proper approach?
2. Can the treatment movement be taken deeper into the range?
3. Is it necessary to go deeper into the range?
4. Should another technique be tried?

If there is no progress, another movement is tried and assessed but if there is a little progress then treatment is either repeated or a second technique is added and the combined movements assessed. If pain is moderate, many different movements can be used during one treatment session. However, assessment of the changes in active movements must be made following each technique.

If improvement in the joint range ceases and pain moderates considerably, the treatment movement is taken deeper into the range to apply some degree of stretch to the resistance. The first time this is carried out the duration of treatment should be short and the depth of range into which the treatment is taken should be limited to avoid reaction. If pain is felt by the patient, very small amplitude oscillatory movements are used at a fairly constant position in the range. If the pain is less troublesome a larger amplitude can be used and this will lessen treatment soreness.

Assessment over 24 hours will reveal whether the rate of progress is adequate and whether undue discomfort has been avoided.

These patients improve in one of two ways. Either the pain and resistance diminish until a painless full range is achieved or the pain recedes and the resistance improves, losing its soft feel and becoming more like a bone-to-bone resistance. As it reaches the latter stage, the amount of treatment and the combination of techniques used at each session is increased. These patients at this stage become part of group 2. It is perhaps unnecessary to mention that active exercises would complement passive treatment at this stage.

As has been mentioned before, the majority of musculo-skeletal patients referred for physiotherapy fit into Group 3. The physiotherapist first needs to determine whether the pain or the stiffness is the dominant problem. If she is in any doubt it is advisable to treat the pain first. This should follow the lines already described under the group 1 heading in which 60% is the dividing line between using accessory or physiological movements. With painful stiff joints the 60% means 60% of the available range of STIFF movement, not 60% of the normal full range. If treating the pain produces no improvement, or if it has only limited success, and the range of active movement ceases to improve, the therapist must change her techniques so that her intention is to treat the stiffness with techniques similar to those described above under the group 2 heading but with a difference (see (3) below). If the patient feels pain (as he most certainly will in these painful/stiff joint structures) then the physiotherapist must appreciate its extent and its site so that she is alert as to what she is subjecting the patient.

Treatment for a stiff painful joint is an important field for the physiotherapist. If firm treatment is done too strongly or at the wrong time, it will be unsuccessful and will cause unnecessary pain and bring the treatment into disrepute. Nevertheless, it is a most important part of manipulation because it can be so dramatically effective when performed accurately.

The following is the routine which should be followed:

1. The initial treatment should be to determine what happens to the joint symptoms and signs when pain alone is treated. The behaviour of the pain and how it may limit any stretching-type techniques that may be used later may be determined.
2. The examination of the patient's joint should reveal the behaviour of the pain, the most restricted movements, and the pain felt when these movements are stretched. The painfully stiff movements should be correlated with the patient's loss of function and it should be determined whether it is the pain or the stiffness that limits the function. The direction of move-

ment selected as the treatment movement should be the one directly associated with the loss of function; it will be the one that has 'comparable signs' described in Chapter 4.
3. When the comparable movement is used as the treatment movement, and where the intention is to stretch stiffness, a gentle grade IV− movement should be applied, the physiotherapist being alert to changes in the patient's symptoms *during* the technique. This first treatment should be firm but not excessively painful though it must reproduce a degree of the patient's symptoms.

While treating stiffness in this group (group 3b) where pain is a factor to be appreciated, both physiological movements and accessory movements are used *but* with a difference when compared with group 2 (stiffness). While performing the accessory movement, the physiological position in which it is performed is decreased in its position in the range, in rhythm with the increasing pressure performing the accessory movement. The more intense the pain the greater the in-rhythm-reduction of the physiological position. As the pain reduces in response to treatment, so the physiological position is not reduced in range. This can be progressed to performing the accessory movement while simultaneously *increasing* the physiological position slightly (Figure 7.16). Obviously this later step is taken only when pain is significantly lowered. Understanding these modifications in treatment is a primary requirement for good technique and effective treatment.

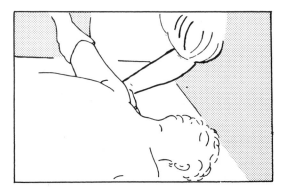

Figure 7.16 Glenohumeral joint; longitudinal movement, in abduction

Figure 7.16 is an example that will help to understand the above text. When the patient has considerable right shoulder pain and treatment has progressed such that the disorder fits the group 3b category. A caudad longitudinal accessory movement, with the glenohumeral joint in abduction, is being used as the treatment of choice. While the therapist's left hand produces the caudad movement of the head of the humerus in the glenoid cavity, her body and left arm follow the movement *and* carry the patient's right elbow further caudad so that the glenohumeral range of abduction is reduced by approximately 5–10°. As pain lessens with this technique the therapist performs the technique with the patient's elbow being moved in parallel, so to speak, with her left hand (which includes the head of this humerus). The next step is that his right elbow is kept stationary as her left hand moves the head of the humerus caudad; that is, the glenohumeral abduction is thus abducted slightly further.

If pain is only reproduced with firm pressure, then it is firm pressure that must be applied. The more easily the pain is reproduced the shorter should be the treatment time and the gentler the technique. If the joint can be stretched strongly with only slight pain then three or more separate stretches, each lasting 1–2 minutes, should be used. The reaction from treatment can be assessed the following day and this will guide the extent of further treatment:

4. If the patient has more than one site of pain arising from different joints or different areas from one joint, each should be treated separately. This situation often exists in the hand and foot.

5. As progress becomes more evident the faulty joint may be treated by more than one movement and stronger grade IV movements may be used. How much is performed at a particular treatment session will be determined by the pain reaction to treatment.

6. As was referred to in the section on 'Treatment of stiffness', treatment soreness can be readily relieved by using large-amplitude movements in the painful direction but short of pain. When stretching joints that are already painful these large-amplitude comfortable movements are an essential part of treatment. Primarily they should be performed in the same direction as the stretching technique but other physiological directions may also be used.

7. When treatment of resistance does not produce an adequate rate of improvement, the next step is to consider manipulation as described on pages 83–84.

It should be realized that muscle spasm may be caused unnecessarily during treatment of painful joints. Spasm often protects a painful joint because it is badly positioned, badly supported, or carelessly held by the physiotherapist. If, in addition to this, the joint is moved unevenly, roughly, or without due respect for pain during treatment, the spasm will further increase. Therefore the first requirement of treatment is careful positioning of the patient, competent handling of the joint and well-controlled technique.

When muscle spasm is a constant minimum

response to movement, no attempt should be made to thrust forcibly through the spasm. Instead, any of the following passive treatment movements could be used. Treatment by tiny amplitude movements that gently nudge at the muscle spasm, gradually attempting to move deeper into the range, millimetre by millimetre, would be the first choice. If there is no improvement, nudging movements should be used in an accessory movement that is slightly restricted by spasm. If this technique does not effect improvement the opposite movement to the physiological movements most restricted by spasm should be used. Grade IV movements should be performed at the limit of the range. Joints exhibiting this type of spasm are characteristically slow in their response to treatment. This variety of spasm does not readily respond to relaxation techniques.

There is one final response by muscle spasm which must be mentioned. It commonly occurs in patients with a mildly and intermittently aching joint. On examination one or more movements may be very slightly stiff. An example of such a restriction of knee extension, together with an estimate of the usual amount of pain felt on movement is shown in Figure 7.17.

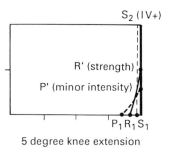

5 degree knee extension

Figure 7.17 Muscle spasm, restriction of knee extension and pain

If passive movements are examined at the usual speed, part of the physical findings may be missed. However, if quick, sharp movements are used at the limit of the range slight muscle spasm may be felt as a response to this testing movement. When this response is present, the treatment movement must be performed so that it almost produces this response. The further away the treatment movement is from producing the response, the less likely is the treatment to be successful.

Muscle spasm (including holding) may be the factor limiting range in the group 3 patients' disorders. The type of muscle spasm referred to in this section is that which occurs at the limit of the available range, is very strong, and occupies only a small part of the range.

Treatment movements

1. Treatment of pain and assessing its effect.
2. Movement through range to spasm then small-amplitude grade IV movements.
3. Manipulation of the conscious patient.

Treatment and assessment of pain

As was mentioned in relation to the treatment of the stiff painful joint, it is wise to begin by treating pain and assessing its effect. Such treatment will give a good indication of the behaviour of the patient's pain and will also show the degree of irritability of the joint disorder. However, when such spasm is the most dominant sign that can be found on examination of the joint's movements, treatment of pain is unlikely to help.

Movement through range to spasm

The next step is to move the joint through a physiological range up to the point where spasm starts and there perform very small-amplitude grade IV movements slowly. These small passive movements can be used in conjunction with active relaxation techniques.

Oscillatory movement is not always desirable (irritability or latent exacerbation) and if the above techniques have proved unsuccessful, the therapist should use a controlled sustained intermittent stretch technique. This applies to treating a painful joint whose range is limited by either structural tightness/adhesions or by protective muscle spasm. Under these circumstances the physiological movement which is restricted and painful, is the movement most often used. It is taken to the comfortable limit of range and, at this point, the physiotherapist adjusts her grasps so that she:

1. Has full control of the movement she will use.
2. Is in the most economical position to be able to sustain the position.
3. Is in a position to be able to prevent the patient from squirming out of her control. Qualification: this does NOT mean, though it may sound to be confirming it, that she is necessarily going to stretch maximally into agonizing pain for the patient; it is merely to augment her control of the technique.

The chosen movement is then moved extremely slowly into the resistance; the physiotherapist should be prepared to retreat instantly 1° or 1 mm as the patient winces. With skill, experience and concentration, this retreat can be performed before the patient winces – the patient then recognizes the skill of this operator and gains confidence in allowing her to go further irrespective of pain.

As this process of moving into and retreating from a resistance, to sustain the stretch position for a half a minute or more, gives the stretched structures, or the protective spasm, time to become less painful and less strong. The movement can then be moved one more degree (or millimetre) and held to await reduction of pain or spasm again. A point in the range will be reached when, if the position is held for even 2 minutes the pain or spasm strength cannot reduce. At this stage small, oscillatory, slow, smooth movements are performed at this range. They are very gradually increased in amplitude, but always reaching the same end position, until a movement of 20–30° can be performed. The passive movement treatment is then over and the patient attempts the same range of stretch actively.

If the range of movement does not improve and if the spasm shows no sign of relaxing it may be necessary to consider manipulation under anaesthesia. However, some orthopaedic surgeons prefer the manipulation to be carried out on the conscious patient because the patient can then provide the manipulator with instant information to direct the kind of technique used. Manipulation under pethidine is a far more preferable choice. However, other factors related to the patient's personality may sway the judgement in favour of manipulation under anaesthesia.

Manipulation of the conscious patient

When the physiotherapist has used further grade IV techniques, coaxing and stretching into muscle spasm or stiffness, she should balance how strongly she needs to push to increase range, against the degree of pain the patient experiences. Then, after consultation with the referring doctor if manipulation is indicated, one of two kinds of technique can be used:

1. The first variety is applicable to small joints such as those in the hand and foot. Here, range is limited by stiffness, not by muscle spasm. The technique is performed as a sudden very small amplitude thrust in the same position and direction as the stretching technique that reproduced the patient's pain. The pressure should be taken up first as a grade IV movement then increased to a grade IV+ and finally, superimposed on this pressure, the thrust is performed.
2. When manipulation of larger joints is contemplated the technique is usually quite different. Here the joint may be protected by some degree of muscle spasm. The manipulation, rather than being a sudden thrust, is a controlled steady stretching technique. The patient must be positioned so that he is unable to move, so that the physiotherapist can feel, in detail, what is happening at the joint during the stretching. A very close watch must be kept on the patient's

hands and eyes as a means of assessing the amount of pain he feels during the technique. Once any tearing is felt the physiotherapist needs to decide instantly whether she is going to push right through the tear or whether she is going to ease her pressure, believing she will be able to have another stretch at a later date. The decision to go on, or ease off, is guided by the amount of pain being felt by the patient (that is, whether the patient is likely to accept further stretching) and the type of tear. If it feels to be one thick adhesion ('dry blotting paper') it is better to push through it as the result is likely to be a good one, in that full range will be restored quickly. On the other hand, the tear may be a soft, weak rupturing ('wet blotting paper') extending through a greater range. When the feeling is present it is better to do little at one stretch.

Learning the skill of this kind of manipulation can be achieved only under close supervision. The instructor, having selected the patient, should perform the manipulation with the novice's eyes and ears wide open. This is necessary so that the juggling necessary to find the right direction for the stretch can be clearly appreciated. The novice should endeavour to feel the slow controlled strength of the technique while also feeling and hearing the structures tear.

The physiotherapist should stabilize the patient with her body and arm, her hand supporting and feeling around the joint being manipulated, while at the same time the other hand stretches the joint. Grade IV stretching is applied to the joint and the pressure is gradually increased until a point is reached when the spasm begins to release. It is usually at this stage that the abnormal structure releases and the range becomes full. The feel and sound of adhesions as they give way vary from a sharp snap which suddenly allows a full range movement, to an extended tearing sound through a short range (dry blotting paper), to a more extended sloppy tearing sound through a slightly bigger range. This last variety does not produce a good result; and the patient needs to exercise most conscientiously, with pain, and on an hourly basis.[3]

This procedure is particularly applicable to the frozen shoulder when stiffness is more dominant than is pain.

Most manipulations after trauma are best done in conjunction with a doctor introducing intravascular pethidine followed by intramuscular pethidine. If a manipulation is done in this way, there is always present a feedback guide (pain) from the patient – this is not present with manipulation under anaesthesia (MUA) which is a procedure to be avoided

whenever possible. However, any MUA should be carried out by the physiotherapist who has an intimate knowledge of the state of the patient's structures derived from her previous treatment of them. Of course the referring doctor and anaesthetist must be present.

Momentary pain

Patients who have 'momentary pain' (Figure 7.18) are discussed separately because they form an important group who are often poorly or unsuccessfully treated. The group is quite large and consists of

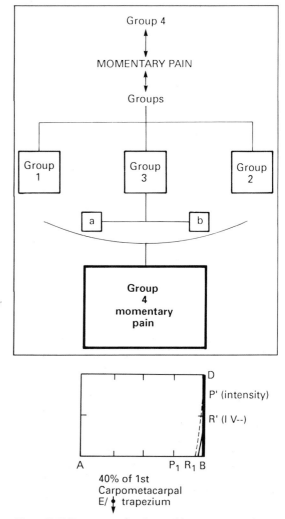

Figure 7.18 Treatment of patients with momentary pain

3. Maitland, G. D. *Mrs. E.: Demonstration of patient I: Shoulder manipulation* (50 mins) and *Demonstration of a patient: Mrs. E. II and III* (55 mins) Videotape Numbers 17 and 18. Postgraduate Teaching Centre Hermitage, Medizinische Abteilung, Bad Ragaz, Switzerland CH7310 (1978)

patients who can be successfully treated if examination detail is accurate and treatment properly applied to the findings.

The examination must divulge the joint sign that is comparable with the patient's symptoms. It is usually a combined physiological and accessory movement. The importance of this joint sign and the method for finding it have been discussed at length and examples have been given. Sometimes it may take two or three sessions to be sure that such a joint sign has been found. Because normal joints can be painful if stretched, it is often difficult to distinguish the painful joint from a normal joint. When a comparable movement is found, it alone should be used in treatment; it should be performed as a mixture of grade IV and grade III movements for approximately 6 or 7 minutes. To employ other grades or directions is usually quite a waste of time. Response to treatment is usually quite rapid; the patient feels the improvement by at least the third treatment.

A good example of this group is the patient who drops things because of momentary pain which is felt on gripping, say, a tea-cup and saucer. The comparable sign may be a posteroanterior movement of the base of the first metacarpal (or the trapezium) at the limit of extension (Figure 7.19).

This brings us to the end of the oversimplified phase 1 (see Table 7.13).

Phase 2
Intra-articular/peri-articular

Treatment related to these two groups comprise (1) techniques of painless oscillatory movements, (2) movements and sustained compression, and (3) stretching into a strong 'bite' of pain.

Intra-articular

(Reproduced from Maitland, G. D. (1985) Passive movement techniques for intra-articular and peri-articular disorders. *Australian Journal of Physiotherapy*, **31**, 3–8, by kind permission of publishers.)

The following gives 'an account of the clinical experiences that relate to Professor Lowther's paper[4] on 'The Effect of Compression and Tension on the Behaviour of Connective Tissues', that is, the metabolic effects of *mechanically* distorting the cell membrane of the chondrocyte cell. He concluded that there are two quite different roles of movement, both of which stimulate the cartilage to

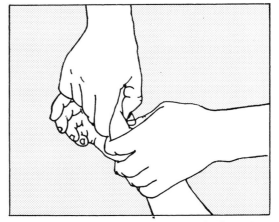

Figure 7.19 Posteroanterior movement at the first carpometacarpal joint

Table 7.13 Phase 1 table

Pain
Accessory neutral without discomfort
Accessory neutral into discomfort
Accessory neutral into pain
Physiological large amplitude without discomfort
Physiological large amplitude into discomfort
Physiological large amplitude into pain
Stiffness
Physiological limit of range
Accessory, limit of physiological range
Pain/stiffness
As for PAIN
As for STIFFNESS (modified)
Momentary pain
Combined physiological/accessory, limit

produce matrix components. The first affects the diffusion of nutrients into the matrix from synovial fluid; the second is a consequence of chondrocyte membrane deformation such as would be produced by the pressure wave due to loading of the joint.

According to Ekholm[5] exercise of the joint appears to increase the penetration of cartilage to nutrients from the synovial fluid. Maroudas *et al.*[6] proposed that the increased flow of nutrients from synovial fluid into cartilage is due more to the

4. Lowther, D. A. The effect of compression and tension on the behaviour of Connective Tissues. In *Aspects of Manipulative Therapy*, Lincoln Institute of Health Sciences, Melbourne, Australia, pp. 15–21 (1979)
5. Ekholm, R. Nutrition of Articular Cartilage. *Acta Anatomica*, **12**, 77 (1955)
6. Maroudas, A., Bullough, P., Swanson, S. A. V. and Freeman, M. A. R. The permeability of articular cartilage. *Journal of Bone and Joint Surgery*, **50B**, 166–177 (1968)

agitation of the fluid film on the cartilage surface during exercise than to cartilage compression and decompression. Lowther (unpublished observations, 1983) referred to this 'agitation' as 'surface stirring', a most eminently suited descriptive term, because it so superbly fits the treatment techniques that will be described in this paper.

Lowther[4] (p. 18) states, and it is this point that relates to the author's clinical experience, that studies on synovial fluid movement 'indicate that the nutrition of articular cartilage could be maintained by passive movement without concomitant loading of the joint surfaces'. From Lowther's work with Catersen[7] on sheep it was concluded that 'alterations in proteoglycan synthesis and content were the result of nutritional changes *directly related to joint movement* and stress'[4] (p. 18). It is interesting to note the comment regarding nutrition being maintained by passive movement, *without* concomitant loading to joint surfaces. The clinical application of the loading (achieved by avoiding or adding joint surface compression) will be evident in the treatment techniques to be described.

Again, to quote an unpublished observation of Professor Lowther (1983), 'One would predict that compression or loading in the joint should be *minimised*, particularly in the very acute stages of inflammation when the polymorphonuclear cell population in synovial fluid is maximal. When this stage has passed, then load bearing should, on balance, be more beneficial than detrimental to recovery of the matrix.'. The two stages referred to here (i.e. 'the acute stage of inflammation' and 'when this stage has passed'), match two circumstances of patients' symptoms which will be discussed.

In relation to passive movement it is appropriate to refer to work carried out by Salter *et al.*[8]. Their findings were that the healing of defects in articular cartilage contains a far higher percentage of hyaline cartilage cells when the affected joint is moved passively and continuously (CPM, continuous passive motion) than if the joint is treated by active movement, and far more than if it is treated by immobilization. It is possible, and perhaps probable, that the fact that treatment using controlled passive movement is more effective (in the author's view) in relieving the pain of intra-articular disorders of the osteoarthrosic type than is active movement, may be related to Salter's finding and Lowther's statement that nutrition could be maintained by passive movement.

Patients whose symptoms arise from intra-articular disorders range between two extremes in their presentation. These are as follows:

1. The first is when a patient has marked restriction of movement due solely to pain felt within the joint (*severe restrictive intra-articular pain*).
2. The second is when a patient has minor symptoms of intermittent aching in a joint, felt only when the joint has had to cope with heavy work or when it has been subjected to passive sustained compressive forces such as lying on the shoulder at night (*minor symptoms with compressive loads*).

Each of the above two particular circumstances require a different and special mode of treatment.

Severe restrictive intra-articular pain

The greater the severity of this pain the greater will be the restriction of joint movement inhibited by pain. The disorder has a high degree of irritability; that is, it takes very little to provoke severe pain, and this increased pain takes considerable time to subside to its usual level. Because of this irritability, both examination and treatment need to be kept to a minimum.

The following principles of the treatment techniques need to be emphasized:

1. The aim of the treatment technique is to perform the largest possible amplitude of movement which the joint can accept without exacerbation, be it an accessory movement or a physiological movement. The larger the amplitude of the treatment movement possible, the better is its effect.
2. Throughout the performing of the passive movement technique, the physiotherapist must:
   (a) Be totally aware of what the patient feels within the joint from the moment the technique is commenced, and
   (b) be totally aware of any changes in what he (the patient) feels as the technique is continued.

Four elements are used in making these assessments. They are:

1. The verbal communication between physiotherapist and patient, achieved by continuously asking questions regarding the effect on the joint symptoms while the technique is being performed.

4. Lowther, D. A. The effect of compression and tension on the behaviour of Connective Tissues. In *Aspects of Manipulative Therapy,* Lincoln Institute of Health Sciences, Melbourne, Australia, pp. 15–21 (1979)
7. Catersen, B. and Lowther, D. A. Changes in the metabolism of the porteoglycan from sheep articular cartilage in response to mechanical stress. *Biochimica et Biophysica Acta,* **540**, 412–422 (1978)
8. Salter, R. B., Simmonds, D. F., Malcolm, B. W., Rumble, E. J., Macmichael, D. and Clements, N. D. The biological effects of continuous passive motion on the healing of full-thickness defects in articular cartilage. *Journal of Bone and Joint Surgery,* **62A**, 1232–1251 (1980)

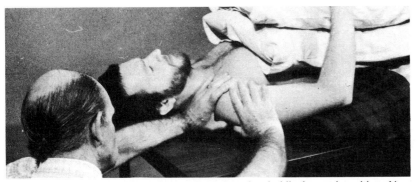

Figure 7.20 Posteroanterior movement of the humeral head while the arm is positioned in its most comfortable neutral position

2. Sufficient awareness to notice any nuances in the non-verbal communication, for example, frowning, squeezing the eyes tightly shut, flinching.
3. While performing the technique the therapist must be aware of even the most minimal muscular protective contraction, brought into play as an automatic subconscious means of protecting the joint from discomfort.
4. The therapist must also be aware of any changes in the feel of friction-free movement while performing the technique.

Treatment

When a movement is *markedly* restricted by pain alone, the first choice of treatment technique is to use an accessory joint movement while the joint is positioned in its most comfortable position.

Figure 7.20 shows a posteroanterior gliding movement of the head of the humerus in relation to the glenoid cavity while the arm is supported with pillows in the comfortable position. This position is usually a mid-range position of all the joint's physiological and accessory movements.

When performing such techniques at the first and second treatment sessions of severely painful and irritable intra-articular disorders, the posteroanterior accessory movement must *not* (1) produce any feeling of discomfort or awareness of uncomfortable joint movement during the performing of the technique; or (2) cause any aching in the joint.

Posteroanterior movement is not the only accessory movement that can be used. Use can also be made of lateral movements of the head of the humerus, longitudinal movements caudad and

anteroposterior movement. To these can be added a rotary movement of the shaft of the humerus in a mid-range 20 degree arc, even though this is not an accessory movement.

Four measures of the effectiveness of the technique can be determined:

1. Subjective changes 'in' the shoulder during the performing of the treatment technique.
2. Subjective symptomatic change 'in' the shoulder following treatment.
3. Objective changes in range and quality of active movement as a result of treatment.
4. The time taken, for any increased symptoms from testing (3), to subside more quickly as compared with the pre-treatment measurement.

These treatment techniques effectively and rapidly reduce pain and improve movement if the selection of the patient is correct. This is not the case if the disorder is an active disease in the acute inflammatory stage. The techniques themselves may be considered to be the 'surface stirring' without loading to which Lowther (unpublished observations, 1983) refers.

Peri-articular

Flint[9] and also Gillard *et al.*[10] have demonstrated the importance of intermittent tensional forces on the maintenance of the structure of the achilles tendon in rabbits. Professor Lowther[4] (p.18) reports that:

It seems likely that . . . tensional forces are important for the maintenance of ligaments and tendons in the joint and perhaps in the joint capsule itself, since Akison *et al.*[11] demonstrated

9. Flint, M. H. The role of environmental factors in connective tissue ultrastructure. *The Ultrastructure of Collagen*, C. C. Thomas, Springfield, Il., pp. 60–66 (1976)
10. Gillard, G. C., Merrilees, M. J., Bell-Booth, P. G., Reilly, H. C. and Flint, M. H. The proteoglycan content and the axial periodicity of collagen in tendon. *Biochemistry Journal,* **163**, 145–151 (1977)
11. Akison, W. H., Woo, S. L. Y., Amiel, D., Coutts, R. D. and Daniel, D. The connective tissue response to immobility: biochemical changes in periarticular connective tissue of the immobilized rabbit knee. *Clinical Orthopaedics,* **93**, 356–422 (1973)

increased stiffness and matrix changes in the joint capsule from immobilized rabbit joints.

Again there is a clinical application to parallel these statements. For patients who have pain from ligamentous or capsular damage or change, their treatment by passive movement ('intermittent tensional forces') is applied in a particular manner. The description of treatment given below will be related to the two extremes of such disorders. These are:

1. Those patients whose damage is recent and quite painful when stretched *(recent peri-articular damage)*.
2. Those patients whose disorder is of a longer standing and more chronic nature *(chronic peri-articular stiffness with minor pain)*.

Recent peri-articular damage

The passive movement treatment for these patients consists of small-amplitude movements, performed slowly, with full awareness of pain response, and repeated in groups of approximately five movements. These movements aim to apply gentle intermittent stretch, provoking only minimal discomfort. These groups of intermittent stretches may be repeated many times, provided there is no increase in the pain response with the movement. Assessment of the effect of the passive movement treatment is made over the 24 hour period following the treatment, and the information thus gained guides how the intermittent stretches should be modified at subsequent treatment sessions. An increase of pain indicates that the technique should be even more gentle; better movement with less pain is a favourable response and calls for performing the movement deeper in the range producing a similar pain response to that of the last treatment.

Chronic peri-articular stiffness with minor pain

Treatment of these patients is almost identical with those described above, but there is a difference in the firmness of the technique. Many physiotherapists are unaware of how strongly our passive movement technique needs to be. As we are sometimes unwilling to apply enough stretch (that is 'intermittent tensional force'), treatment is less effective, and the end result less good for the patient than it might have been had a stronger intermittent tensional force been applied. This then brings us to the question, 'What is going to tell the physiotherapist how strongly this momentary stretch should be applied?' The answer to the question must be qualified by the statement that the kind of peri-articular condition being considered here is not one where the structures are affected by disease, recent surgery or disruption. In the presence of a

chronic disorder the intensity of the momentary mechanical stretch should cause a sharp 'bite' of pain.

It is this 'bite' of pain that must be provoked for the treatment technique to be maximally effective. And it is the achieving of this 'bite' of pain by gradually and progressively increasing the pressure of the stretch, which answers the question 'How hard should I stretch?'

The number of stretches into this 'bite' of pain performed at any one treatment session should:

1. Be few in number.
2. Not be sustained once the 'bite' is provoked.
3. Slowly build up in tension.

When the patient does stretching at home to retain the increased range of movement gained from the treatment, they too must be performed in the same manner, allowing sufficient time between stretches into 'bite' for the discomfort to totally subside. Damage does not occur, despite the 'bite' of pain, provided the passive movement is momentary and intermittent.

Figure 7.21 shows an example of stretching ankle dorsi-flexion where the movement is gradually taken near to the limit of the range, then taken into a momentary 'bite' of pain and immediately released.

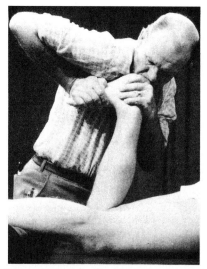

Figure 7.21 Passive dorsiflexion stretch into 'bite'

Figure 7.22(a) shows the position the patient should adopt in stretching into dorsi-flexion as a home exercise. While keeping the heel on the floor, the knee should gradually be pushed further forwards until pain is produced. This position should then be sustained until the pain subsides. The knee is then moved further forwards, again pausing for the pain to subside until the limit of range is reached.

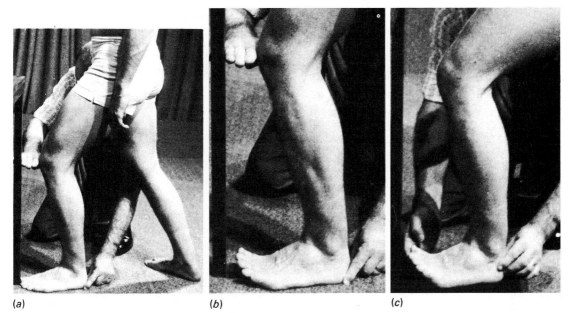

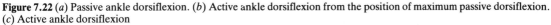

Figure 7.22 (*a*) Passive ankle dorsiflexion. (*b*) Active ankle dorsiflexion from the position of maximum passive dorsiflexion. (*c*) Active ankle dorsiflexion

Having performed this routine of producing 'bite' two or three times, he should then, before releasing his dorsiflexion, attempt to lift the ball of his foot off the floor without uplifting his heel (Figure 7.22(b)).

He should continue endeavouring to lift the ball of his foot until he eventually lifts the whole foot off the floor at the maximum dorsiflexion active range (Figure 7.22(c)).

After completing the routine, when he releases the dorsiflexion, he can expect to experience quite severe sharp pain, but it quickly disappears with repeated active, loosely performed, dorsi/plantar flexion movements.

(End of extract from Maitland (1985).)

Minor symptoms with compressive loads

Patients with minor symptoms on compression fit into the severe restrictive intra-articular group, **but** at a different or less intense stage. Neither the passive movements of the kind described above, nor of the 'continuous passive motion' type described by Salter *et al.*[8], would improve the patient's symptoms or the physical capabilities of his troublesome joint. However, if those same movements are performed with the joint surfaces firmly compressed together, then the techniques can be effective. The following

extract, 'The importance of adding compression when examining and treating synovial joints' in 'Aspects of Manipulative Therapy' 2nd ed., Churchill Livingstone, Melbourne, 1985, is reproduced by kind permission of the publishers.

An hypothesis that there are occasions when a compression component must be added to movements arises from clinical experience. The clinical experience has two separate facets: the first is related to a patient's pain response to such examination and treatment movements; and the second is related to the smoothness of the feeling of passive movement of a synovial joint when joint surfaces are abnormal:

1. The clinical experience related to pain response is demonstrated in the following example. A painful metatarsophalangeal joint of the big toe is passively rotated in a small-amplitude (say 10°) oscillatory manner in mid-range. As the oscillatory movement is performed in mid-range, no ligaments nor any part of the capsule are in any way stretched or put under tension. The important fact about this test is that when the oscillatory movement is performed with the opposing joint surfaces compressed, exquisite pain is provoked; yet when the same movement is performed without the compression component, no pain occurs.

8. Salter, R. B., Simmonds, D. F., Malcolm, B. W., Rumble, E. J., Macmichael, D. and Clements, N. D. The biological effects of continuous passive motion on the healing of full-thickness defects in articular cartilage. *Journal of Bone and Joint Surgery*, **62A**, 1232–1251 (1980)

When the above pain response occurs, the examiner is forced to the conclusion that if a small mid-range movement without compression is painless and the same movement with compression is painful, there must be some mechanisms whereby pain is evoked from the joint surfaces and/or the subchondral tissues.

2. The clinical experience related to smoothness of movement is based on the premise that if a normal synovial joint is moved passively back and forth through even a large arc, irrespective of whether the adjacent joint surfaces are forcibly compressed together or only lightly opposed, the movements will have an identical feel of being smooth and friction free. However, in patients having joint surface abnormalities, a resistance to a movement through range can be felt when the surfaces are moved while being compressed.

The above statement in relation to a normal synovial joint can be demonstrated and appreciated very readily by carrying out the following experiment.

Ask any young person with a normal ankle to lie prone with one knee flexed to a right angle while you face across his or her leg and hold his or her bare foot firmly in both hands. Stabilize the grip against your chest and chin. In this position, rock your trunk from side to side so that the person's ankle is oscillated in a 30 degree mid-range arc of dorsi-plantar flexion. If the test movement is done sufficiently perceptively, the ankle movement can be felt to be just as smooth whether minimal or maximal body weight is transmitted through the foot. The person on whom the experiment is tried is also unaware of any difference in the feel of the dorsi-plantar flexion movement within the ankle. If this same test movement is repeated on an osteoarthritic joint, the loss of the friction-free 'feel' when the joint surfaces are compressed is readily appreciated by the examiner and similarly, the patient is also well aware of the different feeling of movement (Figures 7.23 and 7.24).

On the basis that the two clinical examples presented above are demonstrable, it is interesting to review anatomical and pathological factors which may provide explanations for the examples, thereby adding strength to the proposal that passive movements of a joint should sometimes be performed with the adjacent surfaces compressed.

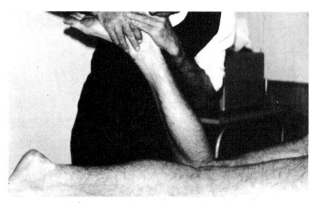

Figure 7.23 30° arc of dorsi-plantar flexion with compression

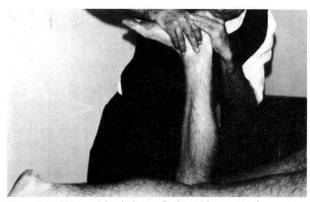

Figure 7.24 30° arc of dorsi-plantar flexion with compression

Joint surface friction

Normal synovial joints

In synovial joints the opposing surfaces consist of hyaline cartilage which in its normal state is macroscopically white, shiny and firm, while microscopically the superficial layer has an unbroken, though rippled, surface. Synovial fluid – which has viscous, elastic, plastic and nutritious properties – plays an important part in the smoothness of movement of the surfaces on each other. The properties of synovial fluid are complex when considered in relation to the part they play in contributing to the low coefficient of friction.

With regard to movement of a synovial joint, the coefficient of friction between adjacent joint surfaces has been presented as 1.002 by Charnley[12], and between 1.013 for normal stresses and 1.2 for higher normal stresses by Malcolm *et al.*[13].

The viscosity of synovial fluid is different in different joints and it also varies within a joint when there are changes in the types of movement being performed. Clarke[14] stated that, as a result of experimental work, the coefficient of friction 'decreased with increased load'.

For a normal synovial joint to function properly it is necessary to have normal hyaline cartilage and normal synovial fluid. When these two components are normal and a joint is moved passively, with or without compression, any variations that may occur in the coefficient of friction will not be perceptible to an examiner when carrying out the second test example described above.

The following figures show the recently dissected hip joint of a heifer being moved through an arc of approximately 30°. This is performed firstly with the joint surfaces gently opposed (Figure 7.25), and secondly the same movement is produced while the joint surfaces are firmly compressed together (Figure 7.26).

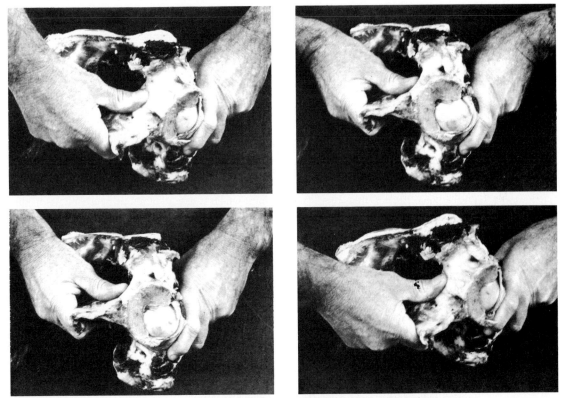

Figure 7.25 Without compression   **Figure 7.26** With compression

12. Charnley, J. Communication to a symposium on biomechanics, Institution of Mechanical Engineers, London (1959) Cited in *Gray's Anatomy,* 35th edn., Longman, London, p. 193 (1973)
13. Malcolm, L. L., Fung, Y. C., Woo, S. L-Y., Akeson, W. H. and Amiel, D. Steady-state dynamic frictional properties of cartilage-cartilage interfaces. *Journal of Bone and Joint Surgery,* **57A**, 567 (1975)
14. Clarke, I. C. Friction and wear of articular cartilage – a pendulum/SES system. *Journal of Bone and Joint Surgery,* **57A**, 567 (1975)

This is the best possible method of manually and mentally appreciating precisely just how smooth joint movement is when the surfaces and synovial fluid are normal, and more importantly, how the feeling of the quality of that smoothness is unchanged in the normal joint when compression is added. The experiment is strongly recommended to prove the credibility of the fact.

Mow and Kuei (1975)[15] reported that they analysed the

> fluid mechanics of the squeeze-film action as a function of the viscoelastic parameters of whole synovial fluid, and hyaluronic acid solutions . . . The theoretical solution . . . showed that normal whole synovial fluid is important in the protection of cartilage, lowering overall pressure in the fluid and increasing the total loaded area of the joint.

The important fact that they determined, which relates directly to this discussion, is stated in their words:

> It was concluded that the viscoelastic behaviour of the whole synovial fluid, attributable to the hyaluronic acid protein complex, *is important in the analysis of the wear of articular cartilage and that lubrication and wear must be considered as two separate but often interrelated phenomena.*

Pathology in synovial joints

Barnett[16] was able to show that by injecting hyaluronic acid into one ankle joint of rabbits, thereby reducing the viscosity of the synovial fluid, and by subjecting the rabbits to long periods of exercising, the injected joints showed much more severe attrition of the articular surface than the control joint.

Broderick *et al.*[17] have shown that there are chemical differences in the synovial fluid of joints affected by rheumatoid arthritis, osteoarthritis, traumatic arthritis, gouty arthritis, Reiter's syndrome, pigmented villonodular synovitis and septic arthritis, when compared with the synovial fluid of the normal joint.

Perhaps, with the chemical changes in synovial fluid that occur with osteoarthritis as stated above, there may also be a change in the viscosity of the synovial fluid. Thus as well as provoking attrition of the articular surfaces, changed viscosity may also increase the coefficient of friction.

In Clarke's experimental work[14], he found that when the joint was 'run dry, the coefficient increased 2 to 10 times.' He also stated that the wear of the cartilaginous surfaces in the dry runs 'was evident as fissuring and flaking of the surface layer similar to osteoarthritic fibrillation'.

McDevitt and Muir[18] carried out an experiment in which osteoarthritis was induced in the right knee of dogs by sectioning the anterior cruciate ligament. Six or more weeks after the operation they found that gross changes in the cartilage of the affected joints were evidenced by the surface being 'less shiny and softer and was noticeably thicker than the control cartilage' which was white, shiny and firm:

> Microscopical changes were noticeable one week after the operation. The cartilage . . . one week after operation, was slightly roughened with occasional small clefts . . . The number and depth of the clefts was greater two weeks after operation . . . Fibrillation . . . gradually progressed with time after the operation until, after 7 weeks, deep clefts were evident and by 16 weeks erosion of the articular surface was complete (Figure 7.27).

Clinical appreciation

With changes in the synovial fluid and the superficial layers of the hyaline cartilage there is an accompanying change in the coefficient of friction. From the time when these changes begin, a stage must be reached when, on physical examination of the joint's movement, the normal feel of friction-free movement is replaced by a perceptively less friction-free feel. This clinical change is more readily appreciated when the joint surfaces are held compressed together and moved.

Everyone is familiar with the feel of moving a joint which is devoid of all, or nearly all, its hyaline cartilage. Similarly, we would all accept that some of these joints have a rougher feel when moved than others. We should, therefore, be able to accept the fact that a stage must exist when this change in friction first becomes perceptible on physical examination. It is the early stages in the changes of friction-free movement that this discussion sets out to show can be assessed by passive movement and that this assessment can be appreciated earlier if joint surface compression is utilized during the test movement. The time at which this change in friction will be perceptible to any particular examiner will depend on his threshold of force perception.

14. Clarke, I. C. Friction and wear of articular cartilage – a pendulum/SES system. *Journal of Bone and Joint Surgery,* **57A,** 567 (1975)
15. Mow Van, C. and Kuei, C. K. The effect of visco-elasticity on the squeeze film action of lubrication of synovial joints. *Journal of Bone and Joint Surgery,* **57A,** 567 (1975)
16. Barnett, C. H. Wear and tear in joints. An experimental study. *Journal of Bone and Joint Surgery,* **38B,** 567–575 (1956)
17. Broderick, P. A., Corvese, N., Pierik, M. G., Pike, R. F. and Mariorenzi, A. L. Exfoliative cytology interpretation of synovial fluid in joint disease. *Journal of Bone and Joint Surgery,* **58A,** 396–399 (1976)
18. McDevitt, C. and Muir, H. An experimental model of osteoarthritis: early morphological and biochemical changes. *Journal of Bone and Joint Surgery,* **59B,** 24–35 (1977)

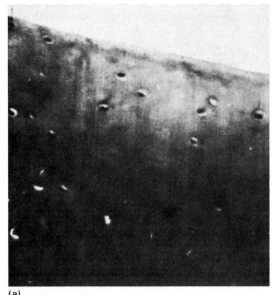 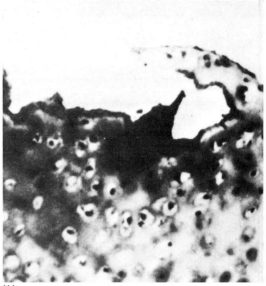

(a) (b)

Figure 7.27 (a) Normal and (b) fibrillated cartilage

Joint surface pain

Goodfellow *et al.*[19] in a paper on patellofemoral pathology, made the statement:

> But how could such a lesion cause pain? Because articular cartilage contains no nerve fibres, and because a smoothly intact articular surface could hardly occasion a local synovial reaction, it is supposed that nerve endings in the subjacent bone transmit the painful stimuli.

Miller and Kasahara[20] found that:

> small myelinated and amyelinated nerve fibres enter the numerous foramina of the epiphyseal and metaphyseal regions of long bones, traverse the thin cortex, and supply the interior of the bone. Small myelinated fibres wind about the trabeculae of the spongiosa or spread out on the under-surface of the articular cartilage.

They also state that 'no function can yet be attributed to any particular type of nerve fibre or nerve ending.'

More recently, Reimann and Christensen[21] reported that 'in the bone marrow, nerves were easily demonstrated, usually closely associated with the vessels'. When histological sections from osteoarthritic femoral heads were undertaken:

> several nerve fibres, in longitudinal as well as cross-sections, were seen in the bone marrow subchondrally where an abundance of vessels was also found. As nerves were also demonstrated in sections with a proliferation of vessels into the calcified layer of articular cartilage, as well as in the subchondral granulation tissue, it was evident that there were more nerves in the osteoarthritic femoral heads than in the control cases.

Aichroth *et al.*[22], in a lecture to the British Orthopaedic Research Society, reported the results of pressure changes within the femoral marrow cavity in two patients with osteoarthritis of the hip, and one control patient. The pressure changes were studied during walking, standing, sitting and lying prone. They stated that 'rapid changes in pressure in both initiating movements and during walking were found in those with osteoarthritis. It was possible that these pressure changes were related to the patient's symptoms, in view of the small change found to produce pain.'

19. Goodfellow, J., Hungerford, D. S. and Woods, C. Patello-femoral joint mechanics and pathology. *Journal of Bone and Joint Surgery,* **58B**, 291–299 (1976)
20. Miller, M. R. and Kasahara, M. Observations on the innervation of human long bones. *Anatomical Record,* **145**, 13–23 (1963)
21. Reimann, I. and Christensen, S. Bach A histological demonstration on nerves in sub-chondral bone. *Acta Orthopaedica Scandinavica,* **48**, 345–352 (1977)
22. Aichroth, P. M., Scott, R. A. P. and Nott, M. Changes in bone marrow pressure on walking in patients with osteoarthritis of the hip. *Journal of Bone and Joint Surgery,* **57B**, 246 (1975)

When is compression required?

Hopefully the above facts provide sufficient evidence to validate the view that symptoms may arise from a joint surface disorder, 'joint surface' in this context referring to all of the tissues and fluid in the section lying between the subchondral section of one bone and the subchondral section of the adjacent bone of a synovial joint.

There are three circumstances under which examination of movement of the synovial joint with its surfaces compressed should be performed:

1. When the usual test movements do not clearly show findings that match the patient's symptoms, test movements through range should be repeated with the joint surfaces compressed firmly, assessing for smoothness of movement and a more matching pain response.
2. When on examination of joint movements it is determined that the patient is aware of pain-through-range, the pain responses through this range should be compared between when the movement is performed with compression and when the movement is performed without compression. If the pain response is much greater when the surfaces are compressed, the indication is that the disorder is probably associated with 'joint surface' abnormality.
3. Even when the coefficient of friction is markedly increased and crepitus may be evident, the patient may suffer no symptoms. However, the more understanding the examiner can have of the state of the joint, the better his evaluation of a patient's disorder can be. Therefore, if the joint surface is thought to be disordered in any way, examination by movement under compression should be performed.

Method of examination

The joints most commonly requiring examination using compression are: the tarsometatarsal joint of the big toe, the patellofemoral joint, the carpometacarpal joint of the thumb, the hip and the glenohumeral joint. The tests for the glenohumeral joint and the patellofemoral joint will be described.

Glenohumeral joint

With the patient's elbow flexed the examiner should fully stabilize the arm against his side with his arm. The palm and heel of the examiner's other hand should be placed around the greater tuberosity of the humerus with the forearm directed at right angles to the glenoid cavity.

The examiner then moves his body so as to abduct and adduct the patient's arm through an arc of 30° from approximately 20° of abduction to 50° of abduction. The arc should be oscillated firstly without any pressure being exerted by the examiner's hand against the tuberosity of the humerus and then repeated with pressure against the tuberosity, compressing the head of the humerus into the glenoid cavity.

Figure 7.28 shows a large amplitude of glenohumeral abduction being performed while maintaining compression of the glenohumeral joint surfaces. Figure 7.28(a) shows that the compression is effected by the physiotherapist's left hand.

As the arm is taken further into abduction, the compression is effected by the left hand and the right thigh pushing from the elbow along the line of the shaft of the humerus (Figure 7.28(b)); the resultant vector of these forces produces a compression of the head of the humerus in the glenoid cavity at right angles to the surface of the fossa.

The smoothness of movement should be compared as also should the pain response in the compressed and non-compressed situations.

Patellofemoral joint

Passive movements of the patella on the femur should be assessed with the tibiofemoral joint in the

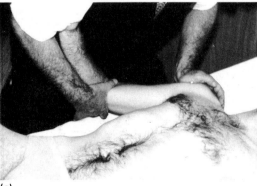

(a)

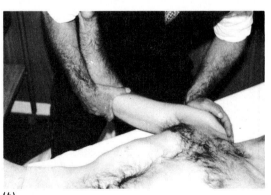

(b)

Figure 7.28 Glenohumeral movement with compression. (*a*) Low angle; (*b*) high angle

extended position and also in different positions of flexion. The reason for this is that in different positions of tibiofemoral flexion, different surfaces of the patella lie against different surfaces of the femoral condyles.

The patella should be moved cephalad, caudad, medially, laterally, and in a direction of axial rotation (especially with the medial border of the patella moving anteroposteriorly into the femoral intercondylar area).

For examination purposes the movements should be performed initially with minimal compression and only progressed to firmer compression if pain is not provoked.

The method is for the examiner to apply pressure to the anterior surface of the patella through one hand while moving the patella with the other hand (Figures 7.29–7.32).

Again, it is the findings regarding smoothness of movement and pain response which are compared with the patient's complaint and his normal knee.

Application in treatment

Patellofemoral syndromes which are mechanical or degenerative in origin respond well to treatment by passive movement of the joint surfaces through a range of movement with a degree of compression which permits the movement to be able to be performed either without pain or with only a small degree of discomfort. The technique is the same as that described previously for examination. However, in treatment, the movement is oscillated back and forth for one or two minutes, following which an assessment of changes in both symptoms and movements is made. The degree of compression used is guided by the assessed response. When a good response is achieved with treatment, stronger compression can be incorporated without increase in discomfort. As this progression becomes possible the patient is also aware of improvement in both symptoms and function.

The following example is of the later stages of treatment of a 20-year-old male with a painful right metatarsophalangeal joint of the big toe. Three months previously, while playing soccer, he kicked the ball while at the same time an opponent blocked the kick. The patient described the injury as a 'stubbed toe' and was able to say that there was no flexion or extension component to the injury. The injury caused severe pain in the metatarsophalangeal joint of the big toe. This pain gradually

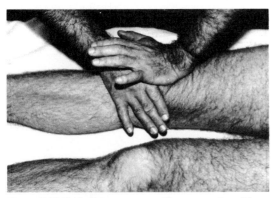

Figure 7.29 Cephalad movement with compression with the knee extended

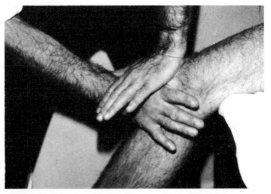

Figure 7.31 Cephalad movement with compression with the knee flexed

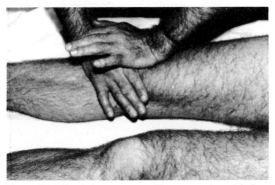

Figure 7.30 Caudad movement with compression with the knee extended

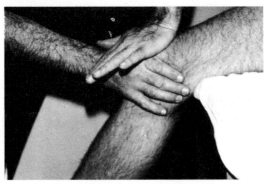

Figure 7.32 Caudad movement with compression with the knee flexed

subsided over the following month but then remained unchanged.

At the time of initial treatment he complained of intermittent severe sharp pain brought on by movement, particularly if he knocked his toe, even lightly. Such pain would last for several minutes before subsiding, and even following this interval he was well aware that symptoms were more easily provoked than at other times. He responded satisfactorily to initial physiotherapy until he reached a stage when the treatment ceased to produce improvement.

On re-examination he commented that he was still mainly aware of his problem if he accidentally stubbed his toe, even lightly. When examining his normal functional movements the ranges were full and comparatively pain-free. However, when the metatarsophalangeal joint was stabilized in a position midway between the limits of flexion, extension, abduction, adduction and the rotations, and the joint surfaces compressed firmly together, his pain could be completely reproduced with small abduction–adduction movements or small rotary movements.

Passive movement treatment was instituted using both abduction–adduction and rotation with the joint surfaces compressed. Initially these were performed with a degree of compression such that only minimal discomfort was provoked with the technique. As the response showed improvement, the techniques were increased progressively from treatment to treatment in both vigour and duration. (The rotary technique is shown in Figure 7.33(a) and (b).)

While taking into account the patient's comments regarding progress, the two main assessments made at each examination session were:

1. Asking the patient to stub his toe gently into the palm of the examiner's hand while the hand was held against the wall.

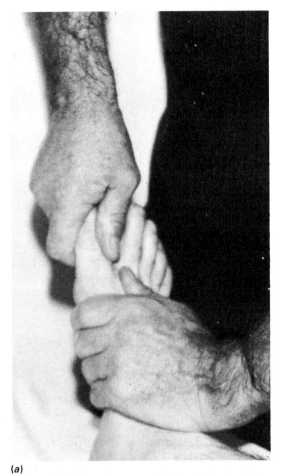

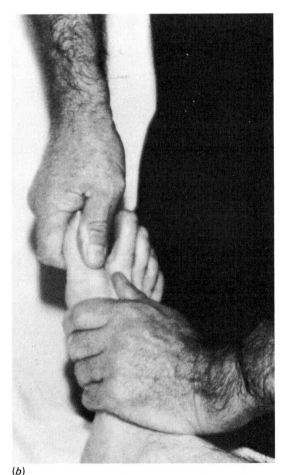

(a)   *(b)*

Figure 7.33 Mid-range rotary mobilizing with compression

2. Assessing at each session the relationship between the pain response and strength of compression possible during treatment.

The response to treatment was very good. After two and a half weeks he could stub his toe firmly with only the slightest discomfort, and treatment was discontinued. (End of extract).

It is worth quoting from experimental work first carried out and presented to the Orthopaedic Research Society by Salter *et al.*[23]:

'In order to study the effects of continuous passive motion on the healing of experimental full-thickness defects in articular cartilage, (they) made a standard experimental injury (four full-thickness drill holes) in the distal joint surface of the femur in twenty immature rabbits which were then treated by one of three methods: immobilization, normal cage activity, or continuous passive motion for periods of up to 4 weeks. Healing of the 280 defects was studied closely and histologically. With immobilization, fibrous tissues filled the defects and there were many joint adhesions. . . . With normal cage activity there was imperfect healing by a combination of fibrous tissues and poorly differentiated cartilage. With continuous passive motion, however, healing through the formation of new hyaline cartilage (chondroneogenesis) occurred in over half of the defects within 4 weeks.'

It is interesting to answer a question posed by Professor Lowther[4] (p. 20): 'How far do these observations (that is the observations he has made in his paper) apply to osteoarthrosic joints?' It is also interesting to relate the question, and the effect of the treatment outlined, to the remaining quotation from his paragraph which is as follows:

'Although the cartilage shows degenerative changes, these tend to be focal. Since inflammation of the synovial membrane is not a major feature, the joint capsule and ligaments are not subject to the same enzymatic damage; continued load-bearing will not affect the capsule and tendons, but may increase the rate of deterioration of the cartilage surface. However, movement of the joint is essential to maintain cartilage nutrition for as long as possible, and to minimize adhesions and bony fusion which tend to increase as the cartilage surface degenerates.'

If the work of Salter *et al.*[8] is to be believed, the relationship between the painful osteoarthrosic joints and the treatment by passive movements may, by improving nutrition, have an advantageous effect on the cartilage (and probably on other associated components), to the extent that the patient's arthrosic joint will function better and be less painful.

Phase 3
Osteoarthritis

The physiotherapist most certainly has a role to play in the treatment of the osteoarthritic joint (Table 7.14). This is so even when the joint (e.g. hip) may in future require surgical replacement.

When a patient has pain within his hip and has marked radiological changes in the hip (loss of joint space and flattening of the head of the humerus) it is still possible to both reduce the pain and improve the quality of its movements and its ranges. In the initial stages while pain is the primary factor, accessory movements produced by pressures applied to the greater trochanter are the first choice. The

Table 7.14 Phase 3 arthritides–treatment

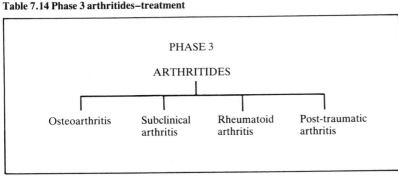

4. Lowther, D. A. The effect of compression and tension on the behaviour of Connective Tissues. In *Aspects of Manipulative Therapy*, Lincoln Institute of Health Sciences, Melbourne, Australia, pp. 15–21 (1979)
8. Salter, R. B., Simmonds, D. F., Malcolm, B. W., Rumble, E. J., Macmichael, D. and Clements, N. D. The biological effects of continuous passive motion on the healing of full-thickness defects in articular cartilage. *Journal of Bone and Joint Surgery*, **62A**, 1232–1251 (1980)
23. Salter, R. B., Simmons, D. F., Malcolm, B. W., Rumble, E. J. and MacMichael, D. The effects of continuous passive motion on the healing of articular cartilage defects – an experimental investigation in rabbits. *Journal of Bone and Joint Surgery*, **57A**, 570–571 (1975)

patient is positioned to lie on his sound side with both hips and knees flexed comfortably and the upper foot and leg fully supported with pillows between the legs. Care needs to be taken to support the foot and ankle so that the femur's shaft-rotation is in a neutral pain-free position. Frequently this is not cared for adequately. The same treatment care is taken as for group 1 or 3a patients. Assessment is carried out impeccably and a written (even graphed) record is kept by the patient as it is an essential component of the analysis of the state of the disorder and its likely prognosis with manipulative physiotherapy.

The ultimate aim with such a disorder is to be able to perform large-amplitude, brisk, shaft rotations in the side lying position described above, or to be able to reach a stage of large-amplitude hip flexion – adduction movements (from an extension adduction or even just an adduction position in the same flexion position). The patient should be taught loose pendular exercises to be carried out three or four times a day, and even at night if he is wakened by pain.

There is another reason for saying that the physiotherapist has a role in treating these patients. An example of a patient will reveal this role.

A woman had a radiologically bad osteoarthritic hip and was having a degree of pain that led the surgeon to say that a hip-replacement operation was necessary. The patient did not want this and was referred to a physiotherapist for treatment. Because the degree of irritability was sufficiently low to allow flexion–adduction movements to be used for treatment, these were performed and progressed as for group 3b patients as described earlier. Shaft rotation as grade III was added in both the flexion–adduction position and the 90° hip/knee flexion position. The result was good and she could walk long distances without discomfort and could use stairs quite well. She was pleased and treatment was discontinued except for her own exercising and a single 6-weekly 'maintenance treatment' session.

One year later she had a fall, landing on her hip. This triggered off an exacerbation of her osteoarthritic symptoms. This time she gained nothing from the same physiotherapist and hip replacement surgery was performed. The surgeon's postoperative comment was particularly poignant: 'I have never seen the structures surrounding the hip in such a healthy state, it was quite remarkable.'

She had a good result from the surgery, responding to treatment and recovering at a decidedly quicker rate than is usual.

This example reveals a second and significantly important aspect to manipulative physiotherapy for the painful osteoarthritic hip. The same applies to other similarly disordered synovial joints.

Another point is raised by this experience. When treating any synovial joint that has radiological evidence of osteoarthritic change, even if a peri-articular structure is the part being treated, the intra-articular changes should also be given the advantage of Grades II or III– treatment which may stimulate nutrition and better function.

Subclinical arthritis

Subclinical arthritis was discussed at length in the previous chapter. Its management, particularly in relation to what the physiotherapist has to offer both in her treatment and in the suggestions for other treatments that she can make, is properly and valuably her role. Its mobilizing treatment would be in the group 1 category as is that for 'jointy people', where the techniques would be directed at the pain. Such a joint disorder is slower in its response than is the mechanical variety of arthritis; in fact it is its slower response that is one of the leading factors in its differentiation. If it responds only slightly in the first four sessions, the improvement may well be enhanced by anti-inflammatory medication. (Mechanical inflammation is often helped less by anti-inflammatory medication.) If the result of combining medication with mobilization is still incomplete, an intra-articular injection of hydrocortisone could be expected to be very successful.

Rheumatoid arthritis

Passive movement techniques are never successful in relieving pain caused by an active rheumatoid arthritis. However, if the rheumatoid arthritis is not active and the patient complains of pain or aching of more recent origin, there may be a mechanical reason or minor recent trauma which is responsible for the pain. Under these circumstances gentle grade II type movements will be beneficial. However, it will be necessary to carry out extremely gentle grade IV– techniques to relieve this pain. Firm techniques should never be used on joints exhibiting rheumatoid arthritic changes because the ligaments and tendons around the joint are structurally weakened by the rheumatoid disorder.

Osteoarthrotic and post-traumatic arthritis

Pain resulting from osteoarthrotic joints or from long-standing traumatic arthritis can be very readily improved by large-amplitude movements within range. When pain is severe, movements of large-amplitude should be used but they should be performed painlessly as accessory or rotary movements in a neutral position. As pain recedes, large-amplitude *physiological* movements should be used, initially without provoking pain. As the condition continues to improve the large-amplitude movements can be taken into pain and probably up to the end of the available range of movement.

Table 7.15 Phase 4 fractures–treatment

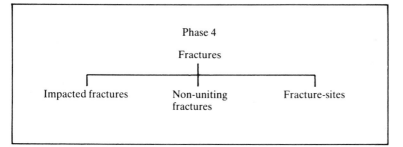

Phase 4
Impacted fractures

Injuries that result in fractures (Table 7.15), for example of the surgical neck of the humerus, are usually severe enough to cause damage to ligaments and capsule, thus laying the basis for a stiff glenohumeral joint. Passive accessory movements of the glenohumeral joint in its neutral and supported position (see Figure 10.34, page 152) can play an extremely vital part in retaining maximum movement without any stress on the fracture. The importance of this early treatment cannot be over-emphasized; it is extremely important to realize that a good functional range can be retained without the fracture being subjected to stress (see page 105).

Abduction is a very important glenohumeral movement. The movement can be performed as part of treatment in all fractures of the humerus if the full length of the humerus is supported throughout the movement with one arm while one of more fingers of the other hand assess movement between the head of the humerus and the acromion process.

Non-uniting fractures

(Reproduced from McNair, J. and Maitland, G. D. (1983) The role of passive mobilization in the treatment of a non-uniting fracture site – a case study. Presented at the *International Conference on Manipulative Therapy*, and reproduced by kind permission of the Manipulative Therapists Association of Australia.)

To date passive mobilization has always been directed towards creating movement at a joint, by applying mechanical pressures to the adjacent bones; the aim being to relieve pain and increase range of movement.

However, since 1982 we have had the opportunity to apply certain passive mobilization techniques to the adjacent bone at a fracture site. Here the aim was to stimulate union at a particular fracture site which was already showing signs of non-union on X-ray and the medical specialist was considering surgical intervention.

This presents a challenge in two areas:

1. That of fracture management which has historically and classically disallowed movement of fractures.
2. That of 'end-feel', where originally there was no predictable concept of 'end-feel' to the movement since we, as physiotherapists, have not as yet developed a bank of knowledge or skill of 'feel' in this area.

Thus the choice of technique in this case did not purely follow our usual principles of applying techniques in that it was not based upon the behaviour of symptoms through range of movement or at rest. Instead it was based upon the following:

1. The recognition of the patient's ability to appreciate 'fracture site pain', as distinct from **all** other types of pain, during movement of the fracture.
2. An academic extension of the concept of accessory movement and 'end-feel', with a knowledge of the orientation of the fracture lines and its internal fixation.

Case study

A 40-year-old man, who had been shot, was admitted to the Royal Adelaide Hospital on 17 September 1981. He had an entry wound just under his xiphisternum and had some bleeding from his left elbow which was unstable.

The bullet had passed through his left elbow joint and entered his chest. He was resuscitated and underwent a laparotomy on the day of admission. The X-rays taken on the day of admission are shown in Figures 7.34 and 7.35.

On the following day (18 September 1981) his elbow was explored in theatre. The findings were a fractured lateral epicondyle and a fractured olecranon with the articular surfaces of the elbow joint

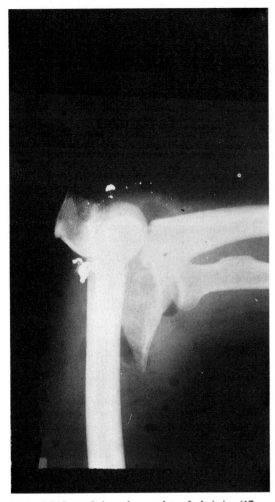

Figure 7.34 Lateral view taken on date of admission (17 September 1981)

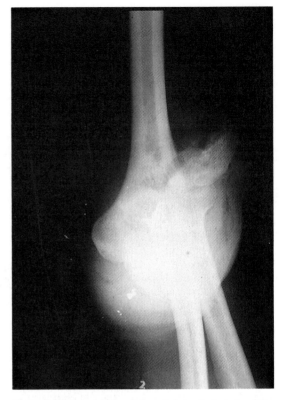

Figure 7.35 Anterior view taken on date of admission (17 September 1981)

slightly scoured. Four pieces of lead and fragment of loose bone and cartilage were found in the area. The lateral epicondylar fracture was reduced 'with a good match of articular surface' and held with K-wire fixation. The fracture olecranon was reduced with 'anatomical apposition of the fragments' and held with tension wire fixation. Figures 7.36 and 7.37 show the X-ray views taken after surgery.

His elbow was then encased in a plaster-of-Paris cast which maintained satisfactory reduction as shown in Figures 7.38 and 7.39.

He made a good recovery and was discharged 10 days later (29 September 1981). An orthopaedic follow-up of his elbow was arranged on 5 November 1981. After removal of the plaster-of-Paris cast, at this follow-up, the patient received treatment for his elbow to improve his range of movement.

At a subsequent orthopaedic follow-up on 10 December 1981, about 4 months after injury, his range of movement was considered to be 'functional' with a fixed flexion deformity of 65° and his active flexion limit was almost full range, at 135°. His range was reported to be improving with physiotherapy.

The follow-up X-ray report (radiographs taken on 10 December 1981) noted that the olecranon fracture showed signs of union, whilst there was some 'rounding off' of the lateral epicondyle fragment, with associated widening of this fracture site. Figures 7.40 and 7.41 show the X-ray views taken at this orthopaedic follow-up.

The senior orthopaedic registrar reported that the epicondylar fracture was progressing to non-union and, upon further discussion with the orthopaedic surgeon in charge of the patient it was decided that in 1 month's time (on 15 January 1982) the K-wires would be removed and replaced with a compression screw. The surgeons were particularly concerned because the fracture was caused by a bullet, which causes heat damage to the bone cells and capillaries

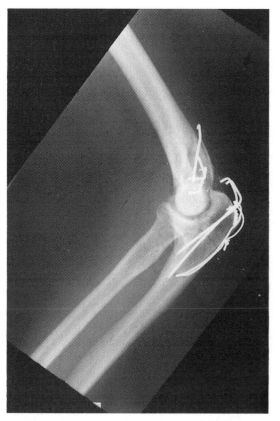

Figure 7.36 Lateral view taken after surgery on 18 September 1981

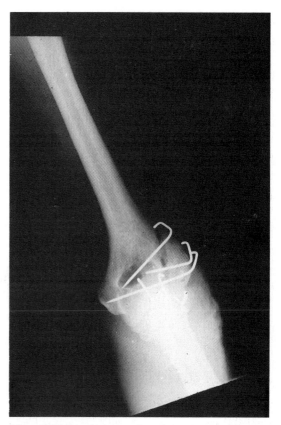

Figure 7.37 Anterior view taken after surgery on 18 September 1981

within the Haversian system, diminishing the usual fracture haematoma and thus the chance of union. Avascular necrosis of the lateral epicondylar fragment was therefore a likely complication.

Meanwhile the orthopaedic surgeon gave his consent to a trial of passive mobilization of the lateral epicondyle while the K-wires were *in situ*, with a view to stimulating union. Passive mobilization commenced on the 16 December 1981. This was 3 months after the incident, when the signs of non-union were present on X-ray.

The patient was treated daily for approximately 1 month. Treatment consisted of supporting his arm in a comfortable degree of flexion (about 65°) with the patient supine; gripping his lateral epicondyle between the thumb and index finger; then mobilizing the epicondyle. The technique used can be described as a combined anteropostero–anterior movement (Figure 7.42), accompanied by compression of the lateral epicondyle into the humerus (Figure 7.43).

The compression was a medially directed grade

IV+++ sustained pressure, while the anteroposterior–anterior pressure was a grade IV glide. This very small amplitude gliding was obviously modified by the presence of the three K-wires, which probably caused the gliding pressure to include a tipping action. The compression component, which was the main component of pressure, was not affected by the presence of the K-wires since it was directed almost parallel to their orientation. There was not a lot of movement present and the 'end-feel' could only be described as tight and slightly 'gritty'. The degree of treatment was influenced by the intention to provoke a small degree of 'fracture site pain' intermittently. This was deemed essential since it confirmed that the technique chosen was effectively creating movement at the fracture site.

On 14 January 1982, about 1 month after passive mobilization was instituted, the patient was readmitted to the Royal Adelaide Hospital and X-rays were taken. These showed signs of union over a small area of the fracture site (Figure 7.44).

The surgeons felt that removal of the K-wires and

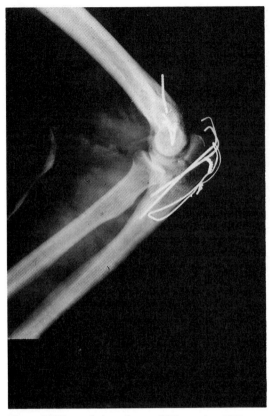

Figure 7.38 Lateral view taken on 25 September 1981

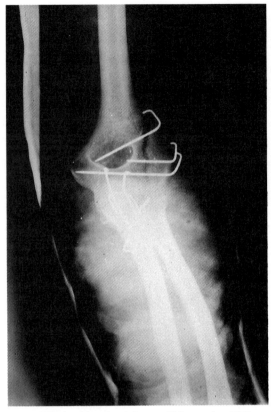

Figure 7.39 Anterior view taken on 25 September 1981

screw fixation was still indicated, but that treatment might be modified dependent upon findings at surgery the next day.

His range of elbow movement was assessed, in theatre, as 10–140° flexion, showing increased range, and upon removal of the K-wires the surgeon *was unable to manually move the lateral epicondyle.* The summary of the surgery stated that there was union throughout and therefore all internal fixation was removed.

Discussion

As mentioned previously, this application of passive mobilization in a controlled way to a fracture site, instead of a joint, challenges the historical and classical management of fractures as advocated by

Hugh Owen Thomas (1834–1891)[24]. He along with his pupil, Robert Jones, laid down the ideals of orthopaedic fracture management as rest, support and immobilization. These ideals influenced orthopaedic practice for the first half of this century.

The concept of compressing fractures by early weight bearing, for internally fixed lower limb fractures, was first advocated by Delbet in 1906[25] but was not universally accepted until 1929 when Bohler[26] in Vienna adopted this practice.

However in recent years, particularly in the last decade, many authors have researched the healing of bone in the presence of compression and electrical currents. Interestingly, authors such as Peacock and Van Winkle[27] ascribe a possible piezoelectric property to the crystalline nature of bone, enabling it to act as a stress transducer. Bone

24. Thomas, H. O. Cited by Osmond-Clarke, H. Half a century of orthopaedic progress in Great Britain. *Journal of Bone and Joint Surgery,* **32B**, 622–623 (1950)
25. Delbet, L. C. Cited by Platt, H. Orthopaedics in Continental Europe 1900–1950. *Journal of Bone and Joint Surgery,* **32B**, 574–584 (1950)
26. Bohler, L. Cited by Platt, H. Orthopaedics in Continental Europe 1900–1950. *Journal of Bone and Joint Surgery,* **32B**, 574–584 (1950)
27. Peacock, E. E. and Van Winkle, W. *Wound Repair,* 2nd edn., W. B. Saunders, Philadelphia (1976)

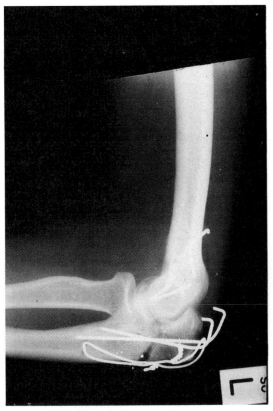

Figure 7.40 Lateral view taken on 10 December 1981

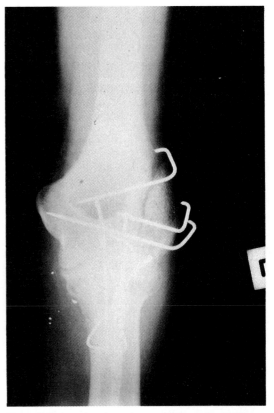

Figure 7.41 Anterior view taken on 10 December 1981

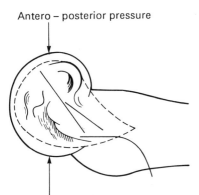

Figure 7.42 Lateral view – lower humerus with K-wires *in situ*

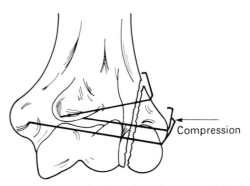

Figure 7.43 Anterior view – lower humerus with K-wires fixation of lateral epicondyle

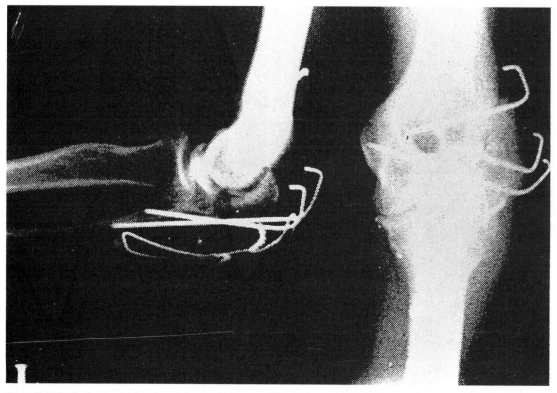

Figure 7.44 Lateral and anterior views taken on 14 January 1982. This was 1 month after passive mobilization and the anterior view appears to show union at the epicondylar fracture site

healing is thought to be enhanced in the presence of small electrical currents which are produced when the crystalline components of bone are distorted by mechanical compression. Many authors have subsequently also studied the effect of electrical currents on bone union[28, 29]. Of particular interest, an article by Panjabi *et al.*[30] outlined a biomechanical study of the effects of constant and cyclic compression on fracture healing in rabbit long bones. Their findings showed that constant compression, as in internal fixation, produced a stronger bone during the early phase of healing. They also found that there was a 27% reduction in the healing time of bone stimulated by cyclic compression.

Conclusion

While the result of union in this case study indicates that passive mobilization of the fracture site, at best, either stimulated or aided union, and at worst, did

not prevent spontaneous union, it is important to emphasize that care was taken to make compression the major component of pressure and that the amplitude of anteroposterior–anterior gliding was minimal. It is also worth emphasizing that passive mobilization was not instituted until 3 months after fracture when signs of non-union were present on X-ray.

Thus the type of technique and the timing of treatment must be considered in any future study of the role of passive mobilization in the management of fractures.

Fractures

The above leads one to treating fracture sites from the beginning. It is the practice in China for fractures to be supported in bucket splints which are removed by the patient on a daily basis when he

28. Hassler, C. R., Rybicki, E. F., Diegle, R. B. and Clark, L. C. Studies of enhanced bone healing via electrical stimuli. *Clinical Orthopaedic and Related Research,* **124**, 9–11 (1977)
29. Yasuda, I. The classic–fundamental aspects of fracture treatment. *Clinical Orthopaedic and Related Research,* **124**, 5–9 (1977)
30. Panjabi, M. M., White, A. A. and Wolf, W. W. Jr. A biochemical comparison of the effects of constant and cyclic compression on fracture healing in rabbit long bones. *Acta Orthopaedica Scandinavica,* **50**, 653–661 (1979)

moves his limb a small number of times. The splint is then replaced for the remainder of the day. With multiple unstable fractures in one limb, such a procedure may not be contemplated. However, it is common practice to have a patient with a fractured femur walking in a plaster or Thomas splint. Therefore, to have the patient in a non-weight bearing (or partial weight bearing) caliper or a bivalve plaster should be acceptable. If then a skilled physiotherapist removes or partially removes the splint and uses passive movement in the manner described above, which is successful with non-uniting fractures, it should shorten the time needed for splinting. Equally importantly, a better range of movement and function of the joints affected by the fracturing incident is achieved if the joints encased in the support would also be moved. Professor Salter's articles[31,32] are a *'must'* in relation to the 'Resters' and 'Movers'. Jull[33] has very clearly described the application of mobilization of joints following fractures.

Treatment of ununited fractures since the example described above have been equally successful and the majority had been unsuccessfully treated by electrical stimulation beforehand.

It is considered in Adelaide by some orthopaedic surgeons that the use of passive movement techniques, such as those described above (McNair and Maitland)[34], would hasten the union of intervertebral fusions, if applied immediately after the surgical procedure.

Phase 5
Hypermobility

Hypermobility is very helpfully discussed by Beighton *et al.*[35]. Hypermobility (general and local), instability, and stable-instability[36] were explained in Chapter 6, as were pain inhibition and apprehension. 'Sprains', including ligamentous tearing and rupture can also be considered under this heading of hypermobility. In terms of treatment, the following should be considered:

1. When a patient who is generally hypermobile has symptoms arising from one of the hypermobile joints, it is treated in exactly the same manner as that described for a hypomobile joint in phase 1 of this chapter.

2. A joint that becomes hypermobile through training, as for a ballet-dancer, may not reach a stage with the training to be sufficiently hypermobile for the expertise required. If the person has great potential in the chosen field, the physiotherapist can help gain the extra range required by techniques described for group 2 patients (phase 1 description). The techniques would be supplemented by training sessions, but a longer period of warm-up is required and also a longer period of time on the one functional movement being treated. Obviously active control of this increased hypermobility is essential and incorporated into the patient's treatment and training sessions.

3. Stable-instability and pain inhibition usually occur together and is common in the knee. When present in the knee, there is an extension-lag, and over-pressure of extension combined with tibial anteroposterior pressure is painful. The treatment consists of:
   (a) Knee extension with anteroposterior movement into a tolerable degree of hurt as a grade IV− progressing to grade IV+ (and later IV++) interspersed with grade III− movements.
   (b) Accessory movements, and especially tibial shaft rotation, are used at the comfortable limit of knee extension, as grade III− movements.

4. Apprehension movement is treated by performing that movement slowly, nudging at the point of the 'apprehension', endeavouring to coerce the range to increase painlessly; that is, without apprehension being provoked. Very slow grade IV− movements are used which are sustained at the position of the point of the apprehension, and then fractionally released. This is the passive movement aspect of the management. To this has to be added re-education of the muscular control of the movement.

5. Sprains can be considered at two levels – those that cause partial ligament tears (e.g. sprained ankle), and those that rupture a ligament (e.g. rupture of medial ligament of the knee):

31. Salter, R. B. Presidental address. *Journal of Bone and Joint Surgery,* **64B**, 251–254 (1982)
32. Salter, R. B. Motion versus rest: why immobilize joints? *Proceedings of the Manipulative Therapists Association of Australia, Brisbane,* 1–11 (1985)
33. Jull, G. The role of passive mobilization in the immediate management of the fractured neck of humerus. *Australian Journal of Physiotherapy,* **25**, 107–114 (1979)
34. McNair, J. and Maitland, G. D. The role of passive mobilization in the treatment of a non-uniting fracture site – a case study. *International Conference on Manipulation Therapy* (1983)
35. Beighton, P., Grahame, R. and Bird, H. *Hypermobility of Joints,* Springer-Verlag, Berlin (1983)
36. Williams, J. G. P. and Sperryn, P. M. (eds.) *Sports Medicine,* London, Edward Arnold, pp. 441 and 586 (1976)

(a) For the sprained ankle variety, as well as 'ice, compression elevation', passive movement should be utilized. The movements should be slow, smooth, grade III−. All directions including all joints from the inferior tibio-fibular joint to the inter-phalangeal joints should be performed but the main emphasis should be placed on the 'injuring movement'. It should be the first movement used in the routine and should be repeatedly performed, being interspersed by the other movements referred to. The 'injuring movement' should be extremely slowly taken to the point where the 'hurt' begins and then held there for some seconds before releasing – this is repeated at least four times hoping to be able to move gradually a little further into the range. If the available range increases well into the procedure, during the holding phase of the technique, a tiny movement may be attempted to gain more movement. This extra added movement should not be held if the hurt increases markedly into a very painful range.

The session of 'injury movement' interspersed with general movements would take as long as 20 minutes. It should be repeated as a slow active home exercise movement in the elevated position at intervals of 1–2 hours. Here it is important that the patient be taught how to monitor the effect of the movement so that an exacerbation is avoided.

(b) The treatment for a complete rupture of the medial ligament of the knee (referred to above), uses much the same as in (a). The aim is to make the unstable abduction of the knee a large range and totally painless. (Other directions of movement would also form part of the treatment.) Once the unstable direction of the knee is painless (and all other movements are painless) re-education can be promoted as rapidly as possible.

Phase 6
Locked joint loose bodies

Although the term 'locked joint' is not ideal, it does serve to differentiate such a disorder from other types of movement restriction. A particular movement(s) of a joint, when it is locked, is blocked from being able to be moved into a range by an obstacle 'in' the joint. The movement cannot be improved by stretching, as would be so if it were stiff. Something is obstructing the movement. To improve or restore the movement, the blocking object has to be moved out of its position. Of course, if it can be moved out of its blocking position it can also move back again, thus to mobilize and successfully free the movement passively is not necessarily going to be a lasting success.

Loose bodies and menisci can be structures that can block movement of a joint and to move them requires specific techniques.

The joint must be distracted or opened to allow movement of the offending mechanical focus within the increased joint space. While the joint is opened on the painful side it should be moved back and forth in directions that will move the bones to which the loose piece is attached. By continuing the movement or varying the movements as dictated by progress, or lack of progress, the obstruction may be moved into a painless position, allowing the joint movement to become free.

Cyriax[37] and Corrigan and Maitland[38] discuss and describe techniques.

37. Cyriax, J. H. and Cyrax, P. J. *Illustrated Manual of Orthopaedic Medicine*, Butterworths, London, pp. 51–98 (1983)
38. Corrigan, B. and Maitland, G. D. *Practical Orthopaedic Medicine*, Butterworths, London, pp. 78–149 (1983)

8

Assessment

The contact between the patient and the therapist should be a pleasant one for the patient. Particularly at the first consultation. Every effort should be made by the therapist to make it so. At all times the questioning of the patient by the therapist should always be in pleasant tones and cheering nuances. It is questioning at the depth of a sympathetic interrogation, an inquisition. It even has touches of the Sherlock Holmes's, noting things that are not as they should be, and so making deductions to ask appropriate questions, to make the features fit, and to make sense out of it all. It really does resemble a detective-like interrogation: the bright lights and intimidation are replaced by pleasantness, giving the patient a feeling of being listened to and believed which leads to a confidence in the therapist.

The word 'assessment' has various meanings, as does its synonym 'evaluation', yet it is the single most critical part of manipulative physiotherapy. The two words include the meanings, examination, comparison and analysis of the abnormalities.

Assessment is subdivided in the following ways:

1. During the first consultation the therapist collates all of the information possible to understand the stage and the stability of a patient's disorder and also to arrive at some kind of diagnosis.
2. It can mean, relating or dissociating a patient's history to the physical findings.
3. It can relate to assessing the patient's personality, his pain threshold and acceptance of pain.
4. At the end of the first consultation, the anticipated prognosis of treatment is assessed as clearly as is possible.
5. At the beginning of each treatment session, the assessment of the previous session should be defined by:
   (a) C/O: asking the patient what he feels has changed.

(b) Objective examination: comparing the asterisked movements.
6. During a treatment session, the effectiveness of each technique is assessed before, **during** and after its application.
7. The behaviour of the symptoms is assessed from one treatment session to the next.
8. Periodically (over a period of four or more treatments) the effect of treatment as a whole is assessed to gain an overall impression of its value.
9. After ten or more treatment sessions (as compared with number (8) above) the effect of treatment is assessed in comparison with:
   (a) The start of the treatment.
   (b) The good treatments and the bad techniques.
   (c) What his body and its disorder tells him about what it needs.
   (d) Assessing comparison of treatment achieved with what was predicted at the first consultation.
10. Analysis of the information derived from number (9) above.
11. As treatment progresses, the changes resulting from each individual technique used, is assessed retrospectively.
12. The long-term effect of treatment is assessed with particular emphasis on the need for prophylactic treatment to lessen likely recurrences.

Summary – the above 12 points can be grouped as follows:

1. At first consultation (numbers 1–7).
2. During treatment from session to session (numbers 5–8).
3. Retrospective assessment and analysis (numbers 9–12).

The area of assessment which is, in general, most *inadequately* covered is COMMUNICATION, especially the in-depth questions that need to be asked.

One of the primary problems with assessing the patient's symptoms is that the therapist has to know what it is she wants to know. The therapist needs to get herself into the patient's skin so that she can know (and therefore feel for him) everything about his symptoms 24 hours of the day. She must know all the subtle nuances of his symptoms from moment to moment, day to day, year in year out. The percentage of therapists who understand what they want to know is small – the best way to learn just what the fussy and subtle things are, and to know what their interrelationships are, is to watch, 'mark, learn and inwardly digest' what the skilled therapist chases up, and try to understand the reasons.

The following is a true example of how the effective questions need to be asked if wrong assessments are to be avoided.

An example of how to avoid making inaccurate assumptions

A young woman has been referred for assessment and treatment of headaches which had resulted from a vehicular accident. Previous treatments had failed and physiotherapy caused 'incredible' pain. The headaches were constant but varied if she used her arms overhead or lifted. Her neck would be stiff on waking in the morning, and at the same time she always had painful eyes. She related the painful eyes to her headaches even though they behaved differently.

Examination and treatment were kept restricted because previous physiotherapy had increased her pain. Palpation revealed tenderness at 0/1 (occipito-atlantal) on the right side, and movements of C2 were both stiff and painful. Cervical extension and rotation right were restricted causing pain in the right upper cervical area.

Assessment: the significant part of relating this story is that at the start of her fourth treatment, she responded to the question:

Q   'How has it been?'
A   'Great, fabulous, I can't believe it.'
ET   Assume nothing – it may have been that her mother-in-law had gone home at last.
Q   'What do you think has produced the improvement?'
A   'The treatment of course because I felt so different immediately after the treatment last time.'
ET   One could assume that all was well and that perhaps treatment could be discontinued.

SO ASSUME NOTHING

Q   'Does that mean you feel cured; 100%; not needing any more treatment?'
A   'I don't know.'
ET   She's either not 'cured' and has some symptoms or signs remaining, she doesn't know what 'cured' means to me, or doesn't know if it will stay cured.
Q   'Your answer makes me feel that you've still got some problems there. What is it that made you make the qualified answer "I don't know"?'
A   And then she commented (among other things) that her neck stiffness had improved but was still present but that it cleared more quickly. Her basis for 'great' was that her previous constant headache had gone.
ET   The most painful movements are greatly improved, but when firm over-pressure was applied, the pain response was very sharp. So, from having at first thought that she might be 90% better, the further probing revealed that further treatment was required to clear the other symptoms and the related signs.

It is this kind of inquisition that is so important – thus avoiding being misled, and making false judgements. *Knowing what you want to know* is the core, or basis, for being able to assess whether more treatment is needed. In fact it is this in-depth assessment of what the patient knows about his symptoms that is the KEY TO ASSESSMENT (C/O is usually more important than objective examination).

Thorough assessments should continue at every treatment session. It is neither tedious nor time consuming, as some people would have one believe. Without assessment, treatment becomes a 'hit and miss' process and is totally against all the rules of proper manipulative treatment.

Communication

Establishing good rapport with a patient is essential, and it is not always easy to achieve. Some people are unable to describe their symptoms, some are stoics, others **complain** excessively. It is often difficult for the therapist to know, on the one hand, what is relative and what can be discarded, and on the other, what *isn't* he telling you that you do need to know. The garrulous patient is usually easier to interpret because when the patient sets forth on a long story of how he stepped off a number 14 bus at the corner of Frome Street and Rundle Street and slipped on a banana skin etc., *ad nauseam* the therapist must gain control.

Example

Q 'How did this happen?'
A 'Well, I was going into town, my wife was out taking the children to school and I was going to work on a number 14 bus.'
ET Here we go, at this rate it's going to take me ages and I'll learn nothing; I'll have to:

1. Gently touch him to distract his line of thinking and ask another question.
2. Ask him another question gradually speaking louder to drown his speaking politely.
3. Distract him by saying 'when was this?' and then take it from that point. The one thing that must not be allowed to happen is for the therapist to lose control.

Q 'Did you actually fall when you slipped?'
Q Touch him and ask, 'How long ago was this?'
Q 'Have you ever had trouble with your shoulder before?'
ET I must keep pouncing on him quickly all the time so as to keep the conversation relevant. In fact, if the therapist knows what she wants to know and has good communication skills, the garrulous patient is much easier to handle than the non-complainer. The patient who is non-communicative and has a high pain threshold and pain acceptance is very difficult. With these people the therapist has to work under very adverse conditions. When it is recognized, the therapist should explain what is required early.

Example

Q 'Would I be right in saying that you don't really like talking about your complaints?'
A 'Well, yes, I suppose that's so.'
ET At least I have got him to say something useful, but I *must* get him 'on-side' by explaining what I need. There are three things I must explain to him:

1. 'I realize it is difficult for you, but can you see, that what you don't tell me, I don't know?'
2. 'Can you see that telling me about your symptoms is not complaining – it is *informing* and I need to have this information.'
3. 'Can you see that you may leave out something important, and so make me make a wrong judgement?'

Q 'You may or may not realize this, but your body can tell you things about your symptoms that I cannot find out unless you tell me – does that sound reasonable?'
Q 'There are three of us in the treating of your disorder – they are (1) the cause of your symptoms; (2) you (as the person who has the symptoms); and (3) me, and I'm trying to help reduce the disability. So, can *you* see the part *you* have to *play*?'

Statement: 'You can't tell me too much, but you can tell me too little. Too little can lead to failure of treatment – THEN THE FAULT IS YOURS, *NOT MINE.*' This statement is not strictly true, but it puts a lot of responsibility on the patient and helps him to be cooperative.

Recording assessments

Assessment requires an in-depth written record of the findings at each session. The value of this is that committing thoughts to paper forces the therapist to think more precisely and accurately. It is not necessary to follow the guidelines and abbreviations set out later in this book (see page 127) but some method must be determined to suit the patient's comments and the therapist's pattern of thinking (see Chapter 9).

With each patient there are many questions and answers that need to be entered in the recording even if it is only to show that the question, which was important, and had to be asked, has in fact been answered.

During the subjective examination the patient may state certain facts related to his disability which may prove to be valuable assessments.

Example

The patient has a right shoulder disorder.

A 'I am able to lie on my left side but I can't stay lying on my right side for long.'
ET This statement calls for an 'immediate response question'. There are two paths to follow – how *long* and *why?* can he not lie on his right side?
Q 'Why can't you lie on your right side?'
A 1. 'I don't know – it may be because I have always slept on the left side and that it has become a habit.'
 2. 'The right hip aches if I lie on it for long.'
 3. 'The pain in my right shoulder increases and I have to get off it.'

These three answers indicate the important fact:

ASSUME NOTHING

ET If the 'number 3' is given, then it is necessary to know how long he *can* lie on his right shoulder before he has to change position, and to know the time the pain takes to subside to the previous level.

Q 'How long can you lie on your right shoulder?'

A 'Well, it hurts straight away, but I suppose I can make myself stay there for 10 minutes or so.'

ET To 'parallel' his line of thought, the next question would be:

Q 'How long does it take for that induced right shoulder pain to subside to its previous level?'

ET The answer to this question will provide an idea of the nature of the disorder.

A 'Oh, only a few minutes, unless I have been on the right shoulder a much longer time.'

Q 'How long would it take to settle then?'

A 'No more than about 10 minutes.'

ET This is not a 'movement' (see irritability 'planning sheet') but it does give some guide to the care needed during treatment ('Nature' of the presentation - planning sheet).

Asterisks

Asterisks (*) are not mandatory for treatment by passive movement to be quickly successful. Their only purpose is to highlight the important aspects that can be used to guide the assessment of the effectiveness of the treatment – it speeds up the whole process.

It is better to asterisk the facts at the time of recording rather than leaving it to the end of the consultation and then putting in the asterisks. The spontaneity is lost, and some facts may be forgotten.

If they are used at the time of recording the aspect, important pointers are not left out, and the asterisks can be made large or small, or drawn in a different colour, so as to indicate the degree of importance of the facts and their relationships to each other.

Using asterisks is just as valuable for the objective examination as it is for the subjective examination. Similarly it is better to make the use of the asterisks progressively *during* the objective examinations rather than *after*. The same applies to both the first consultation and at each treatment session.

Asterisks are neither mandatory nor compulsory jargon. They are time savers, reminders and indicators of highly important facts for the particular person.

Statements and comparisons

At each treatment session, it is mandatory to determine the effects of the previous session. Most patients will make statements about different things that have happened; rarely do they make *compari-*

sons. A 'statement of fact' is rarely of value to the therapist, therefore she has to ask questions that convert these statements into comparisons.

Statement: 'It wakened me three times last night' (this is a fact, not a comparison).

Q 'How many times would it have wakened you before?'

ET I have deliberately left out the qualifying *'before when'* so as to allow for spontaneous comments.

A 'Probably only once on some nights.'

Q 'How many nights?'

A 'About three times a week.'

Q 'And how long ago was that?'

A or three years ago.'

Q 'So how often was it waking you prior to our starting treatment?'

A 'About two or three times.'

Q 'Every night?'

A 'Yes.'

Q 'So the three times last night was approximately the same?'

A 'No, not really, the treatment has lessened the amount of pain I have compared with what I had when I was wakened by it before.'

With some patients it can take a long time to gain accurate useful information, but once started on the question it should be followed through to the needed answer. It is very easy to be side-tracked, and then the information that was in the examiner's mind can be lost.

Initial assessments

The goal of assessment is to know the effect, both subjective and objective, which every technique has on the patient's disorder. At the first consultation it is only possible to relate the irritability to activities that exacerbate the patient's symptoms (see page 23), whereas what is really needed is the reaction to *treatment* techniques.

1. This cannot be achieved (as a general rule) during the first consultation because it includes both examination movements and treatment movements.

2. The therapist therefore has to weigh-up the information and physical examination findings to make a qualified assessment of the treatments effect. During the second session a partial assessment can be made of techniques.

3. At the outset of the third treatment the therapist is in a position to be able to assess the effectiveness of treatment because there will not have been the first consultation examination to take into account.

Subjective assessments

As was stated earlier, 'subjective assessment' is the weak link in the work of most practitioners.

LISTEN
UNDERSTAND
BELIEVE/PROVE/CONFIRM
BE CONSTRUCTIVE
MAKE IT A CHALLENGE
THE PATIENT'S STORY IS TRUE UNTIL PROVEN GUILTY

The following statements underline the main points affecting assessment. The dialogue is an attempt to highlight the kinds of errors that easily creep in if they are not watched for.

What follows is an example of a 'retrospective assessment' comparing at the twelfth treatment spread over 16 days. (As an abbreviation the following can be used R 12, D16.)

Q 'How do you feel now, before we start this treatment session, compared with immediately before the first treatment?'
ET This is seeking spontaneous unbiased answers. (In this example it is assumed he has improved.)
A 'Oh, definitely better.'
ET Four channels are opened:

1. In what way are you better?
2. How much better are you?
3. What do you feel has made you better?
4. What do you still have remaining which still needs to be made better?

Speed of answer

As his response was made crisply and quickly, the improvement is probably substantial so I try to jump a stage or two: I might even get some answers to other questions yet to be asked without having to ask them.

Q 'So, what symptoms do you still have before being 100%?';
A 'Well, I can now throw the javelin at three-quarter pace painlessly, provided I keep my throwing elbow lower than shoulder level.'
Q 'And you couldn't have done that before we started treatment?'
A 'No, no hope. I couldn't even hold a cup of tea.'
Q 'Is that your only remaining symptom? If you could throw above shoulder level would you be cured?'
ET The word 'cured' puts them 'on the spot' so to speak, and makes them think more deeply. It

is surprising how much a patient can have left in terms of symptoms and not mention them because the main symptom is so much better.
A 'As far as I'm concerned yes, but I do still get the occasional twinge, but it is less frequent and less painful.'
Q 'Are there any specific things that will make it twinge?'
A 'No not really.'

Immediate response question

ET The 'not really' indicates that there *ARE* other factors. They are not bothering him because he is so pleased his javelin throwing has improved.
Q 'When you say 'not really' it sounds to me as if there might be something?'
A 'Well, I have noticed the shoulder two or three times when I've stretched over the front seat of the car to lift a small parcel off the back seat, but it's only a trivial thing, especially as the twinge goes immediately.'

One half of 1%

Q 'This is that "one half of 1%" that I mentioned earlier which is so important in my making judgements. So what other things are there?'
A 'I suppose I could say that at the end of a long training session my shoulder and upper arm feel heavy and achey, but it doesn't last long.'
Q 'How long is long?'
A 'It has always gone by the time I get up the next morning.'
Q 'So can you still have some heaviness or aching the next morning?'
A 'Yes, but it's nothing really.' Statement: 'It might be 'nothing' to you but it is a very definite 'something' to me.'
ET He is much better than at the first consultation, but his shoulder has not improved enough if recurrences are to be avoided. This information now becomes a heavy asterisk for me. And he has answered some of the questions I would have needed to ask.
ET It's like getting blood out of a stone – he is a reliable witness but his pain acceptance is so high that the therapist has to work hard to get the information.
Q 'Before this incident 6 months ago were you still training?'
A 'Yes.'
Q 'And did you have any hint of shoulder symptoms?'
A 'No.'

Q   'Are you quite sure of that? – I know some people would consider I was turning you into a hypochondriac – also you're tending to hold back with your answers, but remember my stating that I am interested in "one half of 1%"? And, what you don't tell me, I don't know.'

A   'Well. Yes; if you consider that, when I was about 7 I had a heavy fall onto my shoulder – but that cleared up pretty quickly.'

Q   'What do you call quickly?'

. . . and so it continues.

Assessment guidelines to be explained to the patient

As some patient's feel that they are unable to criticize the therapist or to speak about things that might seem silly, unrelated or trivial, they should be put at ease by explaining the situations that can occur, such as the difference between complaining and informing.

Informing – complaining

1. 'Even if you feel you are complaining, don't feel that, you are not *complaining* you are *'informing'*.
   'And what you don't tell me, I don't know and thus can make wrong judgements.'
2. 'Your body can tell you things which I can't know unless you tell me.' 'I can't hear too much – I *CAN* hear too little.' 'I can stop your comments gently, if you are telling me far too much, but I can't know what you don't tell me.'
3. 'The patient who talks on and on "like a babbling brook" is easier to assess than the one who is reticent to talk or complain.'
4. 'There is a big difference between *"not much"* and *"nothing at all"* when you describe what you feel while we test your movements. Ninety five per cent is not 100%.' Many patients need to be reminded of this many times.

One half of 1%

Patients often find it difficult to know what is relevant. Applying this difficulty to the first examination, it is helpful to say at an appropriate stage (and it must certainly be repeated at the end of the first consultation), 'I am interested in anything and everything, even to the extent of one half of 1%. Your body can tell you things I can only find out if you tell me. Also, nothing is too trivial to tell me – let me make the judgement as to its relevance, don't you make it.'

At the commencement of each treatment session this statement may need to be reiterated especially if the patient finds it difficult to talk about his problems.

Interrogation
Key words/phrases

Q   'What do you call quickly?'
A   'It was a long time ago.'
ET 1. 'Quickly' or 'pretty quickly' are statements of fact, not comparisons;
    2. The word quickly is also a KEY WORD in communication.
    3. To get a useful answer, give him two opposite choices.
Q   'Was it one day or a month?'

Depth of interrogation

This dialogue is a continuation of the patient above who fell on his shoulder when he was 7 years old.

ET This may seem petty questioning but it may turn up factors that will influence an analytical assessment (prognosis of treatment and his future in competitive sport).
A   'It would only be a guess at this stage but I would say about a month or two.'
Q   'And you had nothing – nothing at all – between then and now?'
A   'No.'
ET He's making assessing very difficult.
Q   'Remembering my half of 1%, do you still say you have had nothing in between?'
A   'Well I suppose my shoulder would ache during the baseball season but only minor, nothing to think about.'
Q   'And was the ache in the same area as now, or associated with it?'
A   'Well I suppose it was, but I've always played a lot of sport and I considered it was just a normal thing.'
Statement: 'WELL NOW YOU KNOW IT WASN'T.'
Q   'Gee, you're being a bit fussy aren't you?'
A   'Yes, but if you want to know how much better I can make your shoulder, or whether it will recur, I *have* to be fussy; I do need your help.'

In relation to the objective examination (OE) at the first consultation, the first thing to find is an action he can perform to reproduce his symptoms. His suggestion is throwing something.

OE 'Would you take this pillow in your hand and go over to the wall (7 m away) and throw this pillow GENTLY to me.'

Q 'Did you feel anything – ANYTHING (don't forget the half of 1%) with that throw?'
A 'No – nothing.'
Q 'Now repeat the throw but do it harder and see if you feel your shoulder?'
A (Throws) 'No.'

Confirm

Q 'No what?'
A 'No, I didn't feel anything.'
Q 'This time throw it and try to make it hurt a bit,' which he does.
A 'Yes I could feel it then, but it wasn't much.'
Q 'Has it gone now?'
A 'Yes.'
Q 'Now remember how *hard* you threw the pillow and its response – (throw it again if you need to) – because I'm going to do some treatment to your shoulder, after which I want you to throw with the same power and compare the 'before and after' response following the treatment.'

(Treatment – adequate mobilizing of the acromio-humeral area (as grades IV+, PAs, followed by a lot of grade III).)

Q 'Now throw it at the same power and compare it with before.'

He throws the pillow again from the same distance.

Q 'Any change?'
A 'I don't think I could feel it.'
Q 'Has the hurt gone?'

Does it again – again no pain, and he is throwing above shoulder level.

A 'Yes.'
ET The disorder is obviously not irritable so I will test him more vigorously.
Q 'So, throw it again – maximum effort and try to hurt your shoulder.'
A 'It feels quite different, I didn't feel I had to throw below the shoulder level.'

This is followed by testing the asterisked objective findings to analyse and try to predict:

1. How much more treatment is likely to be required?
2. How close will it be possible to make his javelin throwing normal?
3. Is he going to be able to get back to competitive javelin throwing?

One might ask 'Is all this questioning necessary?'

YES

It certainly is ***. If it had not been taken as far as this, this sportsman would probably not be able to participate in the high ranks of his chosen sport.

WHY?

HOW DO YOU KNOW?

WHY? Because treatment would have been discontinued following the answer to the first question. He would be considered to be almost cured and that the rest of it should get better on its own.
HOW DO YOU KNOW? Because the problem probably had its origin at age 7. It probably had been relatively painless, bu' the underlying damage is still present.

It is impossible to know whether the movements can be freed completely, except in retrospect, but it is possible to get a hint of expectation by the next fourth treatment.

Factors that can affect the assessment

There are many factors other than faulty treatment that can influence the patient's symptoms for better or for worse. Thus it becomes necessary to take account of these factors when judging the symptomatic effect of treatment:

1. It is good practice to tell the patient to avoid doing anything different from his normal routine. Explain that any added or subtracted new thing can make the assessing of changes due to treatment difficult or impossible. By 'thing' is meant:
   (a) Starting or stopping a new medication.
   (b) Going to exercise classes for the first time.
   (c) Being in a very stressful argument in an otherwise peaceful existence.
   (d) And so on.
2. Some patient's symptoms are affected by menstruation. Therefore it is necessary to establish the relationship between:
   (a) what the effect is; and
   (b) does the effect of menstruation occur before menstruation, during it, or after?
3. Changes in weather conditions often worsen a patient's symptoms (but not usually his examination signs).
4. Different ethnic groups react to symptoms in different ways. This being so, the therapist should take it into account when attempting to assess changes in the test movements. This factor applies to those people who over-play rather than understate the disorder. In making the assessment, the therapist should be understanding and accepting rather than being critical.
5. People are different and each person has developed his own 'frames-of-reference'; it is the responsibility of the therapist to judge the assessment with skill.

The assessment

At the beginning of this chapter twelve points were made about the application of assessment. There is assessment *at the first consultation* which is different from the normal *'treatment to treatment' assessments*. Those two examples are different in type to both the *retrospective assessment* and the *'analytical assessments'*.

Assessment at first consultation

The first consultation includes having the patient's story of:

1. How the problem began and progressed.
2. The present behaviour of the symptoms.
3. The effect the symptoms have on the patient.

When the subjective examination with its many parts is completed, assessment is then made of the individual parts of the physical examination.

Assessment here has two aspects:

1. The first is determining the quality, and the range, of movement of the various structures, and the interrelationships between resistance of any kind, and pain. This process provides information that can be used for comparisons during treatment thus guiding the therapist as to what treatment technique changes should be made during treatment.
2. The second aspect is much more important: it helps to discern the diagnosis, and the stage the disorder is in at the time of the first treatment session (analysis). The therapist needs accurate asterisks to determine, by comparing these asterisks before, during and after treatment, if any changes are occurring.

Assessing differences of:
The pain/range response.
The stiffness.
The muscle spasm.
The quality of movement.
A crucial part of this comparing includes what the therapist predicted should happen with the treatment technique used.

This procedure should be used with all physiotherapy treatment whether it is ultra-sound, interferential, exercises or anything else: **but it isn't,** (see example with ultra-sound treatment on page 127), and this is an indictment on the practitioner and the profession.

Subjective assessment

Pain is the most common symptom of the patients whom the physiotherapist is asked to treat. Therefore assessment *changes* in the pain pattern are the most important part. Although the neurophysiology of pain is very complex, in the situations being described here, changes in the pain are not complex (though they may be subtle). They do not require the latest opinions of the neurophysiology of pain. Neither is it essential to know precisely which structure(s) are causing the pain. Many readers will disagree with these views; they will consider that the structures should be identified and must precede treatment – if they cannot be identified, treatment by passive movement should not be applied. Although it would be agreed that to know the structures at fault could enhance the selection of treatment techniques, they should not contraindicate the treatment *per se*.

The more that can be learned about structures and diagnosis, the more constructive the physiotherapist can be, but it is more important to realize that it is the 'examination/treatment/assessment – effect' which guides all aspects; with research work and increased knowledge to follow. Rarely does it evolve in the reverse order. Earlier in this text the two-compartment method of thinking, planning and executing was expounded. One compartment was for the theory, the hypotheses and the speculative ideas; while the other compartment was for the clinical presentation of the patient's disorder (see 'two compartment thinking' aspect of the concept, page 2).

The theory can only be correct if it fits with the clinical presentation. If they do not relate or agree, it is the theory that is wrong, not the clinical. The clinical findings are never wrong; provided of course that the examination is accurately carried out.

There are uncountable numbers of different kinds of pain and it is essential to realize, to believe, and to accept, that this is so. Recognizing the subtle difference in the 'kinds of pain' is not as simple and straightforward as one might expect:

1. Are we agreed that a patient can have at least two kinds of pain? For example, one could be a constant ache and the other a sharp pain in certain positions or unguarded movements.
2. Are we agreed that a patient can have at least two areas of pain arising from very closely related parts of one structure? A common example is

seen with a glenohumeral disorder which is responsible for (a) a constant dull ache *at the insertion of* the deltoid to the humerus as well as (b) a sharp pain felt *in the glenohumeral joint* provoked by an unguarded movement.

Q The reader may say 'why do we need to know these things, and anyway, aren't they obvious?'

A **NO** they aren't obvious – if they were, therapists would be more successful with their treatment because their assessments would be precise and would provide more explicit guidelines for treatment.

If we knew more about the different symptoms, each disorder could have an accurate diagnostic title and its phase would be precisely understood, making the response to treatment predictable.

3. Latent pain is another consideration. When a patient has pain **after** either treatment or examination, as compared with having pain at the time of testing joint movements, this pain is 'latent pain'. The following details of the 'latent pain' need to be known if that latent pain is going to be used for assessment purposes. They are as follows:

(a) The relationship of the intensity of the pain caused by an activity related to the *vigour* of the activity, needs to be determined.

(b) The *timing* relationships between (i) the length of time between the activity causing the latent pain and the onset of the symptoms; (ii) the time taken for the latent pain to subside; and (iii) the factors that are used to make it subside (medication, rest, time).

(c) Pain can commence in a local area and then gradually spread from that point. Timing and behaviour should be determined in very fine detail, especially if the vertebral column is part of the disorder.

(d) Pain may occur in rhythm with particular movements and when so, three aspects are important: (i) Does the *site* of that pain change with continued movement? (ii) Does the intensity of the 'in-rhythm' symptoms decrease or remain unchanged? (iii) Does the 'in-rhythm' pain change to being an *ache* or does an ache become superimposed on top of the 'in-rhythm' pain.

4. The quality of pain can change following the use of a technique. Using, say shoulder flexion as an example of this assessment, a *favourable change* may be assessed even if the patent says 'it's just the same'. For example, the patient may be able to flex his shoulder more quickly, or move easily before reaching the same limit of range where the intensity of the pain has not changed. In other

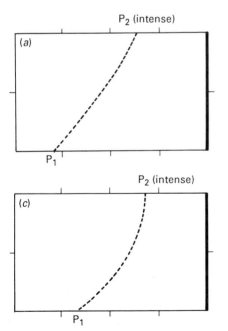
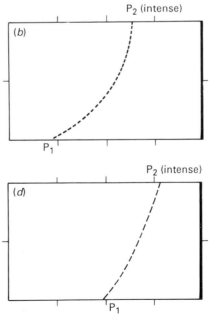

Figure 8.1 Examples of assessed pain changes favourable, yet the patient states that 'pain is the same' following a treatment technique. (*a*) The pre-treatment representation of the pain behaviour. (*b*) Pain is less intense through the same range. (*c*) Pain starts later in the range. The same intensity, P_2, is later in the range. (*d*) The behaviour of pain through the range is similar to (*a*): pain starts later in the range, the same 'P_2 intensity' is much later in the range

words, the range and intensity of pain are unchanged while the quality of the movement up to that point has improved (Figure 8.1). To the patient, 'the pain is the same' because it is equally intense at P2 in all examples shown. This highlights the care required in assessing P1 and also the P1P2 line if favourable changes are not to be missed, or if 'pain is the same' is not to be misinterpreted.

5. An arc of pain is a common finding when examining peripheral joints. The shoulder is a very common example, the pain being felt during mid-range abduction to the fully flexed position with the arm alongside the head. The same arc is usually felt on lowering the arm. Its significance is important[1].

6. 'After' pain is a phenomenon that is less common in peripheral joints than it is in the spine. It is a pain that is not felt until well after the time of its cause. This latent response is discussed fully in *Vertebral Manipulation*[2].

7. 'Release' pain, felt when a painful joint is released from a position of stretch, is common in all joints. This is also discussed in *Vertebral Manipulation*[3] where it has greater significance.

Physical examination assessment

The symptoms felt during test movements are assessed and thought is given to both the 'through-range' and 'end-of-range' responses for their implication of intra-articular and peri-articular disorders respectively (see Chapter 6).

The physical examination must also seek to differentiate out the sources of the patient's symptoms. The fact of having more than one component to the disorder has been discussed in Chapter 4, as have the differentiation tests.

The progression of the disorder at the current episode combined with an understanding of the total history of other related episodes, provides the material required to be able to make an assessment as to the 'stage of the disorder'. Also, the careful examination of the present history of the *changes* in movement or resting capabilities, will guide the assessment of the degree of 'stability of the disorder'. The *disorder* is unstable if the presentation of the site of symptoms varies considerably from day to day, or if the pain responses to a movement (or movements) varies widely from day to day. If the disorder were stable there would be very little change, from day to day, in the patient's symptoms, no matter what he were to do. This

'stability of the disorder' at the time of commencing treatment is a most important assessment.

MAKE FEATURES FIT

Ideally, the end result of this assessment is that the manipulating physiotherapist will have:

1. A diagnostic title.
2. An appreciation of the aetiology of the diagnosed disorder.
3. An understanding of its present stage and stability.
4. An idea of the most effective treatment and its prognosis.

These four pieces of information will be more easily analysed (analytical assessment at first consultation) if all elements fit into a recognizable pattern. They will be harder to assess if the whole story and findings are atypical.

'Treatment to treatment' assessments

This section refers to:

1. Assessment of the state of affairs at the beginning of a treatment session before actually carrying out any treatment. This includes an assessment of the effect of the previous treatment.
2. Assessment of what is happening during the performance of a treatment technique in comparison with what was expected to be happening (as listed in the 'plan' – see page 118).
3. Assessment of the effect of the treatment technique.

Assessing the effect of the previous treatment

This is made by asking questions and testing movements (both being helped by the use of asterisks).

The patient's interpretation of the effect of treatment at three specific times are very valuable. These times are:

1. Immediately following treatment.
2. During the evening of the day of treatment.
3. On first getting out of bed the morning following treatment.

However, it is quite wrong to ask the patient initially about his symptoms at these times. Questioning should be so planned that the physiotherapist can

1. Corrigan, B. and Maitland, G. D. *Practical Orthopaedic Medicine,* Butterworths, London, p. 34 (1983)
2. Maitland, G. D. *Vertebral Manipulation,* 5th edn., Butterworths, London, p. 152 (1986)
3. Maitland, G. D. *Vertebral Manipulation,* 5th edn., Butterworths, London, p. 151 (1986)

evoke spontaneous remarks which are then more informative. This can be achieved with the use of non-directive questions. For example, 'How has it been?' or 'How has it felt since I last saw you?', or one can be somewhat more direct and ask 'What effect do you think the last treatment has had?' If the patient feels he is 'better' or 'worse', further clarification is needed. In wishing to emphasize his present pain the patient may give the impression that he is worse, whereas on closer questioning it may be shown that he was better after his treatment until he performed some activity which aggravated his pain. In these circumstances the treatment helped his disorder rather than made it worse. This kind of information may be gained through the following questions:

1. 'In what way is the pain worse? (Is it more severe, sharper, changed to a throbbing pain, or has it increased in area, etc., etc.)?' Then ask:
2. 'When did it start to become worse?'
3. 'What do you think made it worse?' 'Was it related to treatment or did something else happen that may have aggravated it?'

It is important to make the patient feel comfortable about criticizing the treatment, such as in 'I felt terrible when I left here – that stretching you did was very painful and really stirred things up'. It isn't always easy for a patient to criticize the treatment, nor is it easy for practitioners to be on the receiving end, but is something to be encouraged by both sides: in fact it should be sought:

Q 'Do you feel that what I did last time was the cause of the increased pain?'
A 'Well, I don't like to say it, especially as you have been so thorough, but yes, I did feel stirred up after the treatment.'

We must train ourselves to be comfortable with a criticism and learn how to handle it (as well as how to handle ourselves). Nevertheless, our treatment should be so well assessed that we don't cause bad exacerbations. This is not always easy as patients often withhold information thinking that treatment is supposed to hurt if it is going to be effective.

The difference between 'treatment soreness' and 'disorder soreness' is an important assessment; it is one that the patient can often state if the question is asked – 'Was it just my hands or was it your problem that is more sore?' A treatment soreness will only be felt where the physiotherapist's hands have been in contact with the patient, usually over a tender area. However, if referred symptoms or deeply felt symptoms have been made sore, that soreness cannot be a 'treatment soreness' it must be a 'disorder soreness'. Again it is our responsibility to seek conscientiously the information regarding the possibility that WE have CAUSED increased soreness. This seeking becomes easier as one

becomes more experienced; the causing also becomes less common.

To reiterate a point, *ad nauseam*, which has been spelled out through every edition of both this book and *Vertebral Manipulation*, accurate assessment is absolutely essential. Yet still the message fails to make adequate impact.

1st priority: Spontaneous comparison.
2nd priority: Comparisons from nondirect questions.
3rd priority: More direct through vague questions.
4th priority: Reversed direct questions.

Then the:

5th priority: How did you feel when you left here last time compared with when you came in – before the treatment that day?
'How did you feel over the next few hours?'
'How did you feel that night compared with other nights? As a result of treatment I mean?'
'How did it feel during the night when you were in bed, compared with other nights?'
'What was it like the next morning compared with other mornings?'
'How was it during the early part of that next day?'

Does the message get across in 1990 after many years of saying it? It is so very important: it is vital for successful assessment to lead to the most informative and effective treatment.

Assessment of movement changes, though it too is important, is much easier to judge. As well as assessing the range/pain response comparisons in figures (movement diagrams) and words, the assessment also involves a comparison with:

1. What would be expected recalling what was the treatment and its degree of hurt (and therefore anticipated reaction).
2. The patient's comments regarding the effect of the last treatment.

From this combined assessment of the effect of the last treatment, the 'plan' is made for the current session.

Assessing what is happening during the performance of the treatment technique

This is essential because it must achieve what is planned to happen. It may be that the plan is to use the technique that reproduces the local symptoms but with a minimal intensity of reproduction. The technique must be juggled until it achieves that.

A technique is performed at a chosen grade and the patient is asked whether the technique is causing any alteration to the symptoms. This information is helpful from three points of view:

1. The patient may have referred pain while positioning for treatment. As the treatment technique is performed this pain may gradually lessen and disappear, it may remain at the same level throughout, or it may worsen. Assessment during the performance of the technique will guide whether to continue with the technique, to perform it more gently, or whether a change of technique is indicated. For example, if in the early stages of treatment of a patient who has shoulder pain, performing the technique initially causes an increase of pain, and this pain worsens as the technique is continued, then that technique should be discontinued. The physiotherapist should stand the patient and reassess the movement signs before going on to the next technique.
   On the other hand, if the condition is chronic in nature, it may be necessary to provoke some pain with treatment technique if treatment is to be successful. Hopefully, reassessing the provocation will have brought about a definite improvement in the pain-free range of movement.
2. The patient may have no pain while positioned prior to performing the technique. Then during performance he may feel pain. The physiotherapist may choose to continue with the same technique at the same grade and ask the patient three, four, five or six times during the performance whether the pain remains the same, improves or worsens. If pain increases she may then lessen the grade of the technique, or stop. However, she may do it more firmly if there is no change in the symptoms or if they improve.
3. There is one other response that can be determined during treatment. It is a difficult assessment to make but it is useful to know, when performing a technique, whether the pain is provoked only at the limit of oscillation. The easiest way to make this assessment is to ask the patient while performing the technique, *'Does-it-hurt-each-time-I-push?'* These words are said in rhythm with the strongest part of the treatment technique. The patient easily understands the question if it is put this way and has no hesitation in answering informatively.

In Chapter 9, the section on recording treatment (see page 126) states emphatically 'Record what the patient feels while the technique is being performed.'

Assessment of the effect of the treatment technique

This also requires a balancing of what is anticipated will be achieved by the technique (bearing treatment soreness in mind) against what the patient feels has happened.

To determine the effect of the technique, the patient sits up or stands and is encouraged to move about to loosen any feelings of stiffness or soreness before being asked, 'How does it feel now *compared with* how it felt when you were last sitting up just before I did that last bit of stretching?' It is important to make sure that the patient knows exactly what the comparison is to be made with; it is far from uncommon, even with the use of such a seemingly clear question as is quoted above, for the patient to make all manner of wildly different comparisons. Therefore it is often necessary to ask the question again but using different wording and by gesticulations to express and emphasize the precise comparison being sought. Perhaps it may be necessary for the therapist to confirm her interpretation by asking, 'So what you are saying is that what I have just been doing has made those symptoms ... is that correct?' (And still there will be people who can't be clear.)

When it is more important to assess any changes in *symptoms* rather than changes of physical test movements, the patient should be assisted by saying 'Take particular notice of what you can feel in your —— now, and also the aching you have down here [demonstrate by touching the areas and pause] . . . can you feel them? Well I want you to be clear about what you can feel because after I have done such and such I am going to ask you to see if what I do changes what you feel now.' Question: 'Can you understand what I'm needing from you? It is very important to me, and obviously to you too, but you're the only one who can make the judgements; I'm interested in even the most trivial changes, even to the extent of that one half of 1% difference I talked about with you before. OK?' 'Right, well just lie down on your left side again and I'll do the same thing again.'

If he is still muddled in his thinking, don't give up, rather correct his errors, explain again, and try again.

The patient's movements are retested and a comparison made with those present before the treatment technique was used. When reassessing the movement signs *the same sequence* of movements must be used each time. The reason for this is that one movement that provokes pain may alter the pain felt with the next movement tested. It is inconsistent to test movements one time in standing, another sitting in a chair, and a third time with the patient sitting on a treatment couch without foot support.

Hopefully the subjective and objective examination assessments will agree. If they do not agree, the reason for the discrepancy must be sought.

In principle, when a physiotherapist is in the learning stages of 'treatment by passive movement', the above assessments should be made following each use of every technique. As experience is gained she learns to expect a certain degree of improvement when particular techniques are applied to particular disorders. However, when a patient has movements that are almost painless but stiff she can assume that there will be little change during one treatment session though there may be considerable improvement over two treatment sessions. In these circumstances it would be unnecessary to assess after each technique but comparison of the symptoms and signs at the end of the second treatment session should be made with those at the beginning of the first treatment.

If the physiotherapist is able to judge that changes in symptoms and signs may be expected to take place quickly, she should assess these after each application of a technique and if the *rate* of change is not as much as hoped for, then a change in technique should be made. This procedure should be maintained throughout the treatment, changing from technique to technique to find the one, or ones, that produces the quickest and best improvement.

Retrospective assessment

There are three main times for making retrospective assessments, and although they each seek to determine changes taking place over periods of time, rather than from treatment to treatment, they have slight differences in their functions. The times are:

1. After each few treatments.
2. When progress has slowed.
3. After a planned break from treatment.

After each few treatments

Although careful assessments are made of the effect of each treatment session, it is wise after each few sessions to make an additional assessment determining what the patient feels the overall effect of the last few treatments has been. This gives him the opportunity to think, with hindsight, over a longer period of time and larger number of treatments. The process helps the physiotherapist to get things into a clearer perspective, and to know how helpful the treatment is, or is not, being.

When the physical findings of a patient's disorder are either inconclusive or extremely sensitive, the main assessment lies in the patient's ability to express how he feels his symptoms are changing. This may not be easy for him to do from treatment to treatment. However comparing over a period of say 2 weeks, a patient can more readily state whether he has improved or not, and what particular aspects have changed.

The retrospective assessment is another instance when the using of asterisks is shown to be valuable. For example, after the patient has given his impressions of changes, the therapist can say:

Q 'You said when I first saw you 2 weeks ago, that you were being wakened by this pain four or five times a night, – is this still the same?'

A 'No, that's a good point: I had forgotten about that. It only wakes me once or twice a night at the most now – so it must be getting better, mustn't it?'

To be asking this same question from treatment to treatment may not reveal the degree of change that *is* evident over a longer period.

In the second edition of this book I stated:

'At the beginning of treatment it is not uncommon for a patient to reply, day after day, that he is feeling much better. Then, when asked after say four treatments, "How do you feel now compared with before we started treatment?", he may say cautiously, and after a long period of thought, "I'm sure it's a little better – at least it certainly isn't any worse." Such retrospective assessment alerts the therapist so that she does not fall into the trap of believing she is making as much daily progress as she might have thought she was.'

As stated in the heading, these assessments should be made every few treatments. It should form part of the questioning at each fourth or fifth session:

Q 'You have just said that since I saw you last time you have only been wakened twice each night by this pain, how does that compare with 2 weeks ago?'

A 'I think I would have to say that at night it has been gradually getting less painful. I can't tell from treatment to treatment as clearly as I can in retrospect.'

In terms of MAKING FEATURES FIT, changes in the patient's symptoms should be matched by comparable changes in his asterisked movements. If they do not match, the therapist must endeavour to find the reasons. They can nearly always be found in either the patient's comments related to his symptoms, or in his complaint of symptoms felt on assessing and comparing the asterisked test movements. Patients gradually learn to know the fineness of the detail of their symptoms that is expected of them, and the important role they play in understanding what is being achieved by the treatment.

When progress has slowed

If the first treatment or two produces noticeable improvement, repetition of the same treatment at the next two sessions commonly does not produce the same rate of progress. This is so common as to be the normal expectation. It may be that whatever the cause of the pain may be, the body tends to overprotect it, and that it is this overprotection that the first two treatments relieves. When that has been relieved the next two treatments are directly facing the disorder. This is not the kind of 'when progress has slowed' which is intended by the title. Rather it is that a stage in treatment is reached when progress, which had initially been satisfactory, has slowed down considerably or has ceased. Under these circumstances a reappraisal of the situation (that is, a retrospective assessment) needs to be made.

First it is necessary to clarify with the patient that there had in fact, been progress with the earlier treatment. Assuming that there had been progress, the questions to be answered are:

1. How much progress had been made?
2. What were the changes both physical and subjective?
3. What produced the favourable changes?
4. Did any particular technique seem to help more than others, and had the technique been used again later and what was its effect then?
5. Did any technique seem to aggravate the symptoms at any stage?
6. When did the progressive improvement cease?
7. Does he know why it ceased to improve?
8. *Does his body give him any clues as to why progress ceased? (To answer this he needs to know that his body can provide information which only he can assess.)
9. Does he feel that treatment since progress has slowed down has been too gentle?
10. Does he feel he has reached a stage which he classes as being his normal or does he feel he should be able to improve further?
11. Can he, or does his body, suggest any particular technique or treatment approach that should help?

Following this probing investigation, the current state of the disorder is established.

Q   'What is your MAIN remaining problem?
Q   'Can you do anything now to show me how the symptoms can be provoked?'
Q   'Is that the aspect that has not improved with this more recent treatment?'

From this information, a re-examination is made (the therapist having a totally fresh and open minded new attitude) regarding the next step in treatment.

After a planned break from treatment

A stage can be reached in treatment when it is difficult to assess whether the disorder is being irritated, or the symptoms perpetuated, by treatment. The only way to determine this is to discontinue treatment for approximately 2 weeks and then review the situation with a retrospective assessment. A similar approach is required if it is thought that a stage has been reached when the disorder may continue to improve of its own accord. In both cases a planned break from treatment is required followed by the review. At the end of the break from treatment the following information is sought.

(It will be assumed that there has been some improvement.)

Q   'I'm pleased to hear you are better than when I last saw you. What is it that has improved?' (or 'In what way has it improved?')
ET An open-ended question seeking the valuable spontaneous emphasis from the patient's reply.
A   'I find the aching at the end of the day is getting less.'
ET The critical thing is whether it is still improving. He has said 'getting less'.
Q   'Has that been a steady daily improvement over the 2 weeks?'
A   'Yes, I think so.'
ET Not positive enough for the information being sought.
Q   'You *think* so: do you think there has been any improvement over, say, the last 4 days?'
A   'It's hard to say really.'
Q   'Well, think back to when I last saw you, do you feel there was any improvement over the first 4 days?'
A   'It's hard to tell because it was sore for the first day, I can remember that. Then, yes, I would say that it did improve after that. In fact it was towards the end of that week that I felt better.'
Q   'And now, is it feeling even better than then?'
A   'Probably.'
Q   'Definitely? or perhaps?'
A   'I think I would have to say perhaps.'
Q   'Do *you* feel it would be more constructive for me to treat it again say four times and then leave it alone for *three* weeks or should I leave it alone and review it in two weeks time from now?'
ET One of the hardest treatments to give patients is to NOT TREAT them. However, it is not uncommon for this to be necessary if an informative assessment is to be made. The 'informative assessment' is what this is all about.

A 'I don't know – you're the doc. You tell me. I don't mind. I'll do whatever you say.'

Q 'Well if I treat you four times and then leave it alone for 3 weeks we may be treating it unnecessarily, whereas if we leave it alone now and review it two weeks from now we will both know definitely if it needs treatment or not. If it does need treatment then, all we will have lost is 2 weeks of time. Are you able to put up with it for 2 weeks or would you like it treated now?'

ET The patient has to be part of the decision, especially if he is going to be *happy* with the decision.

A 'I can certainly put up with it, but I want it to be better than this too.'

Q 'But it has improved without treatment during this last 2 weeks hasn't it?'

A 'Yes.'

Q 'So it may improve further over the next two weeks also?'

A 'Yes, I suppose it could.'

Q 'And if it doesn't then we know definitely that it needs more treatment?'

A 'Agreed.'
Statement: 'Well, before we decide, let me re-examine your movements and then we can decide.'

Other subjective assessments could be made which would help with making the decision. It is not necessary to list their dialogue here as it would follow the same pattern, but it is the depth of certainty needed by the questioning that has been emphasized here. Unless the re-examination of the asterisked test movements indicates a worsening of the disorder over the 2 weeks, the most informative action would be to NOT TREAT and review in a further 2 weeks.

It is important to remember than whenever a patient comes in for a treatment, the most difficult treatment to give is *not to treat them*. It is only by a retrospective assessment that such a decision can ever be properly made.

The pattern of 'treatment – break – retrospective assessment' etc. is the ideal approach for the treatment of recurring exacerbation of disorder such as post-traumatic arthritis or degenerative arthritis.

Table 8.1

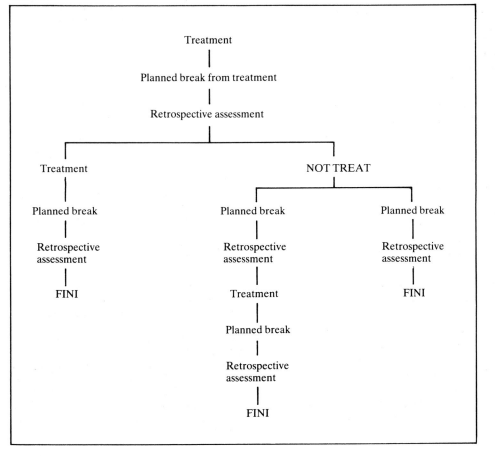

During such assessments it is necessary to try to learn what the patient's normal is. The patient will know what his subjective symptomatic norm is and he may also know what his limitations are. When treatment of his exacerbation has reduced his symptoms to the level of his normal, the therapist can use this same 'planned break/retrospective assessment' approach to determine whether the objective movements can be further improved. If they can be improved, the exacerbations will be less easily provoked and should not require as much treatment to gain the improvement. The end result of treatment is always a compromise rather than a 'cure' because of the underlying pathology.

Analytical assessment

Analytical assessment is the drawing together of:

1. All the patient's symptoms and their history with the details of all the examination findings.
2. The ability to assess the wearer of the problem in terms of frame-of-reference and thresholds.
3. Recognizing relationships between these details and known patterns of disorders, being able to pick out the typical from the atypical, the exotic from the ordinary.
4. Determining the presenting phase of the disorder and the changes that are currently taking place in relation to the degree of stability or otherwise.
5. Knowing what there is to be known about the diagnosed disorder and what its likely pattern of progression would be if it were not treated and then relating this to the changes that can be effected by specific treatments.

None of this is easy, nor is the drawing of it all together and weighing up the prognosis of treatment and its end result. However, it is made easier by the two-compartment method of thinking and treatment: where the history, symptoms and signs dominate one compartment of one's thoughts and can always be correct. In the other compartment are the diagnostic knowns and unknowns, the hypotheses and speculations, which are woven into the clinical compartment; they are used during the examination, treatment and assessments as applicable.

Although the terms 'clinical' and 'theoretical' for titles of the two compartments are not ideal, it is important to know what the compartments are about. One is knowledge, the other is examination of the patient. Treatment of the patient and his disorder can be enhanced by the knowledge, but its assessments have to be based on the 'clinical' (with qualifications from the theoretical).

In conclusion

Assessment is the keystone of effective and informative treatment. It requires an open mind which is prepared to accept what it sees yet at the same time questions what it sees and sets about proving it. Mental agility and a methodical approach to treatment are essential qualities of the physiotherapist. She must be very critical of herself and realize the pitfalls into which she can fall from:

1. Assuming things.
2. Not really getting answers to questions.
3. Accepting statements of fact as comparisons.
4. Disbelieving the patient.
5. Prejudging pain thresholds and attitudes.
6. Failing to think, plan, execute to prove.
7. Avoiding retrospective assessments.
8. Avoiding iatrogenic possibilities.

Tied in with all the problems with making 'assessments' is the biggest difficulty of all – COMMUNICATION. It is an essential art-form in itself on which so much is based. Patience and self-criticism are essential in the learning of this vital skill.

9

Recording

The manner by which examination and treatment findings are recorded is very important. It displays the therapist's clarity of thought as well as her ability to extract succinctly the patient's relevant information at depth. Because recording reveals these qualities, the fact of having to make a written recording, according to a pattern, can encourage the qualities of clear thinking to develop within the therapist.

A written record also encourages a methodical approach to the examination of a patient, and it assists in developing communication skills. This latter is especially true, because the recognition of key words and phrases is essential for clear recording.

Examination

It is important to record related information even when the findings indicate normality. By their having been recorded, reference at a later date shows that the particular questions have been asked, and the particular tests carried out. From the point of view of responsibility, it is a safe procedure to utilize the words that the patient has used and to record them in quotation marks. This has value in making assessments at subsequent treatment sessions when you may, for example, be able to say to the patient, following a comment he makes:

Q 'I'm sorry, I'm not sure I'm understanding what you are meaning. I've got written down here that on Monday the 5th you felt that, in your words, your forearm felt "less fat". Are you now saying that it wasn't "less fat" then or at any stage during treatment?'
A 'No, I had forgotten that – you're quite right, I can remember now, it was less fat then and

it remained so for about 3 days until I knocked it on a door.'
Q 'And do you feel, in retrospect, that that being "less fat" as you put it, was as a result of treatment?'
A 'Yes, I do.'
Q 'So, by what you are now saying, the *fatness* (using his phraseology) that you now feel, in *comparison with* at the beginning of treatment, has not changed?'
A 'Yes that's right.'
Q 'But are you also saying that you were improving as a result of the treatment prior to knocking your arm on the door?'
A 'Yes.'
Q 'So would we be doing the right thing to continue with the same kind of treatment and expect to get the same improvement?'
A 'Yes, I think so, but you're the expert.'

This might be recorded thus:

C/O 'Fatness' was less on 5th + 3 days. Knocked arm on door, 'fat' again, and still. He feels ℞ (this symbol means 'treatment') is correct.

Recording normal findings on a 'record-sheet' is a quick and simple procedure. For example, if the patient has pain in the shoulder area and the therapist has examined the acromioclavicular joint and found it to have normal painless movements, all that needs to be recorded is:

A/C √ √

The point is, *it must be recorded.*

The use of two ticks as indicated above, which follows the indication of the joint and its direction of movement tested, represents range of movement first and symptomatic response second. Thus the 'A/C √ √' means that all test movements of the acromioclavicular joint have a normal range with over-pressure at the limit of range (the first tick), and there is no abnormal pain response with the movement (the second tick). Not all people have the same ranges of normal movement ('John Bull' type physiques tend to be stiffer than tall lean people), and a *normal* finding may be recorded as:

A/C, HF, −10% ✓ ✓ or more informatively, as
A/C, HF −10% (Normal) ✓ ✓
(HF = Horizontal flexion)

Recording initial consultation

There is much more detail to be recorded from an initial consultation than for 'subsequent treatment sessions' described above. However, the same detail is required and so the same symbols and other abbreviations can be used. For these symbols different people have different likes and dislikes. This does not matter provided that the criteria are met.

A patient's main complaint, in his terms, is known. Details of the effects on the patient caused by his disorder need to be understood emphatically and recorded. A movement is not normal (i.e. ✓, √) unless adequate over-pressure is able to be used in the test. When pain is dominant, the point in the range (a) where pain is first felt (P1) should be recorded and also (b) the behaviour of that pain just beyond P1. All items listed in the 'planning sheet' are assessed.

'Cheat-sheets', as they are often termed, have advantages and disadvantages. The primary considerations are that they should not be regimented and they should not be detailed. A cheat-sheet that has a list of questions requiring ticks and crosses should not be used; they are inflexible and destroy independent thinking on the part of the examiner, and they completely obliterate any chance of following the patient's line of thought.

During the initial subjective questioning of a patient about his problem, adequate space on the record sheet must be allowed so that recording of bits of history mingled with bits of symptomatic behaviour may be listened to in the sequence that they are said yet recorded under the sections history and behaviour in chronological sequence.

The first space of a cheat-sheet should be something like 'main problem'. The very first question asked of a patient is 'As far as you are concerned . . . [pause] . . . what do YOU feel . . . [pause] . . . is your MAIN problem?' The response to this is the top line of the record and from it flow all the other relationships to it. Space should be allowed for quite a few statements to be fitted in around each other as he mentions them. This space can be enlarged further to put in a small number of questions which must be asked even if he does not

mention them spontaneously. For example, it is necessary to know the effect of short and long rests, both while resting, and on first getting up; the effects of activity generally, and specific activities for selected joints. Then there is the history of the patient's problem, and this is often quite extensive. Here again adequate space is required to allow for present history, first history and intermediate history.

Perhaps an example may help. Dialogue will be used as it would be during the first consultation and the recording will be listed in the 'case notes' (Figure 9.1). Each piece of information in the dialogue that

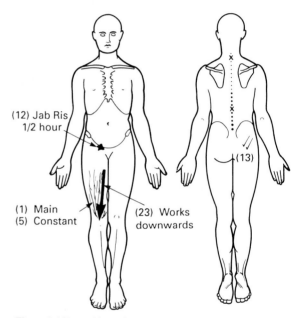

Figure 9.1 Record in patient's case notes

needs to be recorded will be indicated by a number in brackets: by referring to Figure 9.1, the number will show the approximate position on the case-note page where it is placed and the abbreviation used. This placement allows sufficient space to insert information that is gained later in the consultation but which needs to be recorded earlier in the case notes. P represents the patient's dialogue and Th, the therapist's.

Th   'As far as you are concerned . . . [pause] . . . etc.?'

P   'My MAIN problem? Well I suppose I would have to say it's the pain I get here in my thigh and knee.' He indicates it roughly and the therapist ROUGHLY defines it (1).

P   'But I've had it for a long time . . .'

Th   'How long do you mean?'

P   'I suppose about 15 years (2), but not all the time.' (3) Most of the time it's only when I have done a lot of hard cycling (4) but this time it's different.'

Th 'Different in what way?'

P   'Well it's constant this time (5), whereas it used to be intermittent.'

Th 'When you say it used to be intermittent, do you mean in comparison with what you have now?'

P   'It used to be on and off from day to day for about a month at a time (6) and then it would just go away for a year or so (7) but this time it came on about 2 months ago (8) and it's there all the time and gradually getting worse (9).'

Th 'Is it still worsening?'

P   'Yes but not a lot (10).'

Th 'Is the pain at a constant level through the day and night?'

P   'No. It's worse towards the end of the day and when I first go to bed.' (11)

Th 'So what is it like when you first get out of bed in the morning?'

P   'Much better, in fact that's my best time except for a few jabs in my groin with walking but that only lasts for half an hour or so.'

Th 'Show me where.'

P   'Deep in here (12).'

Th 'And do you get anything at all in here (indicating buttock)?'

P   'No.'

Th 'Nothing at all – ever ?'

P   'NO (13).'

Th 'Do you know what makes your leg ache more at the end of the day?'

P   'No, except that I have to go up and down stairs a lot with my job and I don't think that helps it (14).'

Th 'Does it hurt while you are going up or down the stairs?'

P   'Well, I'm conscious of it being tired and heavy going up as the day goes on (15).'

Th 'And what is the problem when you first go to bed?'

P   'I just can't get my leg comfortable, it seems I'm better if I lie on my left side and bend my right knee up and put a pillow under it. But even then I have to wriggle around a fair bit until it settles down (16). I had a fall as a child and I'm told I limped quite badly for a long time, but that was 30 years ago (17), and I haven't had any real problem until this time (18) except of course over the 15 years but then they have been trivial (19).'

Th 'How did this episode begin?'

P   'It just came on.'

Th 'Suddenly?'

P   'Yes quite suddenly, one week it wasn't there and the next week it was' (20).

Th 'So, over how many days did it build up?'

P   'I would say about four or five (21).'

Th 'What did you first notice?'

P   'On the Monday morning when I was getting out of bed I had these jabs in my groin for an hour or so (22) then it cleared up until I went to bed. I couldn't get comfortable because of my groin, and then the next day I was aware of my leg at work (23) and it has just steadily increased since then.'

Th 'Had you been doing anything unusual over the weekend before it started?'

P   'Well, as it happens, yes. I did a lot of skiing which I haven't done for years – and, oh yes, I did have one fall and broke my right ski (24).'

Th 'And are you are able to say whether your present symptoms start from the top and work downwards or the reverse?'

P   'Well my knee is the worst part but I feel it works downwards to the knee (25).' (Figure 9.1).

This is probably enough to show what is meant about the recording of a first consultation and the flexibility that a cheat-sheet should allow for.

Recording treatment sessions

Recording a first consultation obviously contains much more information than does a subsequent treatment session. Also the pattern of recording is not quite the same. The 'subsequent sessions' record the effects of the previous session as an assessment – this does not occur at the first consultation. To simplify the recording of the treatment sessions a regular pattern should be used which will develop the right thinking patterns and avoid forgetting points of importance. The following is the pattern I stick to always – it is reliable, provides consistent assessment markers, and is quick, clear, invaluable to be able to refer back to at later stages when making retrospective assessments:

Date R_x . . D . .
C/O
O/E
Plan
pp
R_x . . . .
. . . .
. . . .
Plan

R_x 3D8: is an example of how it is used and the example means 'treatment number 3 administered on the 8th day since the first consultation.' The record has obvious implications in making assessments. C/O: refers to what the patient 'complains of'. It is used as an assessment of the effect of the last treatment – quotations are used. O/E: refers to what is found during the 'objective examination' (the physical examination) of asterisked findings to determine changes that may have taken place as a result of the last treatment. Other test movements may be rechecked, or new ones may be added. Plan: it is important to make use of this heading to commit to paper progressive thoughts, ideas and plans to prove points. pp: this 'present pain' refers to whatever relative symptoms the patient has before proceeding with the treatment. It is information that is necessary for making an assessment of the patient's symptoms after the treatment technique, compared with what he had before performing the technique. Quotations should be used at this stage. R_x: this is the recording of the treatment, the method will be explained and developed later. Plan: this second 'plan' heading may be utilized at the end of a treatment session or it may be used at stages during the session *as well as* at the end of the session.

At the end of the session it is a record of the therapist's thoughts that have developed during the session as a basis for stating that the 'Plan' for the next treatment should be to do such-and-such provided such-and-such circumstances exist at that time. It is also a very quick memory-retriever. The 'plan' statement is not an unbendable commitment, but there would have to be reasons for changing the plan, and these reasons would have to be recorded in the new plan at that following treatment session.

When 'plan' is interspersed with ' R_x ' it is used to state the reasons for changing to a different technique. The *headings* could look like this:

R_x . . D . .
C/O
O/E
Plan ⎫
pp.   ⎬ (a)
R_x ⎭
Plan ⎫
R_x ⎬ (b)
Plan ⎭
R_x ⎱ (c)
Plan ⎰ (d)

The section identified (a) would be used in the same way as at the beginning of any subsequent session. However, in (b) the effect of the treatment technique both during its performance and on assessment of C/O and O/E after its performance may suggest a change of plan. Such circumstances are common and the new 'plan' needs to be identified. An example of (b) might be:

'Plan: *change to ↻ to avoid discomfort "during"*

So the treatment would be recorded and performed as stated in the plan. The following assessment may indicate a favourable but inadequate change. So, in (c), the plan might say, '*repeat but larger amplitude AND into a small degree of discomfort.*'.

The 'plan' in (d) might then say something like '*too much R_x today.? do lots caud. short of discomf. next time.*'

At the next treatment session it only needs a quick glance at the plan comments to be able to relive the last session and recall what you had in mind.

All of this allows flexibility, reasoning and purpose. The commitment also encourages method, succinctness and thought processes.

Recording the treatment is special. It must be written in the kind of detail that will be brief yet will clearly retrieve the depth needed on re-reading and making assessments.

The record is in two parts, one being the treatment, the other being its effect. For ' R_x and its effect' to be quickly found when reviewing progress as in a retrospective assessment, the two parts should be separated by a thick heavy line. Using a system such as this – where the treatment, its effect and the resulting plan, or change in plan, is recorded – will assist the therapist to visualize her own reasoning.

It *always* disappoints me to see records from people who are trained and endeavouring to follow the concept, not making the use of *this* line as they should. 'Petty' you might say, to which I reply, 'you *can't* make, it is *impossible* to make, the same depth and breadth of assessment without it'; (in a reasonable length of time): if you think you can, then you are not aware of *how deep* and informative in making decisions an assessment can be.

The pattern of recording treatment is as follows:

(i)	R_x Position chosen for the technique (abbreviated words)	effect after R_x
(ii)	The technique used (a symbol)	C/O
(iii)	The grade used (a symbol)	
(iv)	The rhythm used (abbreviated words)	
(v)	The number of times or duration it was performed	O/E
(vi)	**THE EFFECT IT HAD *WHILE* IT WAS BEING PERFORMED**	

It does not matter, not even the tiniest jot, what physiotherapy treatment is being used; think of exercises, think of electrical treatments, of hot pads, of ice, or massage, think of any physiotherapy; it does not matter what it is, it should be recorded in the pattern shown above. As an example, a treatment by ultrasound should be recorded as follows:

pp. tender to touch, spot medial knee
Rx 1 × US 1.0 W/cm² pulsed | C/O 'not tender now'
stationary over tender spot | O/E knee abd ✓ ✓
Without pain

The next example relates the pattern of 'recording treatment' to passive movement techniques for the inferior tibio-fibular joint:

pp. awareness 'in' ankle at front

in – lie on (L), (R) hip/knee F'd,
ankle resting neutral
did ↕ Fib (soft, hands) c̄ sl. compr. · | C/O 'sl. more aware'
| O/E heel gait more DF
| c̄ less p. 'in'

Sl.EOR repro. lessening

What this example is saying is that, before applying the treatment technique, the patient was aware of a feeling within his ankle but anteriorly. The treatment technique was to position him (the word 'in') lying on his left side with his right hip and knee flexed until his lower leg was resting on the treatment couch and his ankle was also able to rest supported in a neutral position; in other words there was no eversion stress at the ankle. The technique used (the word 'did') was an anteroposterior pressure (↕) on the anterior surface of the fibula through the soft parts of the hands (rather than the thumbs) which were comfortably positioned to avoid local discomfort. The anteroposterior pressure, produces an anteroposterior movement of the fibula in relation to the tibia. The pressure also had a slight medial inclination to produce a slight compression of the fibula against the tibia (↕ c̄ sl. compr. meaning with slight compression). The movement was a very large grade III − (III−) as compared with ('III−') movement performed in a smooth rhythm. While it was being performed, the patient was aware that his 'awareness' within the ankle was being reproduced slightly at the end of grade III− range (sl. EOR repro. meaning slight end of range reproduction of 'awareness'). This reproduction of awareness decreased slightly (repro. lessening over the one and a half minutes (1.5′) during which the technique was performed. After that one and a half minutes, the patient felt slightly more aware of the within-the-ankle-anteriorly feeling ('C/O sl. more aware') while in the standing position, but on examination, his walking on his heels showed a greater range of dorsiflexion (O/E heel gait more DF) and he did not feel as much discomfort as he had prior to the technique (' c̄ less p. 'in') – with less pain within his ankle'.

It is easy to see that, crammed into the record of the treatment and its effect, both during and after it, there is a very large amount of material in depth and

in detail. It does not take long to do – it must be written during the treatment session. Making use of symbols (Table 9.1) helps speed the process.

Table 9.1 Symbols

F	Flexion
E	Extension
Ab	Abduction
Ad	Adduction
↻	Medial rotation
↺	Lateral rotation
HF	Horizontal flexion
HE	Horizontal extension
BB	Hand behind back
Inv.	Inversion
Ev.	Eversion
DF	Dorsiflexion
PF	Plantar flexion
Sup.	Supination
Pron.	Pronation
El	Elevation
De	Depression
Pr	Protraction
Re	Retraction
Med.	Medial
Lat.	Lateral
OP	Over-pressure
PPIVM	Passive physiological intervertebral movements
PAIVM	Passive accessory intervertebral movements
ULTT	Upper limb tension tests
LLTT	Lower limb tension tests
Q	Quadrant
Lock	Locking position
F/Ab	Flexion abduction
F/Ad	Flexion adduction
E/Ab	Extension abduction
E/Ad	Extension adduction
Distr.	Distraction
Compr.	Compression
↑	Posteroanterior movement
↓	Anteroposterior movement
→	Transverse movement in the direction indicated
↕	Gliding adjacent joint surfaces
⟶	Longitudinal movement
Ceph	Cephalad
Caud	Caudad

Longitudinal movement is the direction of movement of a joint in line with the longitudinal axis of the body in its anatomical position. When that same joint movement is performed in any other position than the anatomical position, that movement of the joint is still called longitudinal movement even though that part of the body is not now in the anatomical position.

Recording retrospective assessment

Well-managed manipulative physiotherapy depends upon:

1. The initial examination.
2. Continuous assessment.
3. Retrospective assessment.

Numbers (2) and (3) have been explained in detail in Chapter 8 but here, the concern is with how it should be recorded. To be practical, time must be a consideration, but not at the expense of detail and accuracy. The record of a retrospective assessment should stand out from the other parts of the treatment record so that they can be easily traced on reviewing progress at later sessions. This is particularly necessary when a patient has an extensive disorder and considerable treatment. It is immaterial as to how the highlighting and separation of the retrospective assessment is achieved but it should include a statement to show the time with which the assessment is being compared. The important value of spontaneous comments has been emphasized; and not only is this particularly important with a retrospective assessment, but also it must stand out in the written record. We have, therefore, three requirements of the written record:

1. To stand out from other recorded data. To be highlighted so that it is readily seen on checking back through the record.
2. To state with what time the comparison is made.
3. To emphasize the spontaneous information.

The methods one uses to achieve these ends do not matter, but an example may be helpful. The example given should not be thought of as a joke nor should it be seen as unnecessary or ridiculous.

A method is mandatory – without it the importance of assessment in the concept of this text is neither being appreciated nor followed.

Suggested example:

1. Write it in green and reserve the colour green for retrospective assessment alone. (A four-colour biro is a useful tool.)
2. Commence the record with 'cf.' which means 'compared with'.
3. Follow cf. with the date the assessment is being compared with.
4. Such an assessment will start with a question, e.g. 'How do you feel *now* . . . *compared with* . . . when you first came in for treatment?' Aspects of this answer will be spontaneous and should be written in an abbreviated form within quotation marks. As the comparisons unfold the more important or more spontaneous ones can be underlined or highlighted with a green asterisk. When, during the inquiry, a direct question is asked, such as 'How is that pain which you felt was *inside your joint* . . . how does it feel now . . . *compared with* . . . when you first came in?', the patient's answer is prefixed by the letter 'Q' indicating that the answer recorded (not being in quotation marks) came only as a result of a question.
cf. 'Sometimes totally free of p. (constant before);
'can chop wood without jarring now.'
'Thrilled'
Q. can sleep on shoulder now '& clothesline imp'ing' (meaning 'improving')

When recording is accurate and succinct, and can be correctly interpreted by another person reading it, it is an invaluable self-teacher.

10

Shoulder girdle and upper limb

General principles

Before the techniques for each joint are discussed, special features peculiar to the joint will be described and related to examination and assessment. The full examination for each joint will not be dealt with in detail though a Table will be given. Particular reference will be made to 'brief appraisal tests' and 'special tests'. The passive movement tests that form part of *examination* are also movements that can be used in *treatment*.

Examination of passive movements is very important and it is essential for the physiotherapist to know the feel of each joint's movements. This feel is important in two parts of a movement:

1. The first is the friction- and symptom-free quality through its full range.
2. The second is the feel of the movement at the limit of the range.

Symptomatic responses during these movements must be discerned and noted as part of the total test.

Functional demonstration/tests

These consist of a movement or movements which he recognizes demonstrates his disorder (e.g. in a golf swing, his back-swing provokes HIS problem). The therapist analyses (1) the position and (2) the movement involved. This is the first part of the objective examination and is a vital asterisked sign.

Brief appraisal tests

These are among the early tests in the objective examination for the area concerned and consist of asking the patient to perform certain movements against gravity. They provide the physiotherapist with two important guides to examination:

1. They indicate the strength or gentleness required of the movements to determine the abnormalities.
2. They also show the patient's willingness to use the disordered joint. Any abnormal function provides the physiotherapist with a marker against which progress can be evaluated.

Such tests for the shoulder girdle are performed in the standing position. The patient is asked to raise his arms forwards and above his head (flexion), raise his arms sideways to above his head (flexion through abduction), and finally to put alternate arms behind his back reaching as far cephalad as he can. None of these movements, at this stage of the examination, should be performed into a very painful range.

Special tests

Far too often a joint is examined and classed as normal when, if certain special passive movement tests were applied and compared with the normal side, minor faults would not be missed. These special tests are usually movements made up of two physiological movements performed together (such as combining flexion and adduction of the hip) or a combination of a physiological and an accessory movement (such as extension of the carpometacarpal joint of the thumb combined with a postero-anterior movement of the metacarpal on the trapezium or vice versa).

The 'special tests' need only be used when the normal active physiological movements appear to be full range and painless. Before a joint can be classed as 'normal', over-pressure should be able to be applied to these special test movements, and the range and its pain response should be the same as for the sound joint on the other side of the body.

Glenohumeral joint

The glenohumeral joint has large amplitudes of both physiological and accessory movements. These occur in a greater number of directions than in any other joint in the body. As a clinician moves another person's arm passively through a large physiological range, the accessory movements can be felt to be large also. This fact should be borne in mind when considering the selection of treatment techniques[1].

Subjective examination

Accurate pin-pointing of the site of pain for shoulder disorders can be very informative. Pain felt immediately underneath the acromion process is more likely to be arising from the acromiohumeral structures rather than from the glenohumeral joint. Likewise, pain felt at the acromioclavicular area superiorly is unlikely to be a glenohumeral referred pain (Figure 10.1).

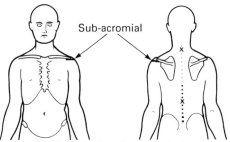

Figure 10.1 Sites of pain, sub-acromial pain

During the subjective examination, it is often useful when attempting to determine the site of pain to grasp around the head of the humerus so that the fingers on one side of the glenohumeral joint can press into the space between the humerus and the glenoid cavity towards the thumb pressing in on the opposite side of the joint. At the same time the physiotherapist can ask the question, 'Is the pain "in" [meaning deep within] here?'. To emphasize the 'within' aspect of the question, the fingers and thumb gently rock the head of the humerus backwards and forwards. It may be necessary to support the acromioclavicular area with the other hand (Figure 10.2). The emphasis with which the patient is able to say 'Yes' or 'No' to the question has very real value.

Pain can be referred both upwards, even as far as the base of the neck (Figure 10.3(a)), or downwards, even as far as the forearm and occasionally into the hand. The referred arm pain is commonly less intense in the distal area.

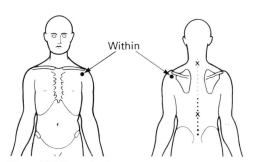

Figure 10.2 Sites of pain within the glenohumeral joint

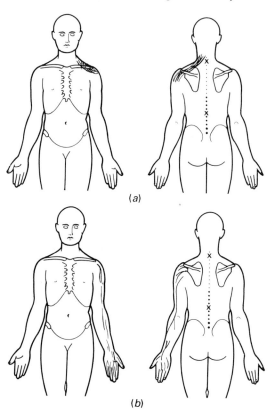

(a)

(b)

Figure 10.3 Sites of pain (a) referred into the neck, (b) referred into the arm

Two common areas of referral, usually associated with chronic disorders, is a patch of pain near the insertion of the deltoid muscle or as a band around the arm at that level (Figure 10.4(a) and 10.4(b)).

Pain felt posteriorly in the upper arm (Figure 10.5(a)) is more commonly cervical in origin than glenohumeral; pain felt in the area medial to the scapula is also more likely to be cervical or thoracic in origin (Figure 10.5(b)). Similarly, pain felt in the

1. Maitland, G. D. *Shoulder Quadrant, Hip Flexion/Adduction,* Video Number 6, (42 mins.) Postgraduate Study Centre Hermitage, Medizinische Abteilung, Bad Ragaz CH7310, Switzerland (1978)

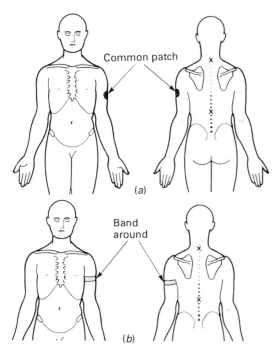

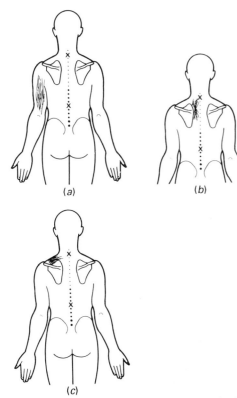

Figures 10.4 Sites of pain (*a*) common patch of pain (*b*) a band around

Figures 10.5 Sites of pain (*a*) posterior arm pain, (*b*) pain medial to scapula, (*c*) supra-spinous fossa pain

supra-spinous fossa, in the absence of any local glenohumeral pain, is unlikely to be glenohumeral in origin; it is more likely to be of cervical origin (Figure 10.5(c)).

When pain or paraesthesia are of a stocking distribution, there is the *possibility* of a causal relationship from the thoracic spine at approximately the junction of the superior and middle thirds of the thoracic spine (Figure 10.6).

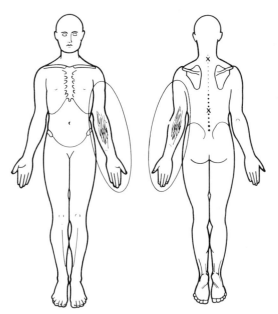

Figure 10.6 Sites of pain, stocking distribution of pain or paraesthesia

Having noted in careful detail the precise site of the symptoms, the next requirement is to determine the behaviour of the symptoms. Remembering that a patient may have both (1) different *kinds* of pain and (2) different yet closely associated *sites* of pain (that is, they may be constantly present or only present with movement – they may be sharp or dull, vague or localized, etc.) it must also be appreciated that the disorder may present with (1) different *behaviours* of pain and (2) different provoking factors for the pain.

By this is meant that the symptoms may be constant and unvarying or constant but exacerbated by certain movements or activities and requiring a calculable period of time to subside – they may only have symptoms following vigorous activities and lying on the shoulder at night or it may be a sharp pain which is only felt with sudden unguarded movement. And so the list goes on.

Objective examination

The full examination for a patient with general shoulder area pain will not be described. However, a plan of the objective examination is given in Table 10.1. The symbols used in this and all subsequent examination tables are defined in Table 9.1, page 127).

Functional demonstration/test

Part of the subjective examination often includes (perhaps even as early as the second or third question) asking the patient if he can demonstrate, here and now, the movement(s) that provokes his symptom(s). A good example of this could be that the patient refers to a throwing action. It is useful to

Table 10.1 Glenohumeral joint – objective examination

What is sometimes referred to as an 'accessory joint', between the head of the humerus and the acromion process, forms part of the examination of the glenohumeral joint.

HIGHLIGHT MAIN FINDINGS WITH ASTERISKS AS YOU GO

Observation
Watch for patient's willingness to move the arm when undressing.

Functional demonstration/tests
As applicable

1. *Their* demonstration of *their* functional movements affected by *their* disorder.
2. Differentiation of their demonstrated functional movement(s).

Brief appraisal
Note abnormalities of appearance, tenderness, temperature and fasciculation. Palpation may be performed here.

Active movements
Active quick tests (+ cervical).
Routinely (with all joints, always modified to suit 'kind of disorder').
F, Ab, (note 'drift'), behind back, HF
Note range, pain, repeated, and behaviour (note scapular rhythm)
As applicable
Speed of test movements
Specific movements which aggravate
The injuring movement

Movements under load
Thoracic outlet tests & ULTT
Muscle power
F & Abd in full medial & lateral rotation

Isometric tests
Rotator cuff
Other muscles in 'plan'

Other structures in 'plan'
Cervical spine
Joints 'above and below'
Thoracic outlet & ULTT

Passive movements

Physiological movements

Routinely

1. If pain severe ↕, ⇢ Caudad, ⇢ lateral; (in neutral pain-free position).
2. F↺, C, Ab, HF, HE, components of hand behind back and ↕ (if active tests positive) or
3. Quadrant and locking position (if active tests negative)

Note range, pain, resistance, spasm and behaviour.

As applicable

1. Canal's slump tests.
2. Differentiation tests.
3. ULTT (upper limb tension tests).

Accessory movements
As applicable
May be assessed at first session or as treatment progresses:

1. By thumb pressures or arm leverage ↕, ↕, caud and ceph. ⇢, laterally:
   (a) In different positions in the range.
   (b) With addition of compression and/or distraction.
2. Mid range Ab/Ad, Rotn, and F/E oscillations:
   (a) With glenohumeral compression.
   (b) With acromiohumeral compression.
3. 1st rib.

Note range, pain, resistance, spasm and behaviour.

Palpation
Temperature   Relevant tenderness (capsule, tendons, bursae, muscles).
Swelling, Wasting   Position
Altered sensation
When 'comparable signs' ill–defined reassess 'injuring movement'.

Check case records and radiographs

Instructions to patients

1. Warning of possible exacerbation.
2. Request to record details.
3. Instruction re 'joint care' if required.

hand the patient something (such as a pillow) and ask him to demonstrate the provoking activity even if it is in the middle of subjective questioning. Such information can provide considerable information which will guide the path of the whole objective examination.

Among the many tests of the active movements, those of flexion and abduction should be done in the same sequence to make the assessments more accurate.

Flexion

The physiotherapist stands behind the patient. She asks him to lift both arms forward and above his head; she is careful not to touch him, so that the spontaneous direction and rhythm of the movement will not be influenced in his manner of lifting them. The movement will be a spontaneous one; he will raise his arm through its most comfortable range to the maximum height he can reach. While the patient is performing this movement, the physiotherapist watches:

1. The scapulothoracic rhythm.
2. The degree of 'drift' laterally from the sagittal plane during the flexion movement.
3. The manner of his movement throughout his range, that is, she assesses whether he has to move the arm slowly because of pain or is able to move quite quickly.
4. The extent of the range.

There is a considerable difference in the appearance of the scapulothoracic movement if the glenohumeral range of flexion is restricted to 40° by a comparatively painless capsular restriction compared with the same range being restricted *solely* by pain. A capsular restriction is demonstrated by (1) hitching of the whole shoulder girdle, (2) rotation of the scapula laterally around the rib cage, and (3) a drift laterally from the sagittal plane of the humerus. In comparison, a pain restriction has none of these features, the 40° flexion being a glenohumeral movement. When both pain *and* stiffness restrict the range of flexion to 40°, there will be an element of 'hitch', 'rotation' and 'drift', but it will be less than is the case stated above, when the movement is painless.

Having noted all that can be seen in relation to the spontaneous flexion, the physiotherapist, while still standing behind the patient, then gently rests her hands on the lateral aspect of his elbows. She asks him to again raise his arms forward and above his head, but this time he keeps his arms closer together. She uses her hand position on his elbows to ensure he flexes in the sagittal plan. That is, she counters his protective rhythm so as to be able to assess the relationship the 'drift' has to the present disorder. His range of flexion and behaviour of pain is then recorded.

Abduction

1. While still standing behind the patient she asks him to raise his arms sideways and above his head while she watches the spontaneous manner in which he performs the movement. She notes the degree of 'drift' forward of the frontal plane, through which the patient moves his arm noting when it begins and the manner in which it increases.
2. The patient is again asked to abduct his arms but this time the physiotherapist gently holds both arms back in the frontal (coronal) plane. This countering of horizontal flexion will probably considerably limit the patient's range of abduction of the painful arm. This new range is noted and recorded.

Hand behind back

Another important functional test movement is to ask the patient to put his hands behind his back as high as he can reach. When he has reached this position the physiotherapist should then hold the patient's arm and endeavour to find out whether his inability to reach a full range is due to limited or painful glenohumeral extension, adduction or medial rotation. Figure 10.24, page 146, shows the test being applied to the patient in lying.

These tests provide valuable markers against which to assess the changes which treatment makes.

Isometric tests (rotator cuff)

The muscles and tendons forming the rotator cuff can be quickly and easily assessed while the patient is standing for the preceding tests. If required, the tests can be performed more finely when the patient is supine.

Special tests

It is not uncommon for a patient with shoulder pain to be able to flex, abduct and place his hand behind his back, in a manner exhibiting an apparent full range. Firm over-pressure should then be applied to these movements.

If the three active tests are normal even when over-pressure is applied, the physiotherapist should then test passively the 'quadrant' and the 'locking position', with the patient lying supine. Only if these tests are negative can the physiotherapist say the glenohumeral joint's movements are normal.

These two tests are unique in that they have not previously been recorded. However, they must be included in the examination for they may be the only movements that indicate that the joint is not fully normal. These movements which will now be described can also be used as treatment movements to relieve a patient's symptoms.

Locking position*** (Appendix 2, photographs S2.1 and S2.2)

To find the locking position the patient lies supine and the physiotherapist abducts the patient's arm from alongside his trunk and endeavours to reach a position of full flexion where his upper arm lies alongside his head.

She places the distal third of her near-side forearm under the medial border of the patient's scapula. Her thumb lies immediately adjacent to the vertebral column and she flexes her fingers over the trapezius to prevent the patient's shoulder from shrugging. She holds his flexed elbow in her left hand, maintaining slight medial rotation and exten sion during abduction.

The patient's upper arm must be maintained in a frontal plan just posterior to the median frontal plane. This posterior frontal plane is only approximately 3 or 4° of horizontal extension behind the median frontal plane. If the horizontal extension is greater than these 3 or 4°, the locking position will not be found. As the abduction movement is continued in the correct frontal plane the humerus will reach a position where it becomes locked. The humerus cannot be moved further towards the patient's head; neither can it be laterally rotated or moved anteriorly from the frontal plane (Figure 10.7)[1].

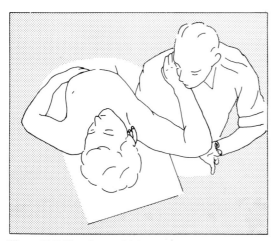

Figure 10.7 Glenohumeral joint: locking position

The line that the point of the elbow traverses, if viewed from the side, is as shown in Figure 10.8 where the locking position is in the shape of a 'cave', the arc of the quadrant is the shape of a small 'mound', and the 'peak' of the quadrant is the highest point of the 'mound'.

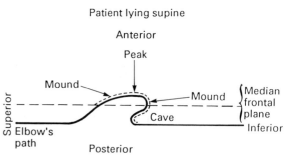

Figure 10.8 A side-on view of the path of the right elbow as seen from his right side looking horizontally towards his left side. The path traverses a line: (*a*)into the 'cave' of the locking position, (*b*)over the 'mound' of the quadrant, (*c*)passing the 'peak' of the quadrant

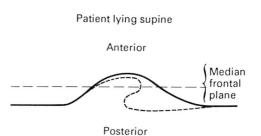

Figure 10.9 A side-on view of the path of a patient's elbow when movements are restricted and the 'locking position' lost

To relate the feel of the 'locking position' to a cave, scouring the normal locking position has the feeling of a rock lined surface of the cave, whereas an abnormal cave is muddy or moss-lined. When glenohumeral movement is obviously restricted, there will be no cave, and the view of the line of the elbow will be as shown in Figure 10.9. This figure should be compared with the normal path shown in Figure 10.8.

A patient whose symptoms are minimal or intermittent may appear to have a full painless range of active movement whereas if the locking position is tested, it may be found to be abnormal and any attempt to push the glenohumeral joint into the locking position will reproduce the patient's pain. This same test movement should be applied to the normal shoulder to compare pain and range and so determine the extent of the disability. The locking position should always be examined when other signs are minimal.

1. Maitland, G. D. *Shoulder Quadrant, Hip Flexion/Adduction,* Video Number 6, (42 mins.) Postgraduate Study Centre Hermitage, Medizinische Abteilung, Bad Ragaz CH7310, Switzerland (1978)

Quadrant**

To reach a fully flexed position from the 'locking position', the pressure maintaining abduction should be relaxed slightly to allow the arm to be moved anteriorly from the frontal plane (which was posterior to the median frontal plane for the locking position). Lateral rotation can then take place as the abduction movement is continued. This anterior and rotary movement takes place in a small arc of the abduction movement. This arc encompasses the peak of the quadrant position. Once past this peak the arm can then drop back behind the median frontal plane again and the abduction movement can be continued until the upper arm reaches the side of the patient's head (Figure 10.10)[1].

The quadrant is that position, approximately 30° lateral to the fully flexed position (Figure 10.12, page 137) where the patient's upper arm has to move anteriorly from the 'locked' position. If the physiotherapist maintains pressure at the centre of the arc of the quadrant, pushing the patient's elbow towards the floor, the upper arm can then be rolled back and forth over the top of the quadrant. To do this successfully it is necessary to control the extent of medial and lateral rotation during the movement through the arc.

To examine the quadrant and locking positions the following procedure should be used:

1. The therapist should put the patient's arm in the quadrant position and apply a reasonable degree of pressure, pushing the patient's elbow towards the floor. She should record the range in this position by observing two things:
   (a) The range of movement in the sagittal plane between the humerus and the anterolateral surface of the scapula.
   (b) The extent of the prominence of the head of the humerus in the axilla.
2. While the patient's arm is oscillated antero-posteriorly in the quadrant position as a grade IV or IV+ the physiotherapist should take note of the site and degree of pain produced by the manoeuvre. The range and pain should then be compared with that present in the normal shoulder. As the position is usually uncomfortable, it is mandatory to compare both shoulders.

The locking position should then be tested on both shoulders, feeling for and comparing the range, the intensity and the site of pain.

The normal 'feel' of these movements must be learnt if small disturbances responsible for minor yet important symptoms are not to be missed.

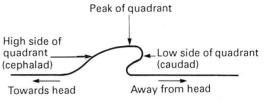

Figure 10.10(a) Glenohumeral joint: quadrant position

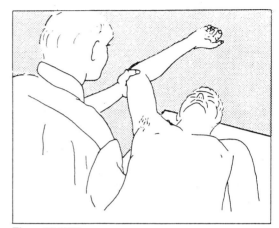

Figure 10.10(b)

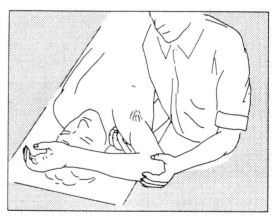

Figure 10.10(c) Peak of Quadrant (b) viewed from caudad position and (c) viewed from cephalad position

Application of the quadrant

There are two shoulder quadrant techniques to be learned. The first is 'rolling over the quadrant' and the second is performing extremely gentle pressure towards all faces of the 'mound' of the quadrant. The first is used when the patient's disorder is minor and chronic, and the second is when the disorder causes subacromial pain which is moderately severe.

1. Maitland, G. D. *Shoulder Quadrant and Hip F/Add,* Videotape No. 6 (42 mins.). Postgraduate Study Centre Hermitage, Medizinische Abteilung, Bad Ragaz, Switzerland CH-7310 (1979)

Rolling over the quadrant

The patient's arm is firstly held very firmly against the 'peak' of the quadrant with his glenohumeral joint slightly medially rotated, that is, his hand is slightly higher (closer to the ceiling) than his elbow. If the arm is positioned exactly on the 'peak' of the mound, the correct rotation position can be maintained accurately and easily with an antero-posterior pressure against the medial epicondyle alone – there will be NO TENDENCY AT ALL for the shaft of the humerus (and therefore the forearm) to roll into a position of medial or lateral rotation. Further proof of being at the right 'peak' position is provided if, when the firm anteroposterior pressure sustained at the medial epicondyle, the glenohumeral joint is adducted 1 or 2°, medial rotation will immediately occur. The opposite is also true: if the humerus is further abducted from the 'peak' of the quadrant, the humeral shaft will immediately rotate laterally allowing the patient's hand to lower towards the floor. Thus one can roll over the 'mound' of the quadrant from one side of the peak to the other by an abduction to adduction and back to abduction of the glenohumeral joint (Appendix 2, S3).

To perform this technique particularly strongly, the back and forth arc of movement occupies a maximum of 6 or 7° while the rotary range occupies 80–90° starting in a slightly medially rotated position on the low side (adducted side) of the quadrant and finishing in an almost fully laterally rotated position on the high side (the abducted side) of the quadrant. This is an extremely difficult technique to perform well, yet it is an extremely important technique, because without the skill, some patients will never be freed of their symptoms.

A vigorous 'roll-over' is even more difficult to perform effectively. It is a painful procedure and requires firm control of the resistance in both the abduction and adduction components, and also to the rotary component. The following is an attempt to describe the technique. To tighten the rotation component of the humeral-shaft rotation during the 'rolling-over' at the 'peak' the abduction or adduction is held back. During this holding-back the rotation is over-pressured and the rotation made to occur *before* the position of the humerus beyond the peak on the side of the 'mound' has been allowed to take place. 'Practice makes perfect', but because it is a painful procedure on even the normal and young model, the opportunities to practise may be limited.

Gentle movements around the quadrant

This technique is equally difficult to perform, yet it is just as essential to acquire this skill as it is for the technique described above. To represent the oscillatory movement of the technique diagrammatically

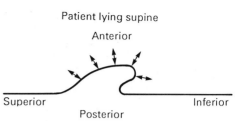

Patient lying supine

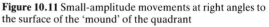

Figure 10.11 Small-amplitude movements at right angles to the surface of the 'mound' of the quadrant

(Figure 10.11) the movements are small in amplitude, slow and smooth in execution, and directed at right angles to the surface of the 'mound' of the quadrant.

The first skill to acquire is the ability:

1. To be able to perform the movements slowly, smoothly and gently at the correct depth.
2. To be able to perform the movements *at right angles* to the particular surface of the 'mound' (Appendix 2, S1 and S2).

The second skill is being able to change the position of the oscillatory movement from one position on the 'mound' to another position. It is a well-known fact that during active abduction of the arm, a lateral rotation of the shaft of the humerus has to take place at approximately 90° of the abduction if it is to be taken beyond that point. In a related way, to change from one position on the 'mound' of the quadrant to another, the humerus has to be lifted far enough away from the 'mound' in the same line as the oscillatory treatment movement was being performed, for the rotary movement of the humeral shaft to be loose, uninhibited and painless. This usually requires a movement away from the 'mound' of approximately 30°.

Moving down the 'low side' (the adducting side or inferior side) of the 'mound' from the 'peak'

Having lifted the humerus the required 30° away from the 'mound', the shaft of the humerus is rotated medially around a stationary and stable axis (the axis *being* the line of the shaft of the humerus). The amount of rotation performed depends on how far *the new* position for the oscillatory treatment movement is going to be from the last position: the greater the distance apart of the positions, the greater is the required degree of medial rotation (Figure 10.12) (Appendix 2, S1).

Having 'lifted away', and having medially rotated the required amount, the shaft of the humerus is lowered towards the floor (Figure 10.13).

Then gently, slowly, and smoothly, move towards 'mound' at right-angles to its surface at this new position. When the appropriate resistance and pain

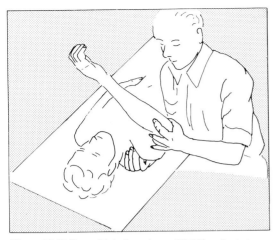

Figure 10.12 'Low side' of quadrant; lift 30° and rotate medially

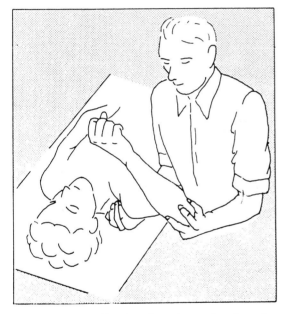

Figure 10.13 'Low side' of quadrant: lower elbow towards floor

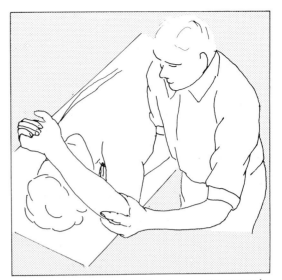

Figure 10.14 'Low side' of quadrant; move elbow towards 'mound'

allowed is dependent upon how far away the new oscillatory treatment position is going to be from the previous position. However, on the high side of the quadrant the rate of change of rotation is greater than on the low side (Figure 10.15) (Appendix 2, S2).

The shaft of the humerus is stabilized in relation to its lateral rotation while the arm (humerus) is *allowed* to slowly lower towards the floor (Figure 10.16).

Then an adduction movement at right-angles to the line of the forearm is directed towards the 'high side' of the quadrant (Figure 10.17).

Other test movements

Flexion

In both examination and treatment of the patient's movements in the supine position flexion must be assessed in all positions between full flexion alongside the head and the quadrant position (approximately 30° lateral to the head). The position of flexion where the main limitation of range or degree of pain is felt is usually the position utilized in treatment (Figure 10.18).

When the glenohumeral joint has obvious limitations of active range the quadrant and locking positions are not required as part of examination.

Horizontal flexion

This is an important movement which should be assessed routinely as it can restrict certain important functional movements.

response is achieved, the oscillatory gentle movement is performed (Figure 10.14).

Moving down the 'high side' (the abducting side, flexing side or superior side) of the 'mound' from the 'peak'

Having lifted the humerus the required 30° away from the 'mound' (see Figure 10.12), the shaft of the humerus is *allowed* to rotate laterally around a stationary and stable axis (the axis *being* the line of the shaft of the humerus). The amount of rotation

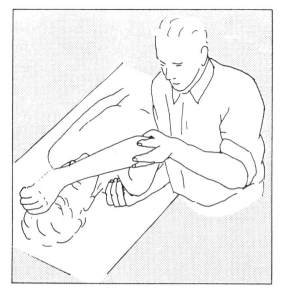

Figure 10.15 'High side' of quadrant; allow humerus to rotate laterally

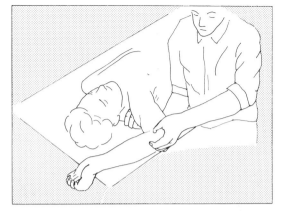

Figure 10.17 'High side' of quadrant; move elbow towards 'mound'

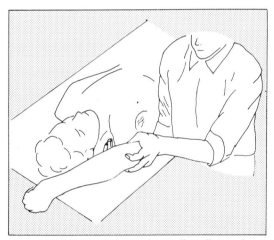

Figure 10.16 'High side' of quadrant; allow elbow to lower towards floor

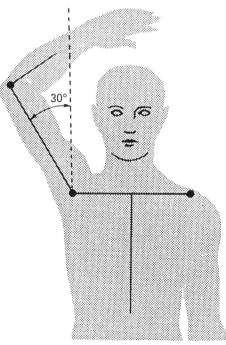

Figure 10.18 Patient supine. Testing by anteroposterior over-pressure on the elbow in positions between flexion and the quadrant

Accessory movements

The accessory movements tested as part of examination are depicted in this chapter. When pain is the primary part of the patient's disorder, these accessory movements must be assessed for range and pain response while the joint is positioned in a 'near neutral/mid-range pain-free position'.

Assessment during treatment

In standing, active abduction without lateral rotation is the movement most commonly used for assessing progress, but when all movements of the glenohumeral joint are limited and painful it is more useful to the physiotherapist to assess active flexion. This is because if treatment effects a 5% improvement, it will be more evident on assessing flexion which has a range of 180° than in the smaller range of abduction.

Techniques
*Flexion and quadrant****

Neither flexion nor the quadrant is used as a grade I movement in treatment because they are end of range positions. Grades II, III and IV, however, are commonly used and the movement may be directed towards any point between full flexion and the quadrant, but it is usually directed towards the limitation or the painful position.

Grade II***
Starting position

The physiotherapist stands beyond the patient's shoulder facing his feet. With his arm flexed, she holds his wrist and hand in her left hand. His hand does not then flap loosely during treatment. She holds his elbow in her right hand with her fingers spreading over the medial aspect of the joint reaching to the upper arm; her thumb is cupped around his forearm just distal to the elbow. She places her right knee on the couch beyond his shoulder. To prevent the movement going beyond an established range of flexion the physiotherapist must position her thigh as a stop for the patient's upper arm as it makes contact across her inner thigh. A pillow or blanket should not be used to form the stop as small variations in the range of flexion cannot properly be controlled. The further laterally away from the patient's head the flexion movement

is directed, the further from the patient's head the physiotherapist needs to stand. Balance is maintained between her standing leg (in this case the left leg) and her right lower leg (Figure 10.19(a)).

Method

The movement, which consists of raising and lowering the patient's arm, through approximately 30°, must be directed in a straight line, it must not swing through an arc. During the treatment movement the patient's wrist traverses the same amplitude as his elbow, thus avoiding humeral rotation. If the flexion is directed towards the quadrant, the movement must be in a line from the opposite hip to the quadrant. The nearer the flexion is directed to the patient's head the more the starting position of the line is directed from the hip of the same side. With this change of treatment direction, the physiotherapist will most probably need to use the other leg to form the stop (Figure 10.19(b)).

Techniques of treatment should never be used nor taught in a set manner. Bearing this in mind, the direction of the quadrant treatment may be required to be directed on the high side or low side as has been described for the small amplitude movements on page 136 (see Figure 10.11). The movement can even be performed in a direction towards the locking position.

There is a further consideration to bear in mind when using very large amplitude movements. When the movement starts with the patient's arm almost

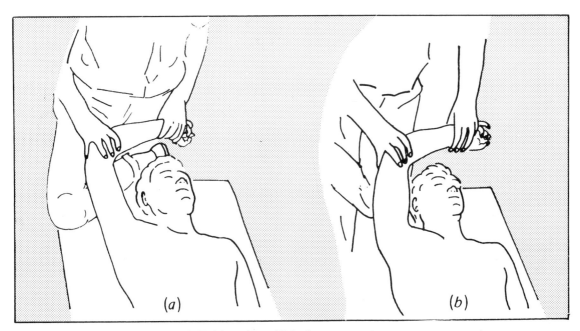

Figure 10.19 Glenohumeral joint, grade II, (*a*) quadrant; (*b*) flexion

touching his chest, and is then taken through and beyond what would be horizontal if the patient were standing, pain or discomfort may be felt at that 90° horizontal position. When this does occur, a gentle lift with the physiotherapist's little finger and thumb holding around the epicondyles, as it passes the horizontal, will avoid any discomfort.

As pain recedes and it becomes necessary to move the arm further into the range, the physiotherapist should lower her thigh which forms the stop. At the same time she must withdraw her knee a little to prevent pressure being exerted against the upper end of the humerus as this would produce an anterior movement of the head of the humerus in the glenoid cavity during mobilization. In fact there are times when the anterior movement should be incorporated with the techniques. This is when glenohumeral flexion is stiff and the head of the humerus needs to be pushed longitudinally or anteriorly to aid gaining improvement in flexion range. Also it may be used when it is desirable to reproduce pain and the addition of the anterior movement does achieve this.

Grade III***

Method

Patients with stiff shoulders will have the same starting position and methods for grade III as described above for grade II, with the physiotherapist's thigh providing the stop at the limit of the range. When the range is only minimally limited, the physiotherapist stands in the same position but uses the treatment couch, not her leg, to provide the

stop. When a III+ movement is used and the range of movement is good, the physiotherapist stands to the left of the patient's head and grasps his right forearm just proximal to the wrist (Figure 10.20(a)). With this grasp she oscillates his arm in the chosen position, through an amplitude of approximately 30°.

If a greater range of flexion is possible, such as with a generally hypermobile person, the physiotherapist places her left hand under his right scapula to raise his shoulder, while controlling the mobilization with her right hand (Figure 10.20(b)).

The incorporation of medial or lateral rotation can be used, as indicated by assessment and examination, to assist improvement of range (when it is stiff in the particular direction) or to reproduce pain.

Grade IV***

Starting position

The starting position is the same as that adopted to find the quadrant position (see Figure 10.10). The physiotherapist's nearside arm supports under the upper rib-angles to raise the shoulder while she holds the patient's elbow in her left hand in a manner which controls a degree of medial rotation.

Method

A firm grasp of the patient's elbow is necessary when the movement is performed at the limit of range in small amplitudes. The mobilization should be performed as an oscillatory movement of 5° or

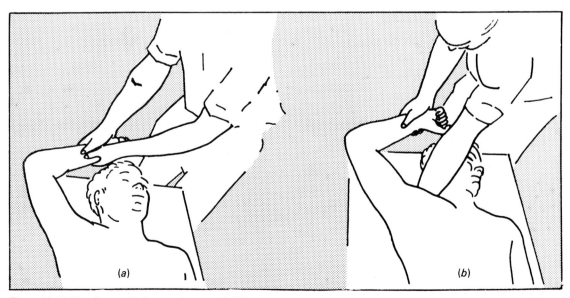

Figure 10.20 Glenohumeral joint; quadrant, grade III

less (Figure 10.10) rather than as a sustained stretch. However, at times, the movement is so small and so slow that it resembles a sustained stretch. This is especially so when muscle spasm restricts the range.

As described for grade III, there are occasions when the physical findings indicate that rotation should be used in conjunction with flexion. When this is necessary, the patient's wrist does not traverse the same amplitude as the elbow, but is controlled so as to rotate the shaft of the humerus to the limit of the range at the moment when full flexion is reached. This can be done with medial or lateral rotation.

Abduction

Abduction is not as commonly used in treatment as is flexion. However, when other mobilizations produce only slow progress the usefulness of abduction as a treatment technique must be assessed.

Grade II**

Starting position

The physiotherapist stands by the patient's right shoulder facing his feet. She cups the web of her left thumb and index finger over his shoulder medial to the acromion process, her fingers extending over the scapula and her thumb extending forwards over the clavicle, or she uses the heel of her hand over the acromioclavicular area. With her right hand she reaches around his forearm to grasp his elbow from the medial side so that his right forearm is supported by her forearm. She stabilizes his shoulder with her left hand while she abducts his arm to the chosen angle. Her thigh, in contact with the lateral surface of his elbow, provides the stop for the movement (Figure 10.21(a)).

Alternative starting positions

The physiotherapist can hold the patient's right forearm by grasping proximal to his wrist. Her index finger extends along the anterior surface of the forearm, her other fingers around the medial border and her thumb around the lateral border. The position requires a tight grasp with the right hand and this may hinder relaxation. The choice of position is guided entirely by the ease with which a relaxed movement can be produced (Figure 10.21(b)).

Method

The patient's arm is moved from adduction until the physiotherapist's thigh stops further abduction. The movement is oscillated back and forth in the amplitude dictated by the patient's signs, usually through an arc of 20° or more. Some patients find it easier to relax their arm as it is moved, pendulum fashion, with the forearm grasp rather than with support under the elbow. The physiotherapist's left hand should be comfortably positioned and maintain an unchanging pressure against the acromion process.

Grade III**

The only variation from the foregoing procedure is that the therapist must hold more firmly with her left

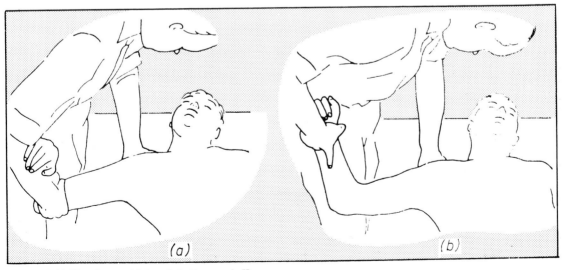

Figure 10.21 Glenohumeral joint; abduction, grade II

hand to stabilize the shoulder girdle when the abduction movement is taken to the limit of the range. This pressure should be constant, rather than being increased in such a way as to serve as an equal and opposite counterpressure at the limit of the abduction. It is not possible to produce grade III movement with the forearm grasp; instead the support must be given under the elbow.

Grade IV

Starting position

When the range is limited and firm stretching mobilizations are required, the therapist changes her position to stand beyond the patient's elbow and faces his shoulder; a straight line from the patient's shoulder to the centre of the therapist's pelvis should pass slightly lateral to the shaft of the humerus when it is abducted to the desired position.

She then crouches over the patient's arm, places her left hand over the acromion process and her right hand under the patient's elbow. This technique can be used to stretch tight structures between the humerus and the scapula on the one hand, and on the other, to emphasize the downward movement of the head of the humerus in the glenoid cavity, a normal action which takes place during abduction of the normal shoulder. If the therapist places her left hand over the acromion process the technique will stretch the structures between the humerus and the scapula. An important change in the technique is made if she places her left hand over the head of the humerus immediately adjacent to the lateral border of the acromion process. Under these circumstances, during abduction of the shoulder, pressure from her left hand will encourage downward movement of the head of the humerus in the glenoid. Her forearms should be positioned in the coronal plane pointing in opposite directions (Figure 10.22). This is glenohumeral abduction combined with longitudinal movement caudad.

Method

The therapist's right arm produces small-amplitude oscillations (2° or 3°) while her left hand maintains a constant pressure against the acromion process. The pressure of the left hand does not increase as the arm reaches the limit of abduction to give an equal and opposite counterpressure, but rather allows the shoulder girdle to rise a limited amount as this allows for better relaxation.

The counterpressure of the therapist's left hand can be on the head of the humerus rather than on the acromion process. When this method is used during the abduction movement the pressure of the left hand on the head of the humerus is an equal and opposite counterpressure so as to push the head of the humerus downwards in the glenoid cavity. This longitudinal movement caudad is described separately on page 150, Figure 10.36.

Abduction with compression***

The technique has two 'starting positions' depending upon whether the abduction is performed below 45–50°, or beyond.

Starting position (0°–50°)

The patient lies supine adjacent to his right hand edge of the table. The physiotherapist grasps his right elbow with her right hand and supports them near the right mid-groin area.

She places the cupped palm of her left hand against the head of the humerus with her fingers pointing medially over his acromioclavicular area (Figure 10.23).

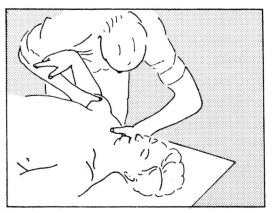

Figure 10.22 Glenohumeral joint; abduction, grade IV

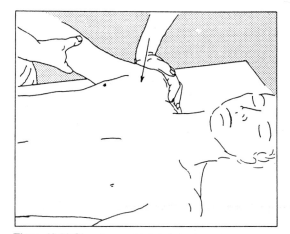

Figure 10.23 Glenohumeral joint abduction with compression 0° to 50°

Method

The therapist applies pressure against the head of the humerus with her left hand to compress the glenohumeral joint surfaces together. This pressure is maintained during the abduction which is produced by a pivoting action of her pelvis on her feet. The supporting position for his elbow enables her to make the pivoting action a single-unit-movement of her right hand and pelvis, and his elbow.

Movements of small amplitude can be performed in any part of the 50° range, or it can be abducted and adducted through the full 50°.

Starting position (50° +)

This is essentially the same as that used for 0°–50° except that more slack needs to be taken up as she firmly adjusts the position of his elbow in her mid-groin: she needs to be in a position to apply pressure through his elbow along the shaft of his humerus (Figure 10.24).

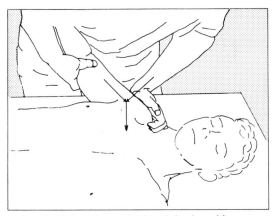

Figure 10.24 Glenohumeral joint; abduction with compression 50°

Method

She pivots her pelvis producing abduction and at the same time she applies pressure along the shaft of his humerus with her right groin in conjunction with her left arm pressure against the head of his humerus. These two directions of pressure are two vectors that combine to compress the articular surface of the head of the humerus into the glenoid cavity.

As stated above, small areas of movement can be utilized or the movement may be performed as a large amplitude of abduction from 50° followed by an adduction return.

Both techniques should be performed slowly if control of the compression during the movement is to be controlled.

Locking position***
Starting position

When the locking position described on page 134 is the only limited movement, the starting position is reached in the same way as that described on that page.

Method

The mobilization consists of either an oscillatory abduction movement or a semicircular movement of the elbow. The dome of the semicircle faces superiorly and the movement is performed as if to scour out the position where the humerus should become locked. The semicircular movement of the elbow is depicted by the double-headed arrow in Figure 10.25.

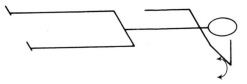

Figure 10.25 Glenohumeral joint; locking position scouring

Lateral rotation**

Because lateral rotation (of the shaft of the humerus) is not commonly used when pain is dominant, grades I and II− are rarely used. Very strong pressures should be used with great care because of its leverage and torsional stress. Grade II is occasionally used and grades II+ and III− are frequently used.

There is one time when lateral rotation is used in conjunction with medial rotation. This is when pain is the dominant factor and the treatment techniques being used are the accessory movements while the joint is positioned in a neutral-mid-pain-free position. Although rotation is not an accessory movement, nevertheless it can be used as an oscillatory medial/lateral rotation of 15–30° positioned as for the accessory movements.

The rotary movement can be performed with the humerus in adduction by the patient's side, in abduction, or in any position between these two limits as dictated by the most painful position or the position exhibiting the greatest limitation.

Grades II+ and III−**

Grades II+ and III− differ only slightly in their end positions when treating pain, with III− being slightly deeper in the range than II+, and reaching the first part of resistance. They can therefore be described together.

Starting position

The therapist stands by the patient's abducted right arm, facing his feet. She cups her left hand laterally around his upper arm near the elbow with her fingers supporting posteriorly and her thumb anteriorly. She positions her left forearm as a stop to prevent his right forearm going further into lateral rotation than the selected range. With her right hand she grasps his slightly pronated wrist, spreading her fingers across his wrist and distal forearm anteriorly while her thumb grasps the back of his wrist (Figure 10.26).

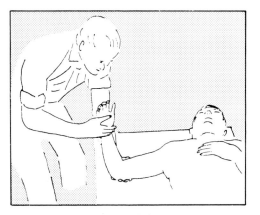

Figure 10.26 Glenohumeral joint; lateral rotation

Method

The oscillatory movement is produced by a to-and-fro movement of the therapist's right hand through approximately 30° around the arc of a circle, the centre of which is his elbow. The movement is taken up to the stop provided by her left forearm. It is important that the patient's wrist should be relaxed during the movement as this will assist relaxation of his shoulder. Her cup-like grasp around his upper arm should be loose, permitting a free rotary movement while at the same time providing a stable pivot point.

If a more vigorous movement is desired, the starting position should be changed to provide greater stability.

Starting position**

The therapist stands beyond the patient's right shoulder. His abducted upper arm is supported in her left hand around the anterior and lateral surfaces of the humerus near the elbow, the point of his elbow extending beyond the edge of the couch. She uses her right thigh, appropriately placed, to form the stop at the limit of the range. She grasps his

right wrist with her index and middle fingers spreading proximally over his pronated wrist anteriorly while grasping through the first interosseous space with her thumb. Her remaining fingers spread around the ulnar border of his hand to reach the dorsum (Figure 10.27).

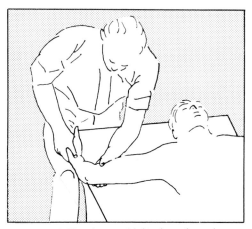

Figure 10.27 Glenohumeral joint; lateral rotation

Method

In this position she can comfortably stabilize around the lower end of his upper arm to form the pivot for the rotation. The rotation is produced through a stable grasp of his wrist pivoting around her grasp of his upper arm. This position aids relaxation because the arm is fully supported, and the firm stop assures the patient that the movement will not be taken beyond the comfortable limit.

Medial rotation***

Medial rotation is usefully employed in movements ranging from grade II with the arm either by the side or in abduction, to grade IV movements in the functional position with the arm behind the back.

With grade II movements oscillating between medial and lateral rotation (see Figure 10.26) through an arc of approximately 25° (plus or minus), the technique forms an essential component for the treatment of pain by accessory movements as described in Chapter 7. It may be performed in various positions of glenohumeral abduction so as to either avoid provoking pain or deliberately wishing to do so as a through-range technique.

Grade II**
Starting position

The therapist stands by the patient's right hip, facing his head. After abducting his arm, she supports

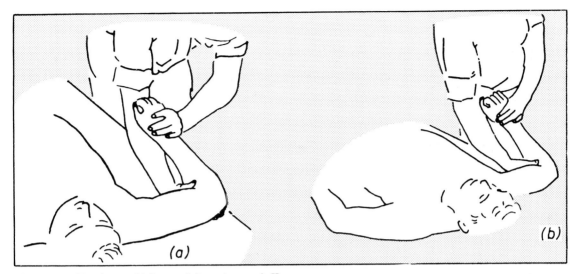

Figure 10.28 Glenohumeral joint; medial rotation, grade II

under the distal end of his humerus with the fingers of her right hand and cups her thumb anteriorly. She grasps over the back of his hand with her left hand, her fingers spreading across the back of his wrist and her thumb grasping anteriorly. When his arm is medially rotated the anterior surface of his forearm contacts the anterior surface of her right forearm to prevent the medial rotation exceeding an established range. She can raise or lower her forearm as necessary (Figure 10.28(a)).

The therapist can use her right thigh to form the stop instead of her right forearm by standing lateral to the patient's arm (Figure 10.28(b)).

Method

The oscillation is produced by the therapist's relaxed grasp of the patient's hand. She extends his wrist slightly as the treatment movement of his forearm reaches the stop provided by her forearm or thigh. Her grasp of his upper arm in her right hand should not be tight, but allow freedom of movement. If the shoulder girdle is not prevented from lifting, it provides a visual assessment of glenohumeral rotation and permits the patient a certain freedom to move if the treatment movement becomes painful.

Grade IV**

Grade IV is not a grade of movement to be used over-enthusiastically, but, as it has a place in treatment, it must be described. When this grade of movement is desired the shoulder girdle must be firmly stabilized.

Starting position

The therapist stands away from the right side of the patient's head facing his feet. She crouches over his right arm, abducted to the chosen range, and supports under his elbow with the fingers of her left hand from the medial side cupping her thumb anteriorly over his biceps tendon. His upper arm rests on the couch with his elbow beyond the edge. She places her left upper arm in front of and just medial to his shoulder. With her right hand she holds his pronated wrist grasping around the ulnar border, her fingers covering the anterior surface of his wrist and adjacent palm and her thenar eminence and thumb, pointing caudally, holding over the posterior surface of his wrist (Figure 10.29).

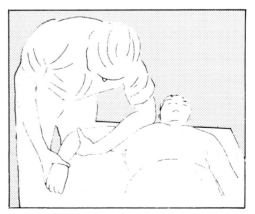

Figure 10.29 Glenohumeral joint; medial rotation, grade IV

Method

The small-amplitude rotary oscillations of approximately 10° are performed by the therapist's right hand on the patient's right wrist at that point in the range which makes the patient's shoulder girdle lift. She limits the lifting of his right shoulder with her left upper arm which moves with the shoulder, providing only enough counterpressure to prevent it lifting too far. With her left hand she prevents his arm drifting into adduction. When the arm requires treatment in this position the movement is usually grade IV.

Hand behind back***

The hand behind the back position, which is functionally very important, is dependent upon medial rotation, extension and, to some extent, adduction. When the arm requires treatment in this position, the movement is usually grade IV. It is not used as a grade I or II movement but can usefully be used as a small amplitude grade III or III− movement alternated with grade IV or IV+.

Starting position**

For movement of the right shoulder the patient lies prone, turned slightly towards his right with his right arm behind his back and the physiotherapist stands behind him:

1. If medial rotation is the component desired, she reaches across to support his elbow with her left hand by grasping posteriorly around the distal part of his upper arm. With her right hand she holds his wrist, her fingers across the posterior surface and her thumb anteriorly (Figure 10.30(a)).
2. If extension is the desired movement, she stabilizes the posterior surface of his scapula in the region of the inferior angle with her left hand and supports under his distal forearm with her right hand (Figure 10.30(b)). She may need to hold his lateral epidondyle in her right hand so as to produce the extension without including any medial rotation.
3. When adduction is the movement desired, she stabilizes his scapula with her left thumb against the medial border inferiorly, and her fingers spread across the adjacent surface of the scapula. With her right hand she grasps around the patient's upper forearm (Figure 10.30(c)). Again, she may need to grasp his elbow to adduct his arm.

Method

In all three of the above positions the small oscillatory movement of the glenohumeral joint is produced by the physiotherapist's right hand. Thus the movement is produced via movement of the humerus. However, the movement can also be produced by stabilizing the humerus and moving the scapula. The adduction movement is achieved by a lateral movement of the inferior angle of the scapula (see left thumb in Figure 10.30(c)). This movement is produced by her left arm acting through her left thumb against the medial border of the scapula near the inferior angle. To produce glenohumeral extension via the moving of the scapula, its inferior angle is moved posteranteriorly by her left hand (see left hand in Figure 10.30(b)).

Although the movements of medial rotation, extension and adduction have been described separately they can be used in any combination. The choice of the combination is guided by the signs found on examination or by the progress achieved with the individual movements. The most painful or restricted direction is the one usually chosen.

Horizontal flexion*

Horizontal flexion is another movement that is not used often in treatment as a technique on its own. However, it is usually incorporated in treatment when movements in several directions are used, as for a stiff glenohumeral joint, or when the movement relates to an acromioclavicular disorder.

Assessment of its value as a solo technique may be necessary if treatment using other movements is not making adequate progress or if horizontal flexion is the main limitation of movement.

Grades II and III***
Starting position

The physiotherapist stands by the patient's left shoulder, facing his right shoulder. She holds his wrist and adjacent forearm with her right hand with his elbow and shoulder flexed 90°. With her left arm she reaches across the patient and grasps the lateral border of his scapula so that her thenar eminence and thumb extend into his axilla overlying the anterior surface of the lateral border of the scapula. Her fingers extend around the lateral margin of the scapula to its posterior surface.

To permit as much freedom in horizontal flexion as possible his arm is positioned midway between medial and lateral glenohumeral rotation. It is only possible to provide a stop for this movement by positioning her body to prevent his right hand continuing its movement (Figure 10.31).

Method

Because horizontal flexion is a difficult movement to perform smoothly in large amplitudes, more care

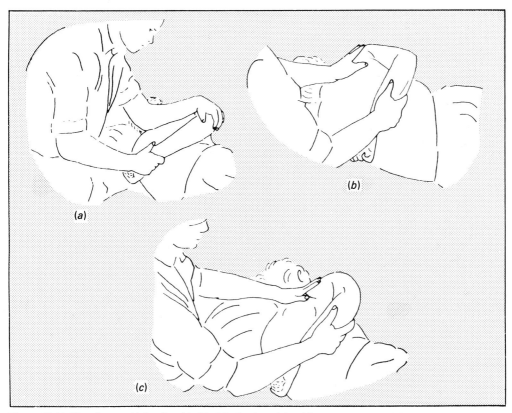

Figure 10.30 Glenohumeral joint; hand behind the back position (*a*) medial rotation; (*b*) extension; (*c*) adduction

than usual is required. The therapist performs it with her right arm while her left hand stabilizes his scapula.

Grade IV**

This grade requires quite a different technique from that used for grades II and III.

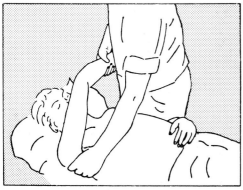

Figure 10.31 Glenohumeral joint; horizontal flexion, grades II and III

Starting position

The therapist stands by the patient's right shoulder facing across his body and places the heel of her left hand under the *medial border* of his right scapula at the level of the spine of the scapula. While holding his right wrist in her right hand, she flexes his elbow and shoulder and carries his arm across into horizontal flexion. She then leans across the patient and places his elbow and adjacent forearm into her right anterior axillary wall. His arm, positioned midway between medial and lateral glenohumeral rotation, is horizontally flexed further until scapular protraction is complete. She then ensures that her left hand position against the medial border of his scapula is correct (Figure 10.32).

Method

The small-amplitude oscillation is produced by the therapist alternately increasing and decreasing her pressure against the patient's upper arm. This pressure is transmitted to her left hand against the vertebral border of the scapula. The horizontal flexion oscillation can be produced by a two-fold

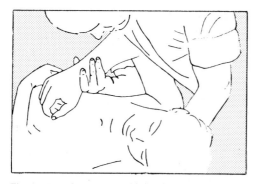

Figure 10.32 Glenohumeral joint; horizontal flexion, grade IV

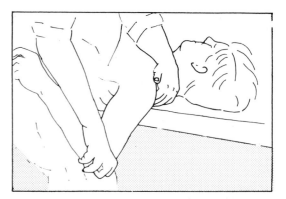

Figure 10.33 Glenohumeral joint; horizontal extension

action. FIRSTLY, the pressure is directed along the line of the shaft of the humerus. This pressure will increase the range of the horizontal flexion because the heel of her left hand will hold the medial border of the scapula against the rib-cage while the lateral border will move posteriorly. SECONDLY, pressure is also exerted against the patient's elbow, but this time the pressure will be directed in a line towards his opposite shoulder. When the technique is used in treatment, the two directions can be used either independently or in conjunction with each other. The choice will depend upon which method produces the strongest horizontal flexion or which of the methods reproduces the patient's symptoms best.

Horizontal extension*

This technique is not often used in treatment but it can be helpful when pain arises from the acromioclavicular joint or when the patient is unable to abduct his arm without bringing it forwards from the frontal plane.

Grade IV*

Starting position

The patient lies on his back with his acromion process at the edge of the couch. The physiotherapist places her fingers under his acromion process to both feel the joint movement and protect the patient against contact with the edge of the couch.

With her other arm she holds around his elbow and stabilizes his forearm against her side or thigh. She then moves the patient's elbow towards the floor so as to produce horizontal extension at the glenohumeral joint (Figure 10.33).

Method

Having taken a patient up to the limit of his horizontal extension the therapist then applies

pressure in this same direction as a small-amplitude oscillatory movement. The degree of abduction of the glenohumeral joint in which this horizontal extension is performed will depend upon the examination findings. If the technique is being used to relieve pain then the degree of abduction chosen would be the one that reproduced the pain. This does not mean that the treatment technique is done in a painful part of that range, but it is done in that direction.

If the technique is aimed at stretching the movement, then the degree of abduction would be the one in which horizontal extension is most limited.

This movement can also be done as a grade II or III movement though it is most commonly performed as a grade IV movement.

Longitudinal movement caudad**

Longitudinal movement is movement of the head of the humerus from the superior extent of the glenoid cavity to its inferior extent. It can be performed with the patient's arm by his side, or with his arm in abduction or flexion in any angle.

Treating pain with the patient's arm by his side will be described first, and this will be followed by the description of the technique being used to increase the range of limited abduction.

Arm-by-side***

The arm-by-side movement can be produced either by the therapist's thumbs on the head of the humerus or by a grasp around the arm. When treating a very painful joint the arm-grasp is better because the head of the humerus is too tender for direct contact. Gentle grade I movements can be very effective in the treatment of very painful glenohumeral joint conditions, and those unaccustomed to using these techniques are usually surprised to find how gently the movement must be performed and how effective the technique then is.

Starting position (grade I)***

The therapist kneels alongside the patient's right elbow. She flexes his elbow and holds his wrist in her right hand while gently hugging his right forearm to her with her right forearm. She places the fingers of her left hand over his upper arm anteriorly with the lateral border of the proximal phalanx of her index finger against the anterior surface of the proximal end of his forearm and her thumb against the lateral surface of the elbow. His right upper arm is lifted fractionally off the couch (Figure 10.34 (see also Figure 7.7, page 76).

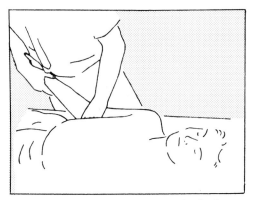

Figure 10.34 Glenohumeral joint; longitudinal movement caudad, arm by side, grades III and IV

Method (grade I)

For grade I movements tiny oscillations are effected by alternating pressures against the patient's forearm through the therapist's index finger. His right upper arm should be held clear of the couch to enable the movement to be free of friction. When extremely gentle techniques are being used it is essential to withdraw the index finger from the patient's forearm far enough to allow the head of the humerus to return to the superior part of the glenoid cavity.

This return movement can be assisted by maintaining the patient's elbow slightly more flexed than a right angle. If the position is maintained it will be natural for the head of the humerus to move upwards in the glenoid cavity once the pressure from the left hand is released.

The degree of elbow flexion is not required for movements that are performed strongly and, in fact, a straighter arm enables the physiotherapist's right hand to assist the longitudinal movement. For this technique she stands alongside the patient, not kneels (Figure 10.34).

Starting position (grades II–IV)**

Grades II, III and IV are performed with very similar starting positions with the variations in amplitude and depth of range being controlled by the physiotherapist.

When direct pressure is used against the head of the humerus the physiotherapist stands beyond the patient's head at the right side and places the pads of her thumbs against the head of the humerus immediately adjacent to the anterior and lateral borders of the acromion process so that caudad movement of the head of the humerus can be felt in relation to them. The fingers of her left hand are spread over the scapular area while the fingers of her right hand spread laterally over the deltoid (Figure 10.35). When it is necessary to avoid pain, as for grade I treatment of pain, the patient's arm is fully supported in a pain-free neutral position.

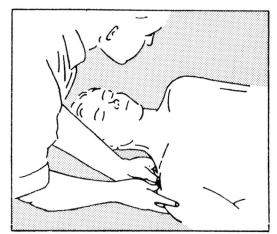

Figure 10.35 Glenohumeral joint; longitudinal movement caudad, arm by side, grades II, III and IV

Method (grades II–IV)

To make the technique more comfortable for the patient, and to enable the therapist to feel the movement of the head of the humerus in relation to the acromion process, the oscillatory movement is produced by the therapist's arm, not by the intrinsic muscles of the thumbs. It is also necessary to use the middle of the pad of the thumb rather than its tip.

In abduction***

The abduction technique is used only when the joint condition requires movement ranging from II+ to IV+.

Starting position

The physiotherapist stands by the patient's right shoulder facing across his body. She abducts his right arm with her right hand while supporting his elbow at a right angle. She supports the distal end of his upper arm medially and posteriorly with the fingers of her right hand while her thumb extends anteriorly around his elbow holding it against her side. Her wrist rests against the anteromedial surface of his forearm and his forearm is supported by her right forearm. The heel of her left hand is placed against the head of his humerus immediately adjacent to the acromion process and her fingers spread over his shoulder towards his neck. For stronger techniques it is necessary to crouch over the patient's arm so that her left forearm, directed caudally, lies in the coronal plane (Figure 10.36).

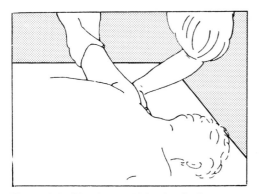

Figure 10.36 Glenohumeral joint; longitudinal movement caudad in abduction

Method

The movement is produced entirely by the pressure of the physiotherapist's left hand against the head of the humerus.

The movement can be performed in three different ways for three different reasons:

1. The first is that as she exerts pressure against the head of the humerus, moving it towards the patient's feet, she can carry his elbow so that the elbow moves as far longitudinally as does the shoulder girdle. This method is used when a maximum range of longitudinal movement is required and pain-response does not inhibit its use. Such is the case in moderately chronic intra-articular disorders or when 'through-range-pain' responses are found when examining active and passive movements.
2. The reason for the second method is the same as the first except that the quality of the pain (e.g. irritability) indicates that the technique must not be painful. This is achieved by carrying the elbow FURTHER distally than the head of the humerus.
3. Thirdly, she can hold his elbow stationary while applying longitudinal movement to the head of

the humerus. This latter technique results in longitudinal movement of the head of the humerus in the glenoid cavity combined with a small degree of abduction of the glenohumeral joint brought about by keeping the elbow stationary.

The amount of movement of the head of the humerus can be felt in relation to the stationary acromion process.

In abduction prone**

The abduction prone technique for this movement has the advantage of stabilizing the patient's arm more firmly and leaving the physiotherapist's two hands free both to control and feel the amount of accessory movement available in the joint.

Starting position

The patient lies prone with his arm abducted and laterally rotated. If the joint range is limited the patient will need to lie more on his left side so that his shoulder will not be horizontally extended. The therapist stands by the right side of his head facing his feet. She places her two thumbs against the head of the humerus immediately adjacent to the acromion process with her fingers spread over the anterior deltoid and lateral scapular area. She then directs her arms caudally in line with the longitudinal movement of the head of the humerus (Figure 10.37). She can use her cupped hand over the head

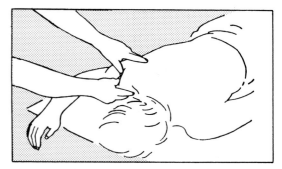

Figure 10.37 Glenohumeral joint; longitudinal movement caudad in abduction prone

of the humerus to produced the caudad movement, or she may use the web of the first interosseous space of each hand, each adjacent to each other and the acromion process.

Method

The oscillatory movement is produced from the therapist's body and arms acting through her thumbs. It must not be produced by her thumb flexors. If gentle movements are required, the point of contact should be through the tips of the thumbs. As stronger movements are desired more of the pad should be brought into contact with the head of the humerus or the hands may be used, as stated above.

In 90° flexion***

The movement in flexion is usually only required as one of a number of techniques used to generally mobilize a moderately painful stiff joint.

Starting position

The physiotherapist stands by the patient's right shoulder facing across his body and supports his right arm, flexed to 90° at the shoulder and elbow, with her right arm. She supports his wrist in her right hand, his forearm on her forearm, and his upper arm against her side. The glenohumeral joint is positioned midway between medial and lateral rotation. Her left hand is placed against the head of the humerus just distal to the acromion process with her fingers directed distally. Her thumb extends laterally round his upper arm (Figure 10.38).

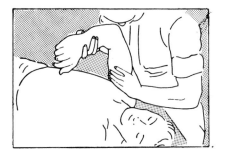

Figure 10.38 Glenohumeral joint; longitudinal movement caudad in 90° flexion

Method

The oscillatory longitudinal movement is produced by pressure against the head of the humerus with the cupped heel of the left hand. The therapist's right hand supports the patient's arm and carries it with the movement so that the angle of flexion at the shoulder is not altered. Alternatively if she holds the elbow stationary a small degree of flexion at the glenohumeral joint will accompany the longitudinal movement as was discussed when the technique is performed in abduction.

In full flexion***

The movement in flexion is of particular use as a grade IV mobilization. It has no place in the treatment of shoulders which are limited in range by pain alone as the pain would be provoked.

Starting position

The physiotherapist stands by the patient's right side beyond his head. She crouches over his shoulder and holds his flexed right arm against her left side. She then places her hands together, behind his deltoid, with the posterior surface of her left index finger against the anterior surface of her right index finger and the two lateral surfaces against the head of the humerus immediately adjacent to the acromion process. Her thumbs extend around the sides of his arm to point towards each other across the axilla. She then has a firm grasp of the upper end of the humerus near the surgical neck (Figure 10.39).

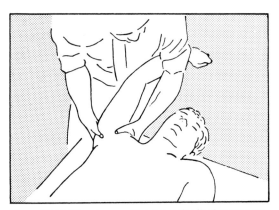

Figure 10.39 Glenohumeral joint; longitudinal movement caudad in full flexion

Method

Before performing the oscillation the therapist applies pressure through the lateral border of her index fingers to take up the slack by raising the shoulder girdle and moving it caudally. Once this slack has been taken up, the oscillation can be performed by alternately increasing and decreasing further pressure to direct the head of the humerus distally in the glenoid cavity.

*Posteroanterior movement***

The posteroanterior movement is one of the most valuable movements in the treatment of extremely painful shoulders. It is not a technique that is hindered by local tenderness as is longitudinal movement. Grade I movements are better produced by direct thumb pressures against the head of the humerus than by using the upper arm as a lever because of the difference in the accuracy of control possible with each method.

Starting position

The patient lies with his elbow flexed and his forearm resting against a pillow(s) on his trunk, and a pillow or blanket should be placed under his elbow. This is to support his forearm so that medial rotation, adduction and extension, are avoided. The position must be adjusted until it is a symptom free position. The therapist kneels laterally and superiorly to the patient's shoulder and positions her two thumbs, back to back, with their tips in contact with the posterior surface of the head of the humerus adjacent to the acromion process and pointing towards the ceiling. The fingers of her left hand are spread over the clavicular area and those of her right hand spread over the deltoid (Figure 10.40).

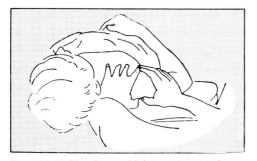

Figure 10.40 Glenohumeral joint; posteroanterior movement

Method

It is of prime importance that the oscillatory movement should be produced by the physiotherapist's arm. If the movement is produced by the thumb flexors the movement becomes uncomfortable for the patient and the physiotherapist loses all feel of movement.

When grades I and II movements are used it is imperative that there should be no pressure against the head of the humerus at the beginning of the movement and that, with each oscillation, the head of the humerus is returned to this relaxed position. As the pressure will be very light the points of the thumbs should be used.

When stronger movements are required (grades III and IV) it is advisable to change the point of contact from the tips of the thumbs to a larger area of the pads.

This anteriorly directed movement of the head of the humerus can be further emphasized by an anteroposterior pressure against the clavicle with the little and ring fingers of the left hand.

Alternative starting position**

When pain is minimal and both accessory and physiological movements are used to mobilize the

joint, it may be more suitable to use the patient's arm as a lever. This change uses a completely different technique.

The physiotherapist stands by the patient's right forearm facing his head. She holds his forearm against her right side and supports under the posterior surface of the head of the humerus with a similar hand grip to that described for 'longitudinal movement caudad in full flexion' (see page 151). The posterior surface of the right hand is placed in the palmar surface of the left hand so that the index fingers overlap and the lateral borders of the index fingers contact the back of the head of the humerus. Her thumbs hold around the humerus to form an encompassing grasp. She may need to crouch if she chooses to position his upper arm in the coronal plane (Figure 10.41). It is most commonly positioned in a small degree of abduction.

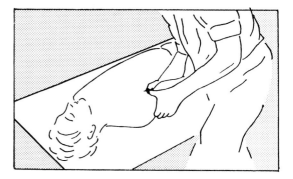

Figure 10.41 Glenohumeral joint; posteroanterior movement (alternative position)

Method

The slack of scapular movement is taken up by lifting the head of the humerus so that any further oscillatory movement will be associated with the posteroanterior glenohumeral movement. Grade III+ movements are performed like a flick, allowing the shoulder girdle to drop an inch or two before countering it with a posteroanterior pressure returning it through the same few inches. The direction of the posteroanterior movement is parallel to the inferior surface of the acromion process. A grade IV+ mobilization is a sustained oscillatory mobilization of small amplitude at the limit of the range.

In abduction***

Treatment in the abduction position is used as grades III or IV when pain is not severe and restoration of range is the primary factor. It is used to restore an accessory movement range which should result in improvement of a physiological range.

Starting position

The physiotherapist stands away from the patient's right shoulder facing across his body. His straight arm is abducted and stabilized by holding his forearm against her right side. The grasp is the same as that described for Figure 10.41 (Figure 10.42).

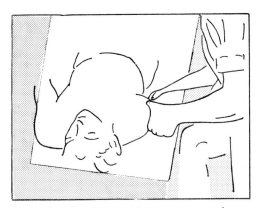

Figure 10.42 Glenohumeral joint; posteroanterior movement in abduction

Method

The movements for grade III and grade IV are performed in an identical manner to that described for producing posteroanterior movements using the patient's arms as a lever (see page 152). Care must be exercised when taking up the slack of scapulothoracic movement.

In abduction prone**

This alternative position provides a greater feel for grade IV movements and leaves the therapist free to use both hands to control the accessory movement.

Starting position

The patient lies prone with his arm abducted and laterally rotated. If the joint range is limited the patient will need to turn slightly towards his right so that his shoulder will not be extended. The therapist stands by his right shoulder facing across his body and places the pads of both thumbs against the posterior surface of the head of the humerus immediately adjacent to the acromion process. She then directs her arms in a posteroanterior direction with her shoulders positioned immediately above the direction of the movement (Figure 10.43).

As with longitudinal movement caudad, the movement can be performed using either the cupped palm of the hand or the web of the first interosseous space of both hands.

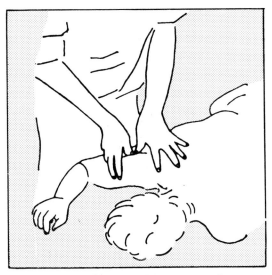

Figure 10.43 Glenohumeral joint; posteroanterior movement in abduction prone

Method

The mobilization is produced by the physiotherapist's arms acting through a spring-like section of the thumbs. The flexors of the thumbs must not produce the movement because the technique then becomes uncomfortable and the thumbs will not be able to appreciate small glenohumeral movements.

In full flexion***

This movement is of particular use as a grade IV mobilization; it has no place in the treatment of very painful shoulder conditions. The starting position is identical with that described for 'longitudinal movement in full flexion' (see page 151). The difference in the method lies in the direction of the oscillation; the head of the humerus is directed anteriorly in the glenoid cavity, not longitudinally.

Anteroposterior movement**
Arm-by-side**

This anteroposterior movement is not as useful as 'longitudinal movement' or 'posteroanterior movement' in the treatment of very painful shoulders. Its main application in treatment lies more in grades III and IV when the joint is stiff and moderately painful.

Starting position

The physiotherapist stands by the patient's right upper arm facing across his body. With the fingers of her right hand she supports the lower end of his humerus posteriorly from the medial side and then rests his forearm on her forearm. She raises his upper arm approximately 20° anteriorly to the coronal plane of the trunk so that the head of the humerus will not impinge against the inferior surface of the acromion process posteriorly.

This position also allows a better anteroposterior movement of the head of the humerus in the glenoid. She places the cupped heel of her left hand anteriorly over the head of the humerus, with her fingers extending superiorly and posteriorly over the acromion process (Figure 10.44).

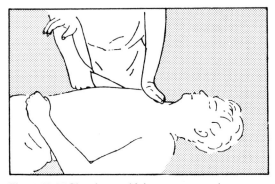

Figure 10.44 Glenohumeral joint; anteroposterior movement arm by side

Method

The anteroposterior oscillation is produced by pressure of the cupped heel of her left hand against the head of the humerus. Her fingers, cupped loosely around the acromion process, do not apply any pressure, but assist in feeling the movement. Different degrees of pressure are required for different grades of movement and greater recoil is permitted for the larger amplitudes.

In abduction***

This movement is only applicable when treatment requires grades III and IV movements.

Starting position

The physiotherapist stands by the patient's right shoulder, facing his feet. She supports the distal end of his humerus posteriorly from the medial side with her right hand, abducts his arm then rests his flexed forearm on her forearm. She places the cupped heel of her left hand anteriorly against the head of the humerus, with her fingers extending medially across the adjacent clavicular area (Figure 10.45).

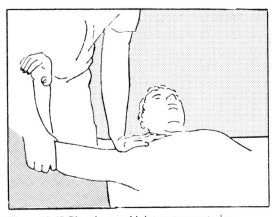

Figure 10.45 Glenohumeral joint; anteroposterior movement in abduction

Method

The oscillatory movement is produced by pressure against the head of the humerus with her left hand.

It may be found that the anteroposterior movement is more effective in different degrees of glenohumeral flexion/extension or horizontal flexion. Anteroposterior movement in the different positions in this horizontal plane should be assessed to find the stiffest or most painful part of the movement before using the technique as a mobilization. This searching for the relevant sign is used with all techniques and is fundamental to effective treatment.

In horizontal flexion**

The horizontal flexion position is only used when general mobilization is being employed for a stiff joint. Only grades III and IV therefore are likely to be used. The starting position is similar to that described for horizontal flexion. The difference is that the humerus is vertical and the hand under the scapula is placed laterally near the posterior rim of the glenoid fossa. The anteroposterior movement is produced by pressure directed down the shaft of the humerus.

Lateral movement

As with all passive accessory movement (except longitudinal movement and posteroanterior movement with the arm by the side), this technique has its main value in the restoration of range rather than in the treatment of the very painful joint which the patient is unable to move because of pain. It is therefore one of many accessory movements used in combination with others in treatment. The movement is performed in two basic positions; one with the arm by the side and the other with the arm in 90° of flexion.

Arm-by-side***
Starting position

The physiotherapist stands by the patient's right side distal to his flexed elbow facing his head. She places her right hand as high as possible to his axilla with the distal aspect of her palm in contact with the medial surface of his humerus. Her fingers spread posteriorly around his arm while her thumb crosses the anterior deltoid. Her left hand supports his elbow, the palm of her hand against the lateral surface of the joint and her fingers supporting posteriorly. She then crouches over his arm so that her forearms can be directed opposite each other in as near the coronal plane as possible (Figure 10.46).

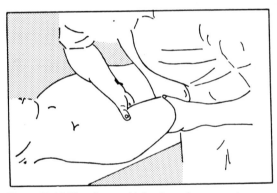

Figure 10.46 Glenohumeral joint; lateral movement arm by side

Method

The mobilization is effected by pressure through her right hand against the upper end of the humerus. If a grade III movement is desired, her pressure must be almost completely released at the end of each oscillation. During grade IV movements, however, some pressure is maintained throughout the technique while an increase and decrease of this pressure produces the oscillation.

In flexion**
Starting position

The physiotherapist stands distal to the patient's right shoulder, facing his head. She grasps the distal end of his upper arm laterally with the fingers of her left hand across the biceps and her thumb across the triceps. With this grasp she flexes his glenohumeral joint 90° allowing his elbow to relax comfortably in flexion. She places her right hand against the medial surface of the upper end of his humerus, high in the axilla, with her fingers and thumb spreading anteriorly. By crouching over his arm she can point her forearm in opposite directions in the horizontal and coronal planes (Figure 10.47).

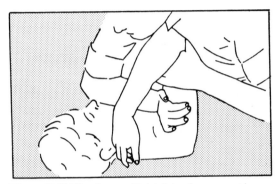

Figure 10.47 Glenohumeral joint; lateral movement in flexion

Method

Movements are produced by her right arm while her left hand either stabilizes the position of his humerus in relation to the scapula by following the movement of the head of the humerus, or it does the opposite by moving the elbow medially. The choice depends on the pain or stiffness found on examination of the movement and the intention to relieve pain or stretch stiffness. This principle of the elbow *following* the humeral head movement equally, or moving further, or in the opposite direction, is the same as has been described for 'longitudinal movement caudad in abduction' (see page 150).

Acromiohumeral joint

This joint space includes the sub-acromial bursa and the supra-spinatus tendon, and as a joint, it moves, whenever the glenohumeral joint moves. This being so, all of the techniques described for the glenohumeral joint (with the exception of 'abduction with compression') apply equally to the acromiohumeral joint.

Differentiation tests

There is one set of techniques that differentiate symptoms that can be provoked by upper arm movements as arising from it (the acromiohumeral structures) rather than the glenohumeral joint. The differentiating procedure is to perform the provoking movement (abduction/adduction, rotations, flexion/extension, horizontal flexion/extension and the accessory movements):

1. Firstly performing it such that it provokes the positive symptomatic signs.

2. Repeating it with a degree of 'longitudinal movement caudad' being sustained so as to keep the humerus away from the inferior surface of the acromion process – pain response is less if the acromiohumeral joint is affected.

3. Repeating it with the acromiohumeral joint compressed – pain response increases if the acromiohumeral joint is affected. This technique will be described.

The differentiating is shown in Appendix 2 Series 4. Photographs S4.1–S4.6 relate to the glenohumeral joint, and S4.7–S4.12 relate to the acromiohumeral joint.

A painful arc of pain during flexion or abduction, even when lowered eccentrically, is a common finding. With the patient lying supine, this arc can be reproduced by resisted movement, especially abduction. To differentiate between supraspinatus tendonitis and the acromiohumeral joint the isometric abduction contraction should be painful whether the head of the humerus is held caudad away from the acromion process or not.

Table 10.2 Acromiohumeral joint – objective examination

The routine examination of this joint must include examination of the acromioclavicular joint and the glenohumeral joint.
 	
HIGHLIGHT MAIN FINDINGS WITH ASTERISKS AS YOU GO
 	
Observation
 	
*Functional demonstration/tests
As applicable
 	
1. *Their* demonstration of *their* Functional movements affected by *their* disorder.
2. Differentiation of *their* demonstrated functional movement(s).
 	
Brief appraisal
Active movements (Move to PAIN or move to LIMIT)
 	
Isometric tests
Other structures in 'plan'
Thoracic outlet
 	
Passive movements (supine)
Test movements 1–3 below should:
(a) Reproduce the symptoms when the humerus is compressed against the inferior surface of the acromion process compared with
(b) Being painless when the head of the humerus is distracted caudad from the acromion process.
 	
1. Oscillatory Abd (from 20° to 50°).
2. Oscillatory F/E, (from 0° to 30°) in slight abd.
3. Oscillatory Rot, in slight abd (30° arc in mid-range).
 	
Differentiation tests (supine)
Differentiating A/H joint:
	1. From rotator cuff. It is A/H if:
	   (a) Isometric 30° abd reproduces symptoms.
	   (b) There is no pain with oscillatory abd at 30° if A/H joint is distracted caudad.
	2. From G/H joint. Oscillatory abd (from 20° to 40°). It is A/H if:
	   (a) Painful when A/H surfaces compressed and moved.
	   (b) Painless when A/H distracted caudad and moved.
	   (c) Painless when G/H compressed and A/H distracted during movement.
	3. From A/C joint. It is A/H if:
	   (a) HF, negative.
	   (b) (↓) clavicular head negative.
	   (c) (→→) caud on acromion or clavicular head: (i) reproduce pain when A/H surface compressed (A/C movement nil); (ii) are painless when A/H surfaces distracted while A/C movement is produced.
	Note range, pain, resistance, spasm and behaviour
	
	As applicable
	1. Canal's Slump tests.
	2. Differentiation tests.
	3. ULTT.
	
	Palpation
	As previously
	+When 'comparable signs' ill defined reassess 'injuring movement'.
	
	Check case records etc.
	
	Instructions to patient
	1. Warning of possible exacerbation.
	2. Request to record details.
	3. Instruction re 'joint care' if required.

Swelling of the bursa can be palpated anterior to the acromion process or posterior to it.

The site of pain is usually local, rarely referred.

Detailed objective examination is given in Table 10.2 and includes the tests for the whole shoulder complex. All of the mobile joints associated with movements of the shoulder girdle must be examined and then the differentiation tests performed to implicate the acromiohumeral joint. The test movements involving the 'quadrant' (and 'rolling-over') and 'locking position' must be clear if the acromiohumeral joint is not causing symptoms.

Techniques

The movements which can be performed that affect the acromiohumeral joint are flexion/extension, abduction/adduction, rotations, anteroposterior and posteroanterior movements, lateral/medial movements and longitudinal movement cephalad/caudad. They have already been described for the glenohumeral joint. However one of the techniques, a combined movement technique, is a little more awkward to perform, and is therefore described.

Rotation with compression***
Starting position

The patient lies supine with his body near the right side of the table. The physiotherapist faces across his upper body from right to left. She holds his right elbow in her right hand with them being comfortably and stably supported in her right groin or against her right thigh. His right hand is firmly supported between her right upper arm and her right side. Her left hand is placed over his acromion process with her fingers pointing posteriorly. Her left elbow is kept away from her trunk so as to enable the caudad pressure to be exerted through her left hand (see Figure 10.48).

Method

To perform a mid range medial/lateral rotation she tilts her trunk to her right (his humeral shaft is then somewhat medially rotated (Figure 10.48(a)) and then smoothly laterally flexes her trunk to the left. With this movement to the left she carries his forearm with her trunk producing a lateral rotation of the humeral shaft (Figure 10.48(b)). His elbow is kept stationary by her right hand and thigh/groin, while the compression of the acromiohumeral space is maintained by an equal and opposite pressure being exerted between her right hand/thigh/groin and her left hand.

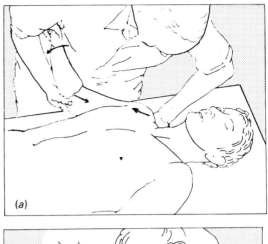

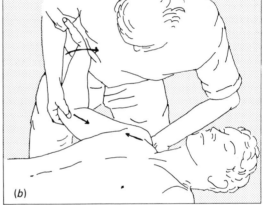

Figure 10.48 Rotation with compression (*a*) medially; (*b*) laterally

Acromioclavicular joint

The movements described later for the scapulothoracic movements all involve movement of the acromioclavicular joint and therefore must be examined. The acromiohumeral joint, because of its close proximity, should also be assessed (Table 10.3). It is surprising, however, how infrequently these scapulothoracic movements reproduce acromioclavicular joint pain. However, pain is readily reproduced during horizontal flexion (the main physiological test), horizontal extension, and flexion. Flexion of the glenohumeral joint is a technique often used in the treatment of the acromioclavicular joint. Other techniques that are more localized to the acromioclavicular joint remain to be described. One such technique involves moving the spine of the scapula and the clavicle towards each other. The remainder involve direct pressure (posteriorly, anteriorly, inferiorly (longitudinal caudad), superiorly, and rotary) against the acromial end of the

Table 10.3 Acromioclavicular joint – objective examination

When examining the acromioclavicular joint (A/C), the G/H, A/H joints or S/Th movements must be examined.

HIGHLIGHT MAIN FINDINGS WITH ASTERISKS AS YOU GO

Observation

*Functional demonstration/tests

1. *Their* demonstration of *their* functional movements affected by *their* disorder.
2. Differentiation of their demonstrated functional movement(s).

Brief appraisal
Active movements (Move to PAIN or move to LIMIT)
Routinely

1. G/H F, Ab, behind back, HF and HE.
2. Scapular elevation, depression, protraction, retraction and rotation. Note range, pain, repeated (note scapular rhythm).

As applicable
Speed of test movements.
Specific movements that aggravate.
The injuring movement.
Movements under load.

Isometric tests
Rotator cuff
Other muscles in 'plan'

Other structures in 'plan'
Thoracic outlet
ULTT

Passive movements
Physiological movements
Routinely

1. G/H, F, Ab (◡), (◠), HF and HE or quadrant and locking position.
2. Scapular elevation, depression, protraction, retraction and rotation. Note range, pain, resistance, spasm and behaviour.

Accessory movements
Routinely

1. By thumb pressures (↓) (↧), (⟶) cephalad, caudad.
   (a) Over acromion.
   (b) Over clavicle.
   (c) On the joint line.
   (d) Repeat with joint compressed.
2. Squeeze clavicle and scapula.
3. Rotation at S/C and A/C joints:
   (a) Transverse axis.
   (b) Vertical axis (by scapular pro/retraction).
4. As for glenohumeral joint.
5. Canal's Slump tests.
6. Differentiation tests.
7. ULTT.
Note range, pain, resistance, spasm and behaviour

Palpation
+When 'comparable signs' ill defined reassess 'injuring movement'.

Check case records etc.

Instructions to patient

1. Warning of possible exacerbation.
2. Request to record details.
3. Instruction re 'joint care' if required.

clavicle. Compression of the joint surfaces can be added to all of these movements by pressing medially against the lateral border of the acromion process. Although pressures can be applied to the acromion process, they do not create as much acromioclavicular movement as do the pressures on the clavicle.

Spontaneous disorders of this joint have thickened soft tissues over the superior joint line and in the acromioclavicular space immediately medial to the articulation. For other disorders see *Practical Orthopaedic Medicine*[2].

On almost all occasions, the site of symptoms is on the top of or deeper within the acromioclavicular joint.

*Anteroposterior movement***
Starting position

The physiotherapist stands by the patient's right shoulder and places the heel of her left hand under the spine of his scapula near its vertebral end pointing her fingers towards the vertebral column. She then places the heel of her right hand over the anterior border of the clavicle near the junction of its middle and lateral thirds pointing her fingers medially (Figure 10.49).

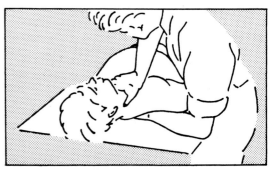

Figure 10.49 Acromioclavicular joint; anteroposterior movement (squeeze)

2. Corrigan, B. and Maitland, G. D. *Practical Orthopaedic Medicine,* Butterworths, London (1983)

Method

Movement is produced by an anteroposterior pressure against the clavicle through the heel of the therapist's right hand countered by the postero-anterior pressure over the medial end of the spine of the scapula.

Alternative starting position**

This method allows for more localized technique.

The physiotherapist stands by the patient's right shoulder, facing his head, and places her thumbs, tip to tip, against the anterior border of the clavicle immediately adjacent to the acromioclavicular joint. Her fingers are spread to provide stability. She then positions her shoulders above her hands to line up with the anteroposterior movement of the joint (Figure 10.50).

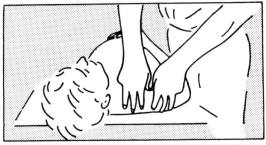

Figure 10.50 Acromioclavicular joint; anteroposterior movement. Alternative starting position

Method

The direction of her pressure must be carefully chosen and the mobilization must be produced by her arms acting through her thumbs, not by the flexor muscles of the thumbs. Movement can be felt through her left thumb as it lies alongside the acromion process.

Posteroanterior movement***

Starting position

The patient rests his elbows and clasps his hands across his abdomen. The physiotherapist kneels by the right side of his head, facing his feet, and places her thumbs, tip to tip, against the posterior border of the lateral end of the clavicle. She should place as much of the pads of her thumbs as possible adjacent to the joint (Figure 10.51).

Method

The posteroanterior movement is produced by the therapist's arms acting through her thumbs. She should position them reasonably close together so

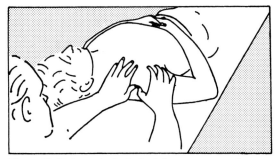

Figure 10.51 Acromioclavicular joint; posteroanterior movement of clavicle

that the line from her shoulders to her thumbs passes through them. The movement must not be produced by the thumb flexors.

Longitudinal movement ***

Longitudinal movement is so named because the movement is in line with longitudinal movement of the glenohumeral joint.

Caudad

Starting position

The physiotherapist stands by the right side of the patient's head, facing his feet. She places the tips of both thumbs on the superior surface of the clavicle adjacent to the acromioclavicular joint and spreads her fingers around her thumbs to provide stability. She should position her thumbs as close as possible to each other. Her forearms must be directed in line with the longitudinal movement of the acromioclavicular joint (Figure 10.52).

Method

The oscillatory mobilization is produced by her arms acting through stable thumbs. She should be able to

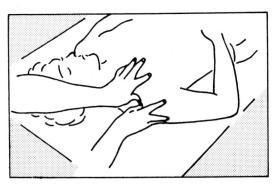

Figure 10.52 Acromioclavicular joint; longitudinal movement caudad

feel movement through the base of the pad of her right thumb, which just overlies the joint, and can compare the movement of the clavicle with the stationary acromion process.

Cephalad

Starting position

The position adopted is the same as that for anteroposterior movement (Figure 10.44) with two exceptions:

1. The physiotherapist places the pad of her thumbs, near their tip, against the inferior surface of the clavicle.
2. She directs her forearms horizontally.

Method

The longitudinal cephalad movement is directed through her thumbs by her body and horizontally directed forearms.

Rotary movements

These are produced by flexion and extension of the patient's arm to which can be added:

1. At the limit of, or during, flexion:
   (a) Longitudinal caudad to inhibit or reduce the rotation.
   (b) Longitudinal cephalad to over-pressure the rotation.
2. At the limit of, or during, extension:
   (a) Caudad to over-pressure the rotation.
   (b) Cephalad to inhibit or reduce the rotation.

Compression

This can be added to movements be exerting pressure directed medially against the lateral border of the acromion process. Its only application is to treat or prevent intra-articular disorders of the acromioclavicular joint.

Sternoclavicular joint

All the movements described above for the acromioclavicular joint, together with glenohumeral and acromiohumeral joints, and all scapulothoracic movements, effect movement of the sternoclavicular joint and must be examined (Table 10.4). Localized mobilization can also be effected at this joint by thumb pressure against the sternal end of the clavicle. The technique will be described for one direction of movement only but mention will be made of the remaining movements.

The sternoclavicular joint is not one to cause much trouble in the spontaneous-onset/trivial-incident group of disorders. There is, however, one qualification that should be made. It is not a joint that is structured to take a lot of work, and it has a tendency to become hypermobile and unstable. Competitive swimming can lead to overuse. The hypermobility is not a problem in itself unless the joint becomes symptomatic. Nevertheless, pain relieving passive movement techniques are just as effective, hypermobile (unstable) or not hypermobile.

*Anteroposterior movement****
Starting position

The physiotherapist stands beyond the left side of the patient's head, facing his feet. She place the tips of her thumbs, pointing towards each other, directly over the sternal end of the clavicle anteriorly and

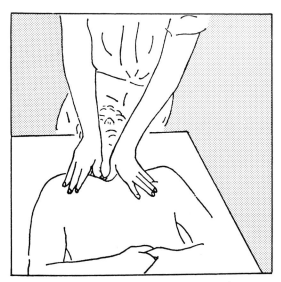

Figure 10.53 Sternoclavicular joint; anteroposterior movement

Table 10.4 Sternoclavicular joint – objective examination

When examining the sternoclavicular (S/C) joint the A/C joint (including relevant G/H, A/H or S/Th movements) must be examined.

HIGHLIGHT MAIN FINDINGS WITH ASTERISKS AS YOU GO

Observation

Functional demonstration/tests
As applicable

1. *Their* demonstration of *their* functional movements affected by *their* disorder.
2. Differentiation of *their* demonstrated functional movement(s).

Brief appraisal

Active movements (Move to PAIN or move to LIMIT)

Routinely

1. G/H F, HF and HE.
2. Scapular elevation, depression, protraction, retraction and rotation. Note range, pain and repeated

Isometric tests

Other structures in 'plan'
Thoracic outlet & ULTT

Passive movements
Physiological movements
Routinely

1. Supine: G/H, HF, HE and F
2. Sidely: scapular elevation, depression, protraction, retraction and rotation. Note range, pain, resistance, spasm and behaviour.

Accessory movements
Routinely

By thumb pressures on clavicle.
($\uparrow$) ($\downarrow$) ($\leftrightarrow$) caudad and cephalad, rotation, distraction and compression.
Note range, pain, resistance, spasm and behaviour.

As applicable Add compression (medial & caud) to above

Palpation

+When 'comparable signs' ill defined reassess 'injuring movement'.

Check case records, etc.

Instructions to patient

1. Warning of possible exacerbation.
2. Request to record details.
3. Instruction re 'joint care' if required.

adjacent to the joint. Her fingers fan around the thumbs to provide stability.

The metacarpophalangeal joints of the thumbs are brought near each other so that the line of the pressure from the shoulders to the thumb tips will pass through them. It is necessary for her to position her shoulders in line with the anteroposterior movement of the joint (Figure 10.53).

Method

The mobilization is produced by the therapist's arms and body, and must not under any circumstances be produced by the flexor muscles of the thumbs. This fact has been mentioned before but it is even more important in the sternoclavicular joint. If fine control of the movement is to be possible, and if the degree of movement is to be clearly felt, the thumbs must only transmit the pressure and not produce it. It is because this joint has such a mobile range of movement that the finesse with which the technique is performed is so important.

Posteroanterior movement*

A posteroanterior movement can be produced by hooking the fingers around the medial end of the clavicle to reach its posterior surface. The movement is then produced by pulling the clavicle forwards and oscillating. Alternatively the thumbs can be placed under the clavicle, similar to the cephalad movement (Figure 10.54) but reaching the posterior surface. By then lowering her forearms she can produce a posteroanterior movement.

Longitudinal movement caudad**

Mobilization in a caudad direction, towards the patient's feet, can be effected by altering the point of contact to the superior surface of the medial end of the clavicle and by the therapist directing her arms caudally. There is very little movement in this direction but occasionally it is more painful than other movements. It may then be the direction chosen for the treatment though it may not necessarily be performed in the painful part of the range.

Longitudinal movement cephalad**

When movement in the opposite direction is required, that is in a cephalad direction, the therapist stands by his right elbow, facing his head. She places her thumbs against the inferior surface of the clavicle adjacent to the sternoclavicular joint. With her forearms lowered to the required angle,

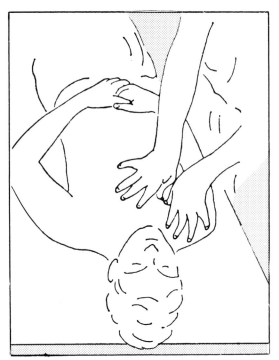

Figure 10.54 Sternoclavicular joint; longitudinal movement cephalad

the oscillatory movement is produced by shoulder and arm movement transmitted through her thumbs (Figure 10.54).

Rotary movements

These movements are performed by flexion and extension of the humerus as described for rotary movements of the acromioclavicular joint. As also described for that joint (A/C), thumb pressures can be applied to the proximal end of the clavicle to inhibit or stretch the rotation.

Compression and distraction

The techniques described for the sternoclavicular joint have been shown with the joint in a relaxed position. From the point of view of both examination and treatment, the same movements can be performed while the joint surfaces are compressed. The compression is produced by the physiotherapist grasping around the patient's humeral head and acromion process and directing a pressure in line with the shaft of the clavicle. This compression can be applied at two extremes of sternoclavicular movement, or at any position between these two extremes. The first extreme is to elevate the patient's shoulder girdle, thus directing the compressive force more towards the patient's opposite hip. The other extreme is to depress the patient's shoulder girdle as much as possible, altering the angle between the clavicle and manubrium so that the compressive force has a slight cephalad direction.

It is also important to realize that the movements can also be performed when the joint surfaces are distracted. The latter technique merely requires the physiotherapist to place one hand on the medial surface of the humerus near its head and then to pull the humerus (and thus the whole shoulder girdle) laterally. As described above for compression, different angles of distraction can be used by elevating or depressing the shoulder girdle.

Both distraction and compression can be used as test movements and mobilizing techniques without being performed in conjunction with the techniques described in the text. Compression is usually of more value than distraction.

Scapulothoracic movement

It is uncommon for scapulothoracic movements to be painful or restricted unless the history includes trauma. The techniques therefore are not commonly used in treatment, but are techniques, which the physiotherapist must be able to handle, even if they are only used for examination purposes (Table 10.5). When treatment is necessary the type of movement is usually a grade III or IV in the direction of the painful limitation. The movements are protraction, retraction, elevation, depression and rotation. Compression of the scapula against the rib cage can be added.

*Protraction***

Starting position

The patient lies on his left side near the forward edge of the couch, his head resting on pillows and his hips and knees comfortably flexed. The physiotherapist stands by his hips, facing his head, and leans across his pelvis to cradle his right ilium in her left axilla. This position aids stability during the large-amplitude scapulothoracic movement. She grasps the medial border of his scapula with the fingers of her left hand.

With her right hand she grasps over the spine of the scapula and cups the heel of her hand anteriorly over the clavicular area. The patient's right arm, flexed at the elbow, must be firmly supported by her right forearm to prevent any glenohumeral movement during the scapulothoracic movement (Figure 10.55).

Table 10.5 Scapulothoracic movement – objective examination

When examining the scapulothoracic disorders the glenohumeral joint must also be examined.

HIGHLIGHT MAIN FINDINGS WITH ASTERISKS AS YOU GO

Observation

*Functional demonstration/tests
As applicable
1. *Their* demonstration of *their* functional movements affected by *their* disorder.
2. Differentiation of *their* demonstrated functional movement(s).

Brief appraisal

Active movements (Move to PAIN or move to LIMIT)
Routinely
1. Glenohumeral (G/H) F, Ab, behind back, HF.
2. Scapular elevation, depression, protraction and retraction. Note range, pain and scapular rhythm.

As applicable
Speed of test movements.
Specific movements that aggravate.
The injuring movement.
Movements under load.
Muscle power.

Isometric tests
Rotator cuff
Other muscles in 'plan'

Other structures in 'plan'
Thoracic outlet & ULTT
Entrapment neuropathy

Passive movements
Physiological movements
Routinely
1. G/H movements.
2. Side lying, scapular elevation, depression, protraction, retraction and rotation (add compression as applicable).
Note range, pain, resistance, spasm and behaviour.

As applicable
1. Canal's slump tests.
2. Differentiation tests.
3. ULTT.

Accessory movements
Routinely
1. Intercostal movements.
2. Lifting scapula off thorax.
Note range, pain resistance spasm and behaviour.

Palpation
+When 'comparable signs' ill defined reassess 'injuring movement'.

Check case records etc.

Instructions to patient
1. Warning of possible exacerbation.
2. Request to record details.
3. Instruction re 'joint care' if required.

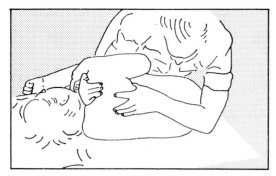

Figure 10.55 Scapulothoracic movement; protraction

Method

The protraction movement, which follows the curve of the rib cage, is produced by the fingers of both hands against the medial border and spine of the scapula. As the scapula moves around the chest wall the physiotherapist lowers the level of her support under his right arm to avoid glenohumeral movement.

Retraction**

Starting position

This position is identical with that used for protraction with one exception: the physiotherapist places her left thumb and thenar eminence very firmly along the lateral border of the scapula (Figure 10.56).

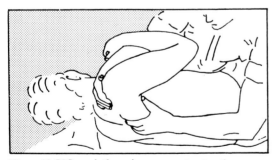

Figure 10.56 Scapulothoracic movement; retraction

Method

Retraction is produced by pressure from (1) the physiotherapist's grasp of the upper scapula and (2) her left thumb against the lateral border of the scapula. Care must be exercised during the movement to see that the patient's arm is carried outwards with the scapula to avoid glenohumeral movement.

Elevation and depression**

Starting position

The starting position for these two movements is identical with that already described above except that the physiotherapist's left hand is placed over the lower half of the patient's scapula with her fingers pointing towards his head. The lower third of his scapula is cupped in her left hand, so that her thenar eminence and thumb grasp the lateral border, and her middle finger grasps the medial border (Figure 10.57).

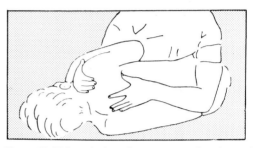

Figure 10.57 Scapulothoracic movement; elevation and depression

Method

During the elevation the upward movement is produced by the physiotherapist's left hand and during depression it is her right hand, cupped over the shoulder girdle, which produces it. The glenohumeral joint is easily stabilized during both elevation and depression.

Rotation**

Starting position

The patient lies on his left side near the forward edge of the couch with pillows to support his head. The physiotherapist stands in front of his pelvis and with her right hand she holds over his acromial area from in front. She flexes his right arm and rests it on her right arm. His arm must be firmly supported to avoid glenohumeral movement taking place during the scapulothoracic movement. With her left hand she grasps the medial and lateral borders of the scapula with her fingers and thumb respectively (Figure 10.58(a)).

Method

Scapular rotation is produced by a combined action of the physiotherapist's two hands. With her left

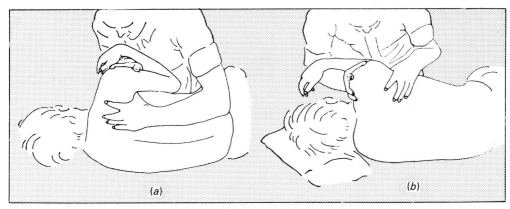

Figures 10.58 Scapulothoracic movement; rotation

hand she moves the inferior angle of the scapula around the thorax while her right hand pivots the scapula from on top. During this pivoting action her right hand stabilizes the shoulder girdle to prevent protraction. The patient's right arm must be stably supported on her left arm and must be flexed in unison with the scapular movement to prevent any glenohumeral movement, and this is, in part, achieved by pivoting her hips from left to right. The position at the limit of the scapular rotation is shown in Figure 10.58(b).

Compression and distraction

During all of the above movements compression of the scapula against the rib cage can be maintained so as to rub firmly the anterior surface of the scapula while moving it in each direction.

For distraction the medial border of the scapula can be lifted off the ribs thus revealing the anterior surface of the scapula for palpation purposes, and for stretching the attached soft tissues. To achieve the maximum range the procedure needs to be performed slowly allowing the patient time to relax.

Condensed examination
Composite shoulder

In the examination of various joints that make up shoulder girdle movements, there is considerable overlap of test movements. Tables have been given for each joint. Table 10.6 aims to bring these together. It remains essential to know which joints are being tested with each individual test movement and to know how *differentiation tests* can reveal the source of the symptoms. Obviously not all of the tests listed have to be performed, but they do provide the complete list.

Chronic/minor symptoms

When chronic minor symptoms occupy any part of the area between a mid-scapular/clavicular line and a line around the mid humerus, the mandatory passive movement tests are as follows:

Supine:G/H, abduction in HE and locking
G/H shaft rotation in HE
Horizontal flexion
Flexion in rotations
Around quadrant & locking
A/C joint, PA & longitudinal caud

Test movements are IV− with observation for pain response. If pain-free, adequate over-pressure is applied until pain is provoked or the movement is judged 'clear'.

When a positive pain response is provoked, that test movement may need to be differentiated to determine the specific joint at fault, or other test movements may need to be tested so as to either exclude or incriminate other joints as contributing to the symptoms.

If all test movements appear 'clear' at first examination, they should be repeated more strongly. If still 'clear', they may prove positive when the tests are repeated at the next consultation.

Proving the shoulder is unaffected

There are occasions when a patient may have a disorder which demands that the shoulder girdle must be examined by passive movements to prove that it is not contributing to his symptoms. However, not all test movements must be done. The following is a short list of those that must be performed:

In standing:
F plus over-pressures at F & Quadrant, locking.
Abd resisted and behind median coronal plane.
BB plus over-pressure.
HF plus over-pressure.
In supine:
Q.
Locking.

Table 10.6 Composite shoulder – objective examination

HIGHLIGHT MAIN FINDINGS WITH ASTERISKS AS YOU GO

Observation

*Functional demonstration/tests
As applicable

1. *Their* demonstration of *their* functional movements affected by *their* disorder.
2. Differentiation of *their* demonstrated functional movement(s).

Brief appraisal
Active movements (Move to PAIN or move to LIMIT)
F (spontaneous then sagittal)
Ab (spontaneous then coronal)
HF, HE
Behind back (wrist mid line)
F and Abd in medial & lateral rotation
Isometric tests
Cuff

Other structures in 'plan'
Thoracic outlet & ULTT
Entrapment neuropathy

Passive movements
As indicated by site of pain and stiffness
Supine

1. G/H joint F, Ab, ($\circlearrowright$) ($\circlearrowleft$), HF, HE.
   or
   Q and locking position.
2. Arm by side (↓) (↓) (↔) caud and ceph, (↔) (gapping G/H joint).
   Arm abducted (↔), caudad, (↕↕).
   Arm in F/Q (↓), (↔), caud (& ceph).
3. A/C joint; Squeeze, (↓), (↓), (↔), caudad and cephalad, Rotn (repeat with compression).
4. S/C joint; As applicable (↔) ceph, caud (↓), (↑) Rotn, distraction and compression (repeat first five with compression).
5. Canal's Slump tests.
6. Differentiation tests.
7. ULTT, and thoracic outlet.

Prone
Hand behind back, E, Ad, ($\circlearrowright$)
Forehead resting in palms G/H. (↓), (↔), caudad, cervical (↓) and (◥) (◤)

Side lying
Scap/Thoracic; as applicable E1, De, Pr, Re, Rotn.
as applicable add compression
Note range, pain, resistance, spasm and behaviour

Palpation
+When 'comparable signs' ill defined reassess 'injuring movement'.

Check case records etc.

Instructions to patient

1. Warning of possible exacerbation.
2. Request to record details.
3. Instruction re 'joint care' if required.

Treatment

The classification of shoulder lesions as presented by Corrigan[2] are:

1. Tendons lesions:
   (a) Rotator-cuff tendons – tendinitis, incomplete and complete rupture, and calcification.
   (b) The biceps tendon – tendinitis, tenosynovitis, subluxation, and rupture.
2. Bursitis.
   (a) Sub-acromial bursitis – chronic or acute calcific bursitis.
   (b) Sub-coracoid bursitis.
3. Capsulitis.
4. Instability of the shoulder joint.
5. The shoulder–hand syndrome.
6. Entrapment neuropathies.

The majority of patient's with shoulder disorders who are referred for physiotherapy have stiffness and pain with arm movement. When examining these patients it is important to test the muscles that make up the rotator cuff as well as the ranges of movement of the individual joints to determine the muscular and capsular components of the pain. For example, it is surprising how often a patient with a diagnosis of 'supraspinatus tendinitis' is found to have also an acromiohumeral joint component. Even when the diagnosis of supraspinatus tendinitis can be made, testing the quadrant and locking positions usually reproduces the patient's symptoms.

Supraspinatus tendinitis

There are two methods for treating this condition by passive movement. Assuming that the quadrant and locking positions reproduce the pain, the first choice would be posteroanterior pressures against the head of the humerus with the patient's elbows by his side and his hands clasped loosely across his abdomen (see Figure 10.40, page 152). Initially, the movements would be performed so as to avoid any pain or discomfort. Usually, the patient notices the pain recede within two or three treatments and then the amplitude of the treatment movement can be increased, aiming to reach a painless grade III movement. Unless there has been a tear affecting the tendon of the supraspinatus, the power of abduction recovers as dramatically as the pain recedes. The posteroanterior movements should be gentle to begin with, and if the assessment is made carefully enough the value of this approach will be quickly evident. It could be expected that progress would enable full-amplitude, gentle, slow, oscillatory movements to be performed rocking the head

of the humerus from a fully posterior position to a fully anterior position.

If the above techniques do not produce improvement quickly, the quadrant movement techniques should be used, performed very gently as grade IV− movements, done either painlessly or with the least possible discomfort (see Figure 10.11, page 136). Assessment of their value is possible after two applications of this technique at the one treatment session. The arc of pain on abduction should improve markedly if the technique achieves the improvement expected. The power of abduction should improve also as it is a pain-inhibition type of weakness. This method of treating supraspinatus tendinitis is quicker in its effect and less painful than transverse friction massage.

Frozen shoulder
First stage

In the early stage of this clearly defined syndrome, pain is the dominant factor, and the patient has little excursion of shoulder movement in any direction. Effective treatment by posteroanterior pressures can be given (see Figure 10.40, page 152) with the patient's arm supported on pillows in a neutral, pain-free position. Great care should be taken to ensure the technique is completely painless, performed slowly and smoothly, and used only for a very short time (30 seconds). At the first treatment the therapist should only assess symptomatic changes, not the joint movements; this assessment should be made over a 24-hour period in these early stages. The patient should experience lessening of symptoms after two treatments, enabling the physiotherapist to increase the amplitude of her technique, and before long, to carry the amplitude into a small degree of discomfort. Standing the patient and asking him to raise his arms forwards in flexion in the sagittal plane should be used for assessment; quite dramatic improvement in range of movement can be anticipated. The stages of treatment progression for pain are detailed in Chapter 7, pages 73–77.

Second stage

In a later stage of the untreated frozen shoulder the patient usually has painful limitation of range, and when the stiff movement is stretched, considerable pain is provoked. When both pain and stiffness are present, the initial method is to treat pain as described previously, going through the stages of accessory and physiological movements. If this approach does not produce improvement, and it should be possible to determine this within two or three treatments, then the resistance itself must be treated. The initial movement should be slow

2. Corrigan, B. and Maitland, G. D. *Practical Orthopaedic Medicine,* Butterworths, London (1983)

smooth oscillatory movements directed towards the quadrant. The therapist must clearly understand how gently she is stretching the supportive structures of the glenohumeral joint and how much pain she is provoking; on releasing a stretch she must determine how quickly the patient's pain subsides. Provided the symptoms subside immediately the stretch is released, more treatment and stronger treatment can be given.

Later in treatment, when treatment of resistance with grade IV and grade IV+ techniques can be used, they should be interspersed with movement in exactly the same direction but performed as a large-amplitude grade III− technique. This will lessen treatment soreness considerably. Alternatively, large amplitude posteroanterior movement (Figure 10.41, page 152) is sometimes more successful in relieving treatment soreness.

It is quite common to reach a stage when the stretching movements (Figure 10.10), as a grade IV movement, page 140), combined with the accessory movements (as described on page 150, Figure 10.38 and on page 151) no longer produce improvement. Even with the inclusion of active exercises undertaken diligently by the patient, the range may not improve. The decision has then to be made whether stronger pressure should be applied, assessing the strength of the resistance and the degree of pain. The patient's temperament should be taken into account and knowledge of the history of the disorder is of value in making the decision. The longer the condition has been in evidence and the less irritable it is, the safer it will be to stretch strongly. After three treatments an attempt to break adhesions may be attempted. Such manipulative procedure is in line with the MUA (manipulation under anaesthesia) procedure used by orthopaedic surgeons. Manipulation carried out on the conscious patient is preferred because under these conditions the patient's reactions can more successfully guide the manipulator. This is a time when intravascular pethidine can be a very valuable adjunct to the manipulation without anaesthesia.

Rarely is manipulation done at a first consultation. The technique is begun gently and repeated several times, gradually increasing in strength, the patient's reaction being watched closely meanwhile. Considerable information can be gained by watching the patient's hands and eyes.

The amount of pain the patient experiences while the structures are being stretched is estimated, thereby calculating how much pain the patient will tolerate if manipulation is attempted. Note is also taken of the strength required to increase the range. Upon release of the stretch, the time the pain or discomfort takes to subside should be ascertained. If the pain lasts for some considerable time then the physiotherapist knows she is limited in how far she can stretch and how many stretches she can apply at one session. In this way she gradually feels her way from treatment to treatment before attempting to manipulate.

The movement used for manipulation is to stretch towards the quadrant position or towards full flexion alongside the patient's head, depending upon which is the stiffer and more painful. It is likely that whichever is the more painful will also be the stiffer one and therefore the more successful direction in which to manipulate. The technique used is shown in Figure 10.10 (page 135), except that the physiotherapist will need to stabilize the patient's chest with her shoulder and trunk so that she will be in the best position to control the technique.

Some therapists consider that the manipulation should be painless and that the accessory movement should be the only movement used, not the physiological movement. However, the author believes that the physiological movement is usually the one that must be used when manipulating the glenohumeral joint.

The procedure of manipulation is one of gradually increasing the strength of the stretch, while remaining fully aware of the pressure being applied and the pain being provoked. It should not be a hasty procedure, neither should it be performed too slowly as this will prolong pain unnecessarily.

When tearing of structures does occur the therapist must instantly appreciate whether the tear is one 'crack' or a series of minor tears. She instantly decides whether she has gone as far as is necessary or whether she must go on to reach a full range. The decision is a difficult one to make – it is better to undo the manipulation than to do too much and cause unwarranted pain. Neither medial nor lateral rotation is suitable to be chosen as the primary technique, the rotary leverage being so great it is difficult to gauge how strongly to proceed.

The feel and sound of the tear can be as follows:
1. A sharp 'snap' sound – this is the most desirable manipulation and requires very little exercise follow-up regimen.
2. A tearing of blotting paper sound – this will require exercises.
3. A wet blotting ripple – effective exercising is vital. Without it the procedure will be useless to say the least.

A patient whose shoulder was manipulated as described above (and without pethidine) is on two videotapes[3], as is her follow-up treatment because of the blotting paper type of tearing.

3. Maitland, G. D. *Mrs Etter: Demonstration of a patient – (1) Shoulder Manipulation.* Number 17, 50 mins. Number 18 (2) and (3), 55 mins. Postgraduate Study Centre Hermitage, Medizinische Abteilung, Bad Ragaz CH7310, Switzerland (1980)

The manipulation should be followed up immediately with repetitive active flexion with the patient lying supine for at least half an hour. This procedure should also be continued hourly at home. At first the patient should concentrate on the gravity-assisted flexion performed supine. This exercise routine performed by the patient should be progressed by the second day to include performing flexion while standing. He should face and stand close to a wall and stretch both arms to a position of maximum flexion. When at the limit of flexion, he should endeavour to lift both arms (with emphasis on the bad arm) off the wall without losing the range of flexion. Flexion should then be exercised actively while the patient lies prone. The patient must be told that if he doesn't exercise properly he will lose his newly acquired range and the fault will be his. Naturally this is not always so, but it does produce conscientious exercising.

The patient should be seen the day following the manipulation to check the effectiveness of the home exercising programme in retaining range. Also, if the patient's shoulder is very painful, mobilizing techniques can be used to reduce this pain.

It should be borne in mind that when a patient has a loss of only 15° of flexion this does not mean that he cannot have adhesions. It may prove necessary, even with this seemingly negligible loss of range, to attempt manipulation if firm mobilizing fails to improve range. Manipulation under these circumstances is rarely unsuccessful.

Third stage

The frozen shoulder has as final stage when the range of movement is restricted but pain-free. If the degree of limitation is such that the patient is unable to carry out any functionally important activities, mobilizing can be used strongly in an endeavour to improve the range. The procedure of stretching, say, flexion with grade IV+ movements interspersed with grade IV+ accessory movements at the limit of flexion has been described earlier. If treatment produces soreness, grade III movements (flexion in this case) can be used to eliminate it.

It is unnecessary, and usually unwise, to continue treatment beyond the stage when the active movements are functional. However, the patient's pain and movements should be reviewed at intervals.

When movements are grossly limited, treatment by passive movement (even MUA) is unlikely to be of any value. It is said that they will regain function with the passage of time.

Painfully stiff shoulder

Many patients are seen who have painful and stiff shoulders which resemble the second stage of a frozen shoulder but who have not had a 'first stage'.

If the range of movement of the glenohumeral joint is limited and very painful when stretched then the treatment is similar to that described earlier ('Second stage, Frozen shoulder'), that is, if treatment of pain fails then the resistance must be treated. Assessment for changes in range and pain must be continued throughout and when a stage of no progress is reached manipulation of the type described above should be considered.

At the initial examination all movements should be assessed for pain and range. The amount by which the pain increases when the movements are stretched is of prime importance. For example, if pain increases rapidly with minor stretching, then gentler techniques and larger amplitudes are needed.

Stretching into the quadrant position is usually the best technique to use initially. As flexion improves, so should all other ranges of movement. However, horizontal flexion or the ability to get the hand behind the back may not progress at the same rate. When this is the case, stretching techniques in three directions (quadrant, horizontal, flexion and hand behind back) can be used at each treatment session. Opposite directions of movement (e.g. Quadrant followed by hand-behind-back) should not follow each other. Whenever stretching techniques are used, accessory movements should also be used at the limit of the particular physiological range being stretched. Accessory or physiological movements should also be used following the stretching but performed more gently and with a large-amplitude to reduce treatment soreness. The effectiveness of these latter movements is dramatic.

Osteoarthritis

It is well documented that osteoarthritis is uncommon in the glenohumeral joint. However, it does occur occasionally and these patients are frequently referred for physiotherapy. The treatment of pain has already been described in detail and it is this treatment that is used for these patients. However, when dealing with the osteoarthritic shoulder the physiotherapist should not hurriedly change from the posteroanterior accessory movement technique to a flexion or quadrant movement, because to do so, may cause an exacerbation. In other words, if there is any indication of even minimal crepitus, or if there are arthritic signs in other joints, treatment of the shoulder is more likely to be successful if the accessory movements alone are used. They might need to be grade I or grade II− initially, but the aim should be to reach a stage when grade III− (or even III+) movements through the full excursion of the accessory range can be performed without pain.

The physiological movements of abduction, medial or lateral rotation in some degree of glenohumeral abduction, may be used as grade II movements with success.

Minimal intermittent minor shoulder pain

Patients who fit this category usually feel sharp pain when the arm is used unexpectedly, vigorously or in an awkward manner. Examination of the normal movements will prove negative but either the quadrant or the locking position will be found to be positive. When such is the case the more dominant one should be used as the treatment technique.

If the quadrant is being used as the treatment technique then initially the treatment technique should not provoke discomfort. It should be performed as very small amplitude grade IV− all around the top of the quadrant position (see page 136).

As the quadrant becomes almost painfree the technique whereby the arm rolls back and forth over the quadrant can be used (see page 135).

If the locking position is to be treated (see Figure 10.7) then gentle oscillatory movements similar to those described for treatment of the quadrant should be used. A scouring type movement as described for Figure 10.61 is also used.

Fractures of the humerus

When a patient fractures his humerus the stress causing the fracture also strains the structures supporting the glenohumeral joint. If the fracture is immobilized by a splint which does not encompass the glenohumeral joint, passive movement of the glenohumeral joint can be performed without moving the fracture. There are passive mobilizing techniques that can be applied to the glenohumeral joint which effectively maintain or improve the range of movement available at the glenohumeral joint. This can be achieved even with fractures of the surgical neck of the humeral joint. If the fracture is impacted, more movements can be used because the fracture is stable.

These techniques are modifications of those in the preceding text of techniques. The patient's upper arm should be comfortably supported near his trunk and the most important technique would be lateral movement of the head of the humerus as shown in Figure 10.46. The modification necessary would be that, instead of using the hand to produce lateral movement at the glenohumeral joint, the therapist would use one or both of her thumbs high in the axilla on the head of the humerus, and the mobilization would be by small amplitude slow oscillatory movements. The second important technique would be posteroanterior movement of the head of the humerus as depicted in Figure 10.40. The third important technique would be produced by longitudinal thumb pressures against the head of the humerus as depicted in Figure 10.35.

Abduction is a most important movement of the glenohumeral joint and should be regained and/or retained as early as possible. Very gentle small amplitude slowly performed oscillatory abduction movements should be performed at the limit of the range. To be sure that there is no movement taking place at the fracture site two rules must be adhered to:

1. The humerus must be supported securely throughout its length.
2. The physiotherapist should firmly imbed her index finger between the lateral border of the acromion process and the head of the humerus so she can freely feel both bones. In this way she can be sure that the humeral head moves in the right proportion as the humerus is abducted.

If the fracture is one that allows the arm to be abducted from the patient's side, then modifications of the techniques depicted in Figures 10.42, 10.36 and 10.37 may be used whereby the thumb is used directly on the head of the humerus rather than the hand. However, the anteroposterior movement of the head of the humerus in the glenoid cavity as shown in Figure 10.44 is best performed with the therapist's hand over the head of the humerus. This is because it spreads the area of contact.

The techniques referred to above are very effective, not only in assisting range, but also in reducing pain.

Acromioclavicular joint pain

Pain arising from the acromioclavicular joint is almost invariably felt locally. Rarely does it refer far from the joint but when it does, the referral is usually towards the neck.

The best techniques for treatment of the acromioclavicular joint are movements of the clavicle produced by the thumbs (shown in Figures 10.50, 10.51 and 10.52). The grades used would be IVs into pain, mixed with grades II and III−.

Sternoclavicular joint

Pain in this joint also causes local pain and the technique performed with the thumbs shown in Figure 10.53 and longitudinal movement caudad are most effective. The direction of treatment movement chosen should be one that reproduces the pain, and the grades would be the same as for the acromioclavicular joint.

Upper limb

Elbow joint

The elbow joint is complex, consisting of the humeroulnar joint, radiohumeral joint and the superior radioulnar joint. Any one of the three can cause pain in the elbow and therefore differential examination of each joint is an important skill. It is also necessary to take into consideration that if the elbow is held 10° short of full extension there is an amplitude of abduction/adduction movement. During this abduction/adduction movement, the olecranon process swings from side to side in the olecranon fossa, the head of the radius is compressed and distracted from the capitulum as the radius moves cephalad and caudad in the superior radioulnar joint (Figure 10.59(a) and (b)).

When the elbow joint is in extension and over-pressure is added to supination and pronation, the olecranon process rotates in the olecranon fossa (Figure 10.60(a) and (b)).

When the wrist is ulnar deviated the radial head moves caudad; during radial deviation it moves cephalad.

Palpation of the soft tissues in the olecranon fossa, especially during passive elbow extension, can reveal indicative signs comparable with the disorder.

It is impossible to produce movement in any one of the three joints without producing movement in the others. Therefore, testing movement of one bone on the other must be done by the physiotherapist's fingers and thumbs rather than resorting to gross movements. When movements are tested, the accurate site of the pain felt by the patient is a guide in determining which of the joints is at fault.

Examination

Subjective examination

When a patient is talking about the behaviour of his symptoms he may, without realizing, give a clue as

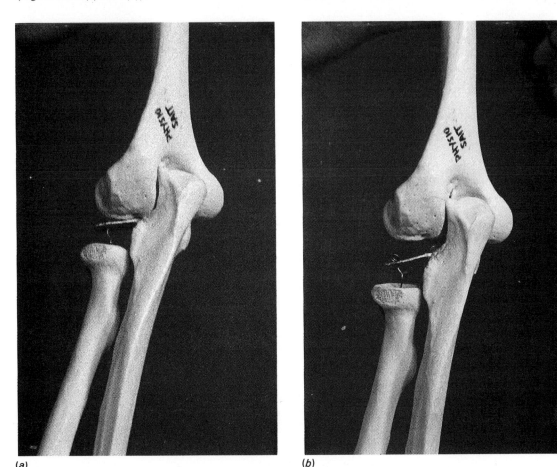

(a)   *(b)*

Figure 10.59 Elbow joint. (*a*) Abduction, humeroulnar approximation and olecranon abduction in olecranon fossa, and (*b*) adduction, humeroulnar distraction and olecranon adduction in olecranon fossa

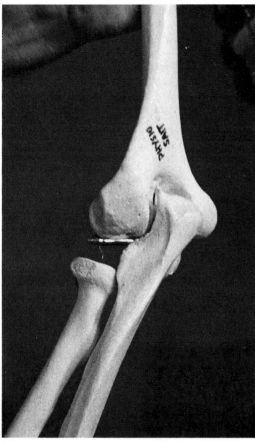
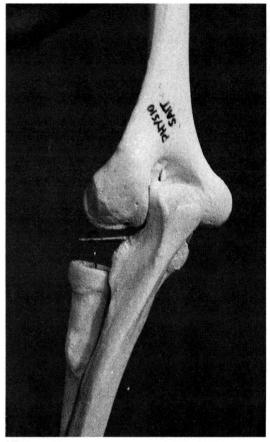

(a)   (b)

Figure 10.60 Elbow joint. (*a*) Supination of olecranon process in olecranon fossa. (*b*) Pronation of olecranon process in olecranon fossa

to the source by instinctively either moving it in a flexion/extension direction or supination/pronation direction. The latter, for example, leads one to think of the radioulnar joint.

Regarding the site of symptoms, it is important to know whether they are palpable and whether they are deeply situated within the joint. If they are deep, time should be taken to know precisely which of the closely associated joints seem to be implicated.

Objective examination[4]

On the whole, the elbow joint is inadequately examined by therapists. This accounts, in part, for poor results obtained in physiotherapy treatment of such conditions as tennis elbow.

Functional demonstration/tests

Analyse the movement he can demonstrate that produces his pain: using a screwdriver.

Brief appraisal

When a patient appears to have a reasonably good range of movement he can be asked to actively flex his elbow fully and then to bounce back and forth at the limit of his flexion range; if he feels pain then the movement should be compared with that on the other side. Extension should be similarly assessed by bouncing movement at the limit of the range. Following the flexion and extension the patient should be asked to supinate and pronate his forearm

4. Maitland, G. D. *Elbow, Knee, Shoulder,* Videotape Number 13, 32 mins. Postgraduate Teaching Centre Hermitage, Medizinische Abteilung, Bad Ragaz CH7310, Switzerland (1978)

as far, as hard and as rapidly as possible. These tests give a useful guide to the extent of elbow joint problems.

Special tests

Examination of the physiological movements of flexion, extension, pronation and supination is insufficient to determine the normality or otherwise of this joint. Full use of accessory joint movement must be made if some disturbances are not to be missed. Other authors, and in particular Mennell[5], have discussed the range of lateral accessory movements which is possible when the elbow is held a few degrees from the extended position. This is not the only position in which accessory movements should be assessed. Extension in adduction and extension in abduction are two movements that must be examined when active extension is normal. Similarly, flexion can be examined in both adduction and abduction.

When the elbow is fully extended the amplitude of accessory movement from adduction to abduction can be represented diagrammatically by a straight line $X_2 Y_2$ (Figure 10.61), where X_2 represents the limit of adduction and Y_2 represents the limit of abduction. If the elbow is now flexed 10° the two positions, adduction and abduction, can be represented respectively by another straight line with the limits X_1, and Y_1. The amplitude of this accessory movement is greater in a few degrees of flexion than in the fully extended position.

If the elbow, while firmly held in adduction, is moved from extension through 10° of flexion, that is from X_2 to X_1, it will be felt that the movement is not a straight line but has a curve near the limit of extension as shown in Figure 10.61. The flexion movement in abduction from Y_2 to Y_1, also follows a slight curve though it is less marked.

The procedures adopted to examine and treat these movements follow.

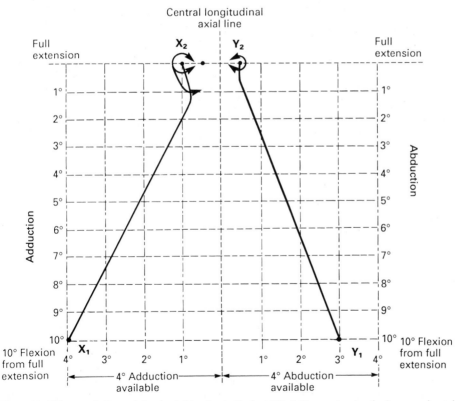

Figure 10.61 Range of elbow abduction/adduction in the last 10° of elbow extension (only approximately degrees used) viewed from the anterior aspect of the wrist in the anatomical position. The complete line represents the path traversed by the wrist during passive extension (*a*) with the elbow pressured into adduction ($X_1 X_2$) and (*b*) with the elbow pressured into abduction ($Y_1 Y_2$). The arrowed circular areas represent the scouring movements (E/Add at X_2; E/Abd at Y_2) used in examination and treatment.

5. Mennell, J. McM. *Joint Pain*, Churchill Livingstone, London; Little Brown & Co., Boston (1964)

Extension/adduction***

The extension/adduction movement is only used in treatment when grade III or IV is required. For the shoulder, the quadrant position was described as a point in the abduction to flexion movement. A similar position occurs at the elbow when it is flexed more than 10° from full extension while held in either adduction or abduction. During the first few degrees of flexion/adduction the forearm moves in a plane almost parallel to the elbow sagittal plane. A point is reached where the elbow abducts slightly and then adducts, and continues to increase the adduction to the X_1 position. Once this point is passed, if the adduction pressure is maintained, the glenohumeral joint will medially rotate. The most important part of the movement is the point near where abduction occurs. The elbow cannot be locked near this roll-over point as can the shoulder (see page 134), yet the movement has a similar feel. The two joints are also similar in that when the elbow joint is the source of minor symptoms and its movements appear to be normal, this accessory range may be diminished and painful. In treatment, the movement of extension/adduction can be scoured in much the same way as was described for the glenohumeral joint. The scouring movement is represented at X_2 by the arrowed circular arcs in Figure 10.61.

Starting position

The patient lies far enough from the edge of the couch for his elbow to lie just beyond the edge when his arm is abducted 30°. The physiotherapist, standing by his right shoulder and facing his feet, rests her left forearm in front of, and just medial to, his shoulder. With the fingers of her left hand she supports his elbow posteriorly from the medial side while her thumb extends around the medial epicondylar ridge of the humerus to reach the front of his elbow. The back of her left hand rests against the surface of the couch at its edge. His elbow should be fixed firmly between her hand medially, her fingers and the couch posteriorly, her thumb anteriorly, and her left thigh laterally. This encircling stabilizing grip is essential if the movement is to be performed accurately.

The therapist then grasps the patient's supinated right wrist with her hand, her thumb over the anterior surface and her fingers over the dorsum. The supination is not held strongly at the limit of the range. Once this position is reached she medially rotates his right glenohumeral joint to stabilize his elbow more easily during the adduction; the abduction counterpressure afforded by her left hand is then assisted by the edge of the couch (Figure 10.62).

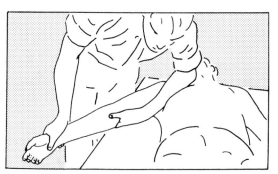

Figure 10.62 Elbow joint; extension/adduction

Method

Whenever this movement is used in treatment, the part of the range that is lost or most painful should first be sought. The treatment movement is then usually directed at this particular part of the range in one or two ways. The limitation can be approached by an adduction or adduction/extension movement, or it can be a scouring circular movement (as depicted in Figure 10.61).

The adduction and adduction/extension directions of the treatment movement can be performed as a grade III or IV. If a grade III movement is used, the pressure maintaining adduction is almost completely released to allow the joint to relax to the position almost midway between abduction and adduction before oscillating back to the adduction position. When a grade IV movement is used, the pressure maintaining adduction limits the oscillation to a small amplitude.

The scouring movement is produced by maintaining the adduction pressure while flexing and extending the elbow across the limitation. This type of movement can be further varied, if the limitation is very painful, by easing the adduction pressure as the pain and limitation are approached. This arc of movement can be performed when extending towards the limitation or adducting towards it.

Extension/abduction***

Similarly, extension/abduction should be checked from the fully extended position through the first 10 or more degrees of flexion. As with extension/adduction, a point is reached during this range of flexion where the arm must be allowed to adduct if the flexion movement is to be continued. Beyond the point of maximum abduction the arm moves laterally again, but this lateral movement will be a lateral rotation of the glenohumeral joint rather than an abduction of the elbow. There is not the same feel of a locking position with this movement as there is with adduction but it is still obvious that the movement from Y_1 to Y_2 in Figure 10.61 is not a straight line but is slightly curved. Any loss of the smooth contour of this curve can be appreciated and can be treated by movement into this position.

Starting position

The starting position is similar to that described for extension/adduction with the exception of the physiotherapist's grip of the patient's wrist. She holds his supinated wrist from the medial side with her fingers spreading over the back of his wrist and her thumb over the front. If his glenohumeral joint is slightly laterally rotated the abduction movement can be directed against her thigh which then acts as the fulcrum (Figure 10.63).

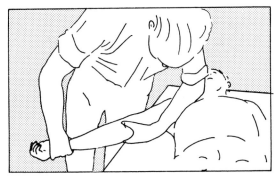

Figure 10.63 Elbow joint; extension/abduction

Method

Movements are performed in the same way as in extension/adduction. Flexion/extension movements or circular movements can be performed while maintaining abduction pressure in much the same way as one would scour a hollow. An abduction movement can be directed at the limitation of the painful part of the range from midway between abduction or adduction using grade III or IV movements. For each method the patient's elbow must be firmly fixed by the physiotherapist's hand against a very firm fulcrum.

The above are examples of extension/abduction and extension/adduction being used as examination procedures and yet also being used for treatment.

Flexion/abduction and flexion/adduction

These two movements should also be used as special tests for the elbow. They are described on pages 180 and 181. They too can be used for examination and treatment. When used for examination purposes a grade IV to grade IV+ is used.

Differentiation tests

When supination or pronation provoke the patient's symptoms and it is necessary to differentiate between the radiohumeral and superior radioulnar joint as the source, the rotary movement is performed with the wrist held in ulnar-deviation (to lessen the stress on the radiohumeral joint) and then repeated with the wrist in radial deviation. Different positions of elbow flexion/extension may also help to make the differentiation. Also, if there is an intra-articular involvement of the superior radio-ulnar joint, adding medially directed pressure against the proximal end of the radius during the rotary movement will increase the pain response.

When flexion or extension provoke the patient's symptoms, the position (of flexion or extension and ulnar deviation) should be held while the head of the radius is moved back and forth (AP-PA). If the disorders lies in the humeroulnar articulation, movement of the radius will not make any difference to the pain response.

Examination for each joint

Tables 10.7 (humeroulnar joint), 10.8 (superior radioulnar joint) and 10.9 (radiohumeral joint) provide the pattern of examination for each of the three joints which comprise the elbow. As mentioned above the site of pain produced by any of the test movements will help to indicate which joint is involved. It is also useful to have a 'composite table' (Table 10.10) as there is considerable overlap in the test movements used for each of the individual joints.

Techniques
Extension

Extension is commonly used in grades II and III– but when the joint is only mildly painful grades III, IV and IV+ may be used.

Grade II***
Starting position

The physiotherapist stands by the patient's right hip, facing his head, and rests her right knee on the couch. With her left hand she supports laterally around his right arm just above his elbow with her thumb anteriorly and her fingers posteriorly. She grasps the palm of his supinated hand with her right hand; her thumb reaches between his thumb and index finger to the back of his hand and her medial three fingers reach around the hypothenar eminence to the back of his hand. Her index finger points

Table 10.7 Humeroulnar joint – objective examination

The routine examination of this joint must also include examination of the superior radioulnar (R/U) joint as supinator/pronator torsion is possible at the humero−ulnar joint.

HIGHLIGHT MAIN FINDINGS WITH ASTERISKS AS YOU GO

Observation

*Functional demonstration/tests

As applicable

1. *Their* demonstration of *their* functional movements affected by *their* disorder.
2. Differentiation of *their* demonstrated functional movement(s).

Brief appraisal

Active movements (move to PAIN or move to LIMIT)
Routinely
F, E, Sup and Pron in F and E
Note range, pain
As applicable
Speed of test movements.
Specific movements which aggravate.
The injuring movement.
Movements under load.
Thoracic outlet tests.
ULTT.
Muscle power.

Isometric tests

Muscles in 'plan' plus clenching fist in different positions of elbow.

Other structures in 'plan'
Thoracic outlet
Entrapment neuropathy

Passive movements
Physiological movements
Routinely
F, E, Sup and Pron in F and E
Note range, pain, resistance, spasm and behaviour
As applicable
E/Ab, E/Ad, F/Ab, F/Ad, Ab and Ad in 5° F and E

Accessory movements
As applicable

1. (→•), (•←)
   (i)   on olecranon.
   (ii) on coronoid.
2. (→•←) caud. (humeral line) in 90° elbow F.
   (i)   on olecranon (thumbs).
   (ii) on coronoid (thumbs).
   (iii) general humeral line.
3. F over wrist in anterior elbow.
4. (→•←) ceph. caud. ulnar line (with wrist deviations) in different angles of elbow F and E.
   Note range, pain, resistance, spasm and behaviour
5. Canal's Slump tests.
6. Differentiation tests.
7. ULTT.
Note range, pain, resistance, spasm and behaviour

Palpation
Temperature.
Swelling and wasting.
Altered sensation.
Relevant tenderness (ulnar, nerve hypersensitivity).
When 'comparable signs' ill defined reassess 'injuring movement'.

Check case records etc.

Instructions to patient

1. Warning of possible exacerbation.
2. Request to record details.
3. Instruction re 'joint care' if required.

proximally over the anterior aspect of his wrist. She moves close to his elbow and uses her thigh to provide the stop at the required angle (Figure 10.64).

Method

The oscillatory movement is performed entirely by the therapist's right arm while her left hand acts as a comfortable support around the patient's elbow. With her grasp of his right wrist she endeavours to encourage relaxation in this area and throughout the arm. The amplitude of movement varies but is usually approximately 20–30°, and is performed smoothly and slowly.

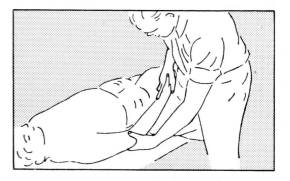

Figure 10.64 Elbow joint; extension, grade II

Table 10.8 Superior radioulnar joint – objective examination

The routine examination of this joint must also include examination of the humeroulnar and radiohumeral joints.

HIGHLIGHT MAIN FINDINGS WITH ASTERISKS AS YOU GO

Observation

*Functional demonstration/tests
As applicable

1. *Their* demonstration of *their* functional movements affected by *their* disorder.
2. Differentiation of *their* demonstrated functional movement(s).

Brief appraisal

Active movements (move to PAIN or move to LIMIT)
As described for the elbow joint

Isometric tests

Other structures in 'plan'

Thoracic outlet
Entrapment neuropathy

Passive movements

Physiological movements
As for elbow joint
Accessory movements
Routinely

1. Ab and Ad of elbow in 5° F (sup. R/U).
2. (↔) cephalad and caudad (ulnar line) in different angles of elbow F and E and different angles of Sup and Pron (using wrist deviations), without compression and with compression.
3. (↓) and (↑), each in full pronation and full supination.
4. Supination/pronation with compression.
Note range, pain, resistance, spasm and behaviour

As applicable

1. Canal's Slump tests.
2. Differentiation tests.
3. ULTT.

Palpation

+When 'comparable signs' ill defined reassess 'injuring movement'.

Check case records etc.

Instructions to patient

1. Warning of possible exacerbation.
2. Request to record details.
3. Instruction re 'joint care' if required.

Table 10.9 Radiohumeral joint – objective examination

The routine examination of this joint must include examination of other joints forming the elbow.

HIGHLIGHT MAIN FINDINGS WITH ASTERISKS AS YOU GO

Observation

*Functional demonstration/tests
As applicable

1. *Their* demonstration of *their* functional movements affected by *their* disorder.
2. Differentiation of *their* demonstrated functional movement(s).

Brief appraisal
Active movements (move to PAIN or move to LIMIT)
Routinely
F, E; Sup and Pron in F and E
Note range, pain

As applicable
Speed of test movements.
Specific movements which aggravate.
The injuring movement.
Movements under load.
Thoracic outlet tests.
Muscle power.

Isometric tests
Muscles in 'plan' plus clenching fist in different positions.

Other structures in 'plan'
Thoracic outlet & ULTT.
Entrapment neuropathy.

Passive movements
Routinely

1. F, E; Sup and Pron in F and E.
2. (↔) ceph and caud (by wrist deviations) in different angles of elbow from full F to full E, and full supination to full pronation.
3. (↓), (↑), in different positions of F, E, Sup., Pro., without compression and with compression.
Note range, pain, resistance, spasm and behaviour

As applicable

1. Canal's Slump tests.
2. Differentiation tests.
3. ULTT.

Palpation
+When 'comparable signs' ill defined reassess 'injuring movement'.

Check case records etc.

Instructions to patient

1. Warning of possible exacerbation.
2. Request to record details.
3. Instruction re 'joint care' if required.

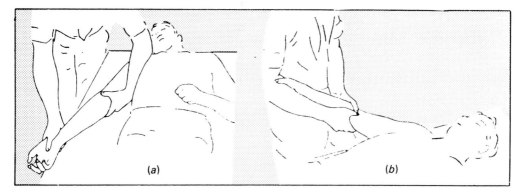

Figures 10.65 Elbow joint; extension, grade III (*a*) and (*b*)

Grade III

If grade III movements are used when the elbow has a limited range of extension the starting position is identical with that described for grade II. However, if the range is nearly full, a different starting position is required.

Starting position**

The patient lies with his arm abducted approximately 15° so that his wrist is clear of the edge of the couch. The therapist stands by his right shoulder, facing his feet, and supports under his elbow from the medial side with her left hand while holding his shoulder down with her left forearm. With her right hand she grasps his partially supinated wrist laterally, her thenar eminence and thumb pointing distally across the front of his wrist and her fingers across the back of his wrist and hand (Figure 10.65(a)).

Method

The oscillation is done entirely by the therapist's right arm, and the patient's right hand is stabilized by her grasp of his wrist. The amplitude of elbow movement is approximately 20–30°. If the treatment is to be directed towards a 'through-range-pain' the technique would be performed smoothly and slowly, but if it is used for a chronic disorder presenting with 'end-of-range' symptoms, it would be performed as a staccato movement flicking gently at the end of the extension range.

Alternative starting position***

There is another technique that sometimes provides a better feeling of the last 30° of extension and it is a technique that allows some patients to relax more easily.

The therapist stands by the patient's right hip, facing his head. She lifts his right arm and holds his hand against her right side. She holds around his elbow with both hands, her thumbs holding anterior to the joint and her fingers overlapping posteriorly (Figure 10.65(b)) or feeling for soft tissue movement (during the extension phase) between the olecranon process and the margins of the olecranon fossa (Figure 10.66(a)).

For examination purposes, this palpation of soft tissue movement should be compared with that present in his normal elbow because the normal has a wide variation from person to person. The normal should allow the finger tips to easily fit into the space between process and fossa margins and feel clean bony margins.

Palpation of these margins, which can be critical in a thorough examination routine, can also be carried out with the patient lying prone, his upper arm supported on the table and his hand and forearm hanging down towards the floor. His elbow is thus flexed to 90° (Figure 10.66(a)).

In the same two positions shown in Figure 10.66(a) and (b)), pressure can be applied to the olecranon process by the therapist's thumbs to produce four movements. These movements are:

1. Medial.
2. Lateral.
3. Longitudinal caudad.
4. Compression.

Alternative method

The oscillation is produced by raising and lowering the patient's elbow 4 or 5 inches (100–130 mm) while his wrist is stabilized. The treatment may be assisted by applying either compression or slight

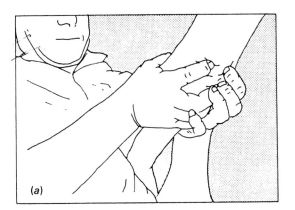

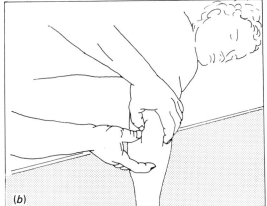

Figures 10.66 Palpation in olecranon fossa (*a*)in extension; (*b*) in flexion

distraction to his elbow by using her body through her grasp of his wrist. Adduction or abduction can also be added to the extension movement by increasing the pressure in either direction by her left or right hand.

Grade IV

This movement should never by performed more strongly than as a grade IV−.

Starting position***

The starting position is identical with that described for Figure 10.66(a) except that the therapist's hand and knee should be the fulcrum for the movement rather than the couch. This position enables a more perceptive feel of the strength of the oscillation.

Flexion

Passive movement in this direction is a very useful treatment procedure, particularly with grade III or IV.

Grade II**

Starting position

The physiotherapist stands by the patient's right shoulder facing his feet and supports under his right elbow from the medial side with her left forearm crossing his right upper arm. With her right hand she grasps his partially supinated wrist from the lateral side with her fingers across the back of his hand, and her thumb between his thumb and index finger into his palm. To provide the stop for the flexion movement, she flexes his elbow to the required

position and then raises her left forearm until it is in firm contact with the front of his right wrist (Figure 10.67).

Method

The oscillatory movement, performed by the physiotherapist's right arm, is taken back and forth through 20–30° slowly and smoothly up to the stop provided by her left forearm. As the range improves her left forearm can be lowered.

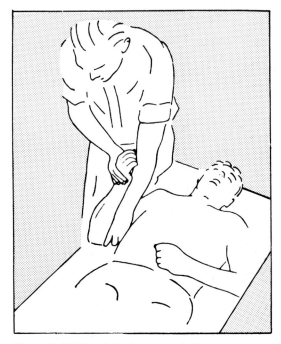

Figure 10.67 Elbow joint;flexion, grade II

Grades III and IV**

When the range of flexion is limited and grades III and IV are required a similar starting position to that adopted for grade II is used. However, if the movement is almost full range a different starting position is required.

Starting position

The physiotherapist stands by the patient's right side, distal to his elbow, facing his head. With her left hand she supports his right upper arm just above the elbow. She flexes and partially supinates his elbow holding the back of his hand with her right hand, her thumb passing through the first interosseous space, her medial three fingers spreading medially around the fifth metacarpal and her index finger extending distally along the back of his hand (Figure 10.68).

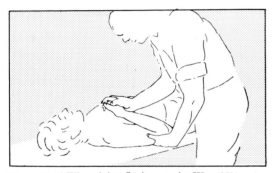

Figure 10.68 Elbow joint; flexion, grades III and IV

Method

The oscillation is produced entirely by moving the patient's right arm while her left hand acts as a support under his elbow. Grade III movements are large with amplitudes of between 10 and 30° reaching the limit of the flexion range, and grade IV movements are small amplitude oscillations of 3 or 4°, or even less.

Flexion with accessory movement

Frequently a joint exhibiting minimal symptoms may have a full range of flexion. It is inadequate under these circumstances to test flexion only as a straight sagittal direction of movement. There are three ways the movement can be varied, and during examination these should be tested with grade IV type movements before determining that flexion has a painless full range. These movements are flexion/adduction, flexion/abduction and flexion with distraction. When employed in treatment they are used only in grades III or IV.

Flexion/adduction***

Starting position

The physiotherapist stands by the patient's right hip, facing his head, and fully pronates his forearm. She holds his fully pronated wrist with her left hand, her fingers over the back of his wrist and her thenar eminence and thumb over the front. She grasps firmly from the medial side around his upper arm at the junction of the middle and lower thirds in such a way as to hold his upper arm laterally rotated. The slack in soft tissue must be taken up fully. Both of the therapist's forearms are then rotated opposite to each other (Figure 10.69).

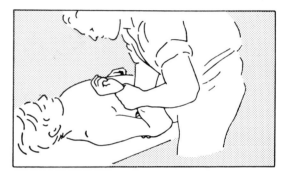

Figure 10.69 Elbow joint; flexion/adduction

Method

The flexion/adduction movement is performed entirely by the therapist's left arm while she prevents any medial rotation of the glenohumeral joint with her firm grasps of his upper arm with her right hand. If medial rotation is not prevented, the adduction strain at his elbow will be lost. The treatment movement can be performed as large-amplitude oscillations through 10–15° (grade III) or as small oscillatory movements through 3 or 4° (grade IV).

Flexion/abduction***

Starting position

The physiotherapist stands by the patient's right hip, facing his head, while supporting under his upper arm with her left hand and flexing his elbow with her right hand. With her left hand she grasps his upper arm at the junction of the middle and lower thirds in such a way as to prevent lateral rotation of the glenohumeral joint. With her right hand she grasps his supinated wrist from the medial side, her fingers spreading across the front of his wrist and her thumb across the back (Figure 10.70).

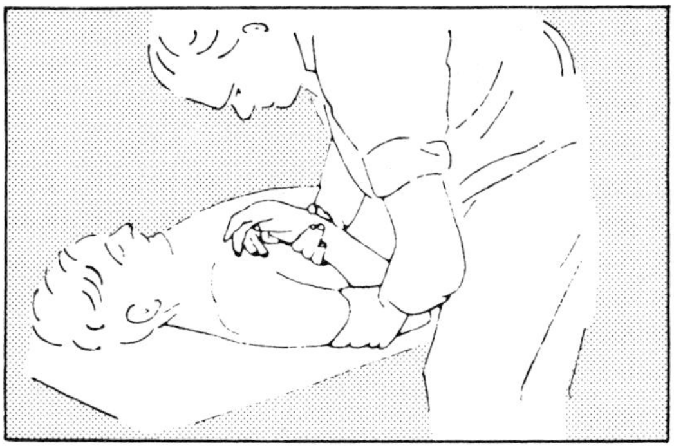

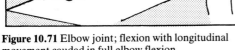

Figure 10.70 Elbow joint; flexion/abduction

Method

She flexes his elbow and displaces the wrist laterally with an abduction movement at the elbow joint, while applying an equal counterpressure with her left hand, preventing any lateral rotation of the glenohumeral joint. If this counterpressure is unsuccessful, the sideways movement of the patient's wrist will consist of lateral rotation of the glenohumeral joint without any abduction at the elbow.

Flexion with longitudinal movement caudad**

This is the least useful of the three combined movements associated with flexion.

Starting position

The physiotherapist stands by the patient's right hip, facing his head. She flexes his elbow with her right hand, grasping around the medial aspect of his supinated wrist, her fingers spreading across the front and her thumb across the back. When his elbow reaches 90° of flexion she places her supinated

left forearm just proximal to her wrist, in the crook of his elbow. Elbow flexion is continued until her left wrist is firmly squeezed between his forearm and upper arm (Figure 10.71).

Method

The movement consists of small oscillations produced by the therapist's right arm. Care is needed to maintain her wedged arm in a *constant proximity to the patient's elbow* because the tendency will be for it to be squeezed out. A wrong degree of supination forming the wedge will make the position very uncomfortable for the patient.

Longitudinal movement caudad (90° flexion)*

This movement should be tested when joint signs are minimal. It is a mobilization used in the treatment of stiff elbows.

Starting position

The physiotherapist stands by the patient's right elbow, facing his left knee, and flexes his right elbow to a right angle or at the limit of his range of flexion. She supports the back of his supinated right wrist by grasping around his medial metacarpals with her fingers and through the first interosseous space with her thumb while maintaining his wrist in a neutral position. She places the heel of her left hand over the anterior aspect of his upper forearm with her fingers spreading distally down the front of his forearm. Her left thumb spreads laterally around his forearm and her three medial fingers spread medially (Figure 10.72).

Method

The slack of scapulothoracic depression must be taken up before alternating pressures are applied

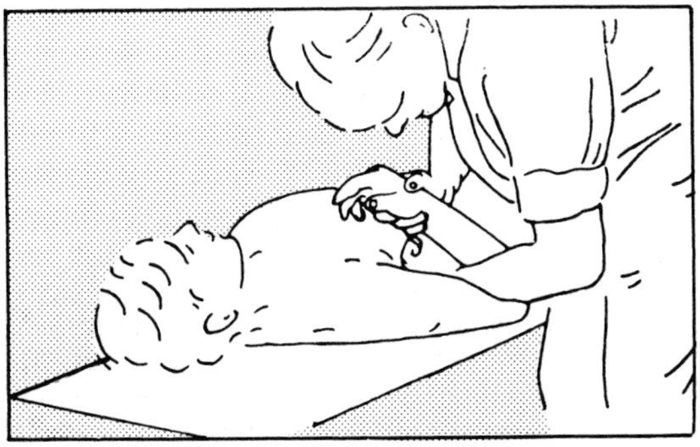

Figure 10.71 Elbow joint; flexion with longitudinal movement caudad in full elbow flexion

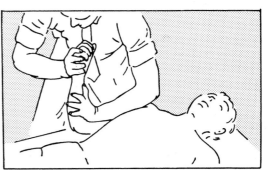

Figure 10.72 Elbow joint; longitudinal movement caudad (90° flexion)

against the forearm to produce the distraction movement. There is very little movement in this direction and it is almost impossible to feel any localized accessory movement unless the 'Alternative method', which follows, is used. The movement can be combined with minimal elbow flexion movement, or the therapist can carry the patient's hand with the movement, maintaining a constant elbow angle.

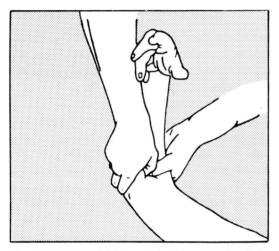

Figure 10.73 Elbow joint; longitudinal movement caudad (90° flexion), alternative position

Sometimes distraction is produced better by thumb pressure against the anterior surface of the coronoid process.

Alternative starting position**

The physiotherapist stands by the patient's right hip, facing his head. His arm is flexed and supported against her right upper quadriceps area. She then grasps his forearm near the elbow, placing the pads of her thumbs against the coronoid process. The fingers of her right hand spread medially around his forearm and those of her left hand spread laterally. She should position her index fingers so that their lateral margins are in contact with the distal margin of the medial and lateral epicondyles (Figure 10.73).

Alternative method

The movement is produced by the arms acting through the pads of the thumbs while counterpressure is exerted through the index fingers against the epicondyles. The pressure must not be created by the thumb flexors as the movement then becomes uncomfortable for the patient and all feeling of movement is lost to therapist.

Distraction can be performed in different positions of elbow flexion, and during treatment it may be necessary to carry out the distraction movement in more than one position of elbow flexion.

Superior radioulnar joint

When a patient has a disorder causing pain-through-range, he frequently will supinate and pronate his forearm unconsciously while talking about his elbow symptoms. This should immediately alert the therapist to the likelihood of radioulnar involvement.

If a patient has pain within his elbow, especially if this is felt posteriorly, and is only reproduced with firm over-pressure of supination or pronation, supination and pronation of the olecranon process in its fossa should be examined by thumb pressures against the process (see Figures 10.65(a) and (b)).

As well as supination and pronation, the superior radioulnar joint has passive accessory movements of the head of the radius on the ulna. These are posteroanterior and anteroposterior movements, which can be performed with the forearm in any degree of elbow supination or pronation, flexion or extension. Longitudinal movements cephalad and caudad are the two remaining accessory movements, though they have limited practical application. All of these movements can be performed with or without compression of the head of the radius against the ulna (Table 10.8).

*Supination****

As the techniques for grades I to IV are similar, whether the range is restricted or not, the movement will only be described as a grade II and IV+ movement in a full range joint.

Starting position

The physiotherapist stands by the patient's right side beyond his flexed elbow, facing his head, and supports under his elbow with her left hand. With her right hand she grasps his supinated wrist from the medial side, her fingers spreading across the front of his wrist and carpus, and her thumb across the back (Figure 10.68).

Method

A grade II movement may require a very flicky action by the physiotherapist's right hand if the disorder is neither severe nor irritable. It is performed from midway between supination and pronation to full supination. The supination is produced by a combined action of the physiotherapist's own supination together with flexion of her wrist and fingers. During the movement the patient's wrist must be stabilized to prevent flapping. If the disorder causes much pain the technique is performed smoothly and slowly.

When grades III and IV are performed, the therapist must support the patient's elbow medially to prevent glenohumeral adduction, or alternatively, she must begin the movement with the patient's elbow adducted against his side.

For stronger grades of movement a different starting position is adopted which places the therapist in a more economical working position.

Grade IV+**

Starting position

The physiotherapist stands by the patient's flexed right elbow and holds the distal end of his fully supinated radius and ulna in her left and right hands respectively holding far enough distally to stabilize the hand. She fully supinates her left forearm and holds the distal end of his radius posteriorly with her lateral surface of the distal phalanx of her index finger and anteriorly with the pad of her thumb. With her right hand she holds the distal end of the ulna, her thumb and thenar eminence pointing distally over the posterior surface of the ulna and her fingers holding anteriorly. Her forearms are directed opposite each other at right angles to the coronal plane of the fully supinated wrist (Figure 10.75).

Method

Keeping her forearm in the same line, she supinates his forearm 2 or 3° by transmitting a rocking action of her pelvis and trunk through her hands to his radius and ulna and then releases the IV+ pressure to a IV or IV−. Repetition of this action produces the oscillatory supination. The amplitude is small and if the joint range is limited she merely turns her body towards the right to change the direction of her forearms. Her body, arms and hands move as a cemented single unit.

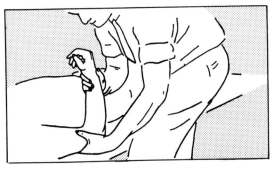

Figure 10.74 Superior radioulnar joint; supination grades I–IV

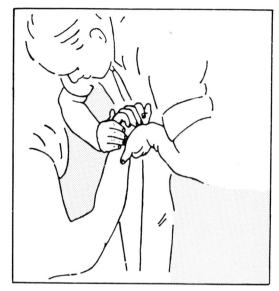

Figure 10.75 Superior radioulnar joint; supination grade IV+

Pronation***

Starting position

The physiotherapist stands by the patient's right hip facing his head, supporting under his flexed elbow with her right hand so that her fingers can reach the lateral surface. With her left hand she grasps his pronated forearm distally, her fingers extending across the dorsum of his wrist and hand to reach the carpus and her thumb extending around the anterior surface. This position is necessary to stabilize the wrist during the pronation movements (Figure 10.76).

Method

The therapist performs the rotary movement by slight glenohumeral flexion combined with slight extension of the left shoulder and elbow to move her arm forward. This action is combined with full flexion of her wrist and fingers to produce the pronation. With her right hand she stabilizes his upper arm, preventing abduction of his shoulder.

A more efficient position for grade IV+ movements can be used.

Grade IV+**

Starting position

The therapist stands by the patient's elbow, facing across his body. His elbow is flexed to 90° and pronated. She grasps the distal end of his radius and ulna with her left and right hands respectively. She

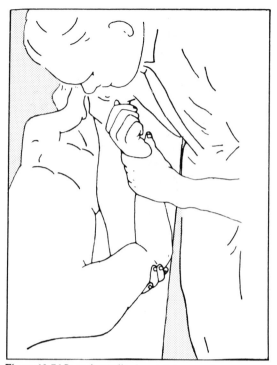

Figure 10.76 Superior radioulnar joint; pronation

places the thenar eminence of her left hand against the dorsal surface of the radius with her thumb extending distally across the back of his wrist while her fingers grasp anteriorly around his radius. With her right hand fully supinated she grasps around the distal end of his ulna, the heel of her hand and her thumb pointing proximally against the anterior surface of the ulna and her fingers grasping around the ulna to reach the posterior surface. She directs her forearms opposite each other (Figure 10.77).

Method

The oscillatory pronation is produced by the same method as that described for supination.

Anteroposterior movement

The anteroposterior movement is the direction the head of the radius moves in relation to the ulna.

Although the range of movement is greatest when the forearm is midway between pronation and supination, the technique is more commonly used in either the fully supinated or pronated position. It is used most when loss of range is more important to the patient than his pain, but it is also important when minor symptoms arise from the joint when the pain can be elicited by this technique. The treatment

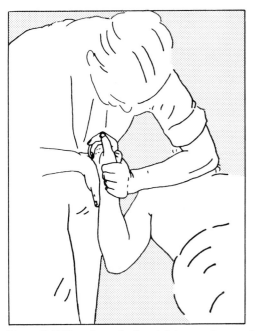

Figure 10.77 Superior radioulnar joint; pronation, grade IV+

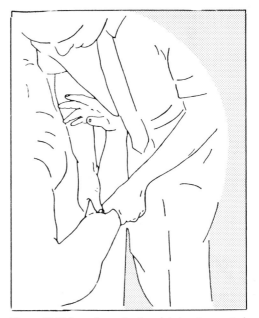

Figure 10.78 Superior radioulnar joint; anteroposterior movement in supination

usually involves grade III or IV movements and it is described here in a position of approximately 30° elbow flexion and full supination and pronation.

However, when pain-through-range is present, or when it is pain that is the dominant element grade II movements are used with the forearm in a mid-position between supination and pronation. It can then be performed as an anteroposterior movement, a posteroanterior movement, or as an oscillatory movement back and forth (AP/PA/AP etc.) in the middle of its range.

In supination***

Starting position

The physiotherapist stands by the patient's right side beyond his slightly flexed right elbow, facing his head. She supports the back of his supinated forearm against her right side and places the pads of her thumbs over the anterior surface of the head of the radius. She should gradually apply pressure with her thumbs so they sink into the relaxed muscle tissue to contact the head of the radius. The fingers of her left and right hands spread over the lateral and medial surfaces of the upper end of the forearm (Figure 10.78).

Method

The oscillations are produced by the therapist's arms and the pressure is transmitted through her thumbs,

which act as springs. The pressure required for the mobilization must not be produced by the thumb flexor muscles.

In pronation

Starting position

The starting position is similar to that described above for supination (Figure 10.78) except that the physiotherapist holds the patient's pronated right wrist around its lateral border with her right hand, her thumb crosses the back of his wrist and her fingers cross the front. It is necessary to hold his forearm in pronation because the anteroposterior pressure tends to produce supination. She supports his forearm against her side and places her left thumb against the head of the radius and her fingers around the lateral surface of the forearm (Figure 10.79).

Method

The mobilization is performed by the therapist's left arm through the stable thumb while maintaining the pronation with her right hand.

Posteroanterior movement

This movement has a similar application in treatment to the anteroposterior movement and there-

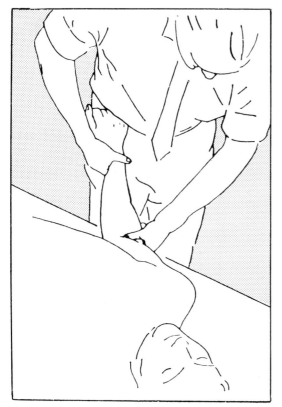

Figure 10.79 Superior radioulnar joint; anteroposterior movement in pronation

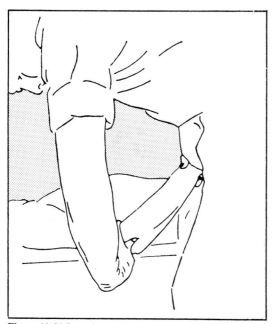

Figure 10.80 Superior radioulnar joint; posteroanterior movement in supination

fore grade III and IV movements are the ones commonly used. Also it can be performed in varying degrees of elbow flexion extension, supination or pronation. Posteroanterior movement will be described with the elbow in approximately 30° of flexion at the limits of both supination and pronation.

In supination***

Starting position

The physiotherapist stands by the patient's right side beyond his slightly flexed elbow, facing his head, and holds his supinated wrist from the medial side with her right hand. She places her thumb across the front of his wrist and her fingers across the back. The pad of her left thumb, pointing distally, is placed against the dorsal surface of the head of the radius. To provide a counterpressure for the movement, her fingers are placed against the front of the distal end of the upper arm. Because this movement tends to produce pronation it is necessary to stabilize the patient's wrist in supination (Figure 10.80).

Method

The therapist produces the movement by small adduction movements of her left shoulder combined with slight forearm supination to exert pressure against the head of the radius with her left thumb. If the pressure is produced by the flexors of the thumb, the feel of the movement will be lost and the pressure will be uncomfortable to both patient and operator.

In pronation***

Starting position

The same starting position and method are adopted as have been described for posteroanterior movement in supination (Figure 10.78) except that the wrist is held with the forearm pronated.

Longitudinal movement caudad*

This movement can, like the other accessory movements, be performed with the elbow in any degree of flexion, extension, supination or pronation. However, if maximum excursion of movement in the normal joint is required the forearm should be positioned midway between flexion and extension and also midway between supination and pronation. The movement will be described in this position but other positions can be used. The position used in treatment is commonly the one found to be most restricted or most painful unless a through-range-technique is required.

Starting position

The physiotherapist stands by the patient's right side just beyond his elbow and rests his right forearm against her right side. She holds across the front of his upper arm, proximal to his elbow, with her left hand, her fingers spreading laterally and her thumb medially. Her main point of contact against his upper arm is the web of her first interosseous space. With her right hand she grasps the anterior surface of his supinated carpus. Her thumb grasps around the radial surface proximal to the base of the fifth metacarpal. The middle finger and thumb must reach as far as possible around the posterior surface of the carpus. Her right forearm must then be brought into the same line as the patient's forearm (Figure 10.81).

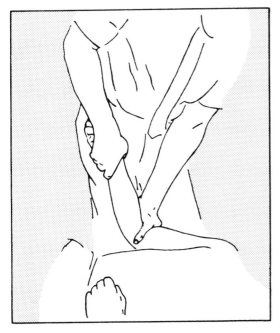

Figure 10.81 Superior radioulnar joint; longitudinal movement caudad

Method

When this technique is used as a grade IV movement, the slack in soft tissue must first be taken up. As the therapist pulls with her right hand her left hand must sink into the patient's flexor muscle tissue to hold his upper arm firmly. Slack must also be taken up at the wrist. Small oscillatory longitudinal movements can then be performed by a pulling action with her right arm counteracted by a stabilizing pressure through her left hand.

The movement caudad can be enhanced by adding ulnar deviation in rhythm with the pulling action.

Longitudinal movement cephalad*

This movement is mainly used as a grade IV movement in positions between 90° flexion and full flexion. The technique will be described with the patient's forearm midway between supination and pronation in 90° of flexion. It is also a technique that can be used for radiohumeral disorders, and thus in 'differentiation tests'.

Starting position

The physiotherapist stands by the patient's right side beyond his flexed elbow facing his head and grasps his right hand in hers as if shaking hands. She then extends her right wrist, and his, and supports under the distal end of his right upper arm with her left hand. She crouches over his hand and supports her right hand against her right hip (Figure 10.82).

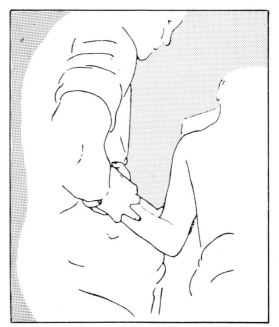

Figure 10.82 Superior radioulnar joint; longitudinal movement cephalad

Method

There is no slack to be taken up with this movement and the small oscillations are produced by pressure through the physiotherapist's wrist along the line of the shaft of the radius together with radial deviation of the wrist joint.

Radiohumeral joint

Symptoms do not commonly arise from this joint unless it has been involved in trauma or unless there is some disorder of the elbow or superior radio-ulnar joint.

The main technique used in examining this joint (Table 10.9) is to apply a compressive force through the patient's hand so as to compress the head of the radius against the capitulum. The technique is shown in Figure 10.82 above, with the elbow in approximately 90° of flexion. To localize the movement as much as possible to the radiohumeral joint the pressure should be transmitted through the patient's thenar eminence with the wrist deviated radially directing the force through the radius. The compression technique should be performed through as large a range of elbow flexion to extension range as is possible.

If the technique described above does not produce any symptoms, then a supination to pronation oscillatory movement should be added to the compressing of the head of the radius against the humerus. Again, this should be performed in various positions of elbow flexion and extension.

Chronic/minor symptoms Examination

When a patient's elbow symptoms are comparatively minor, or are long-standing, there are certain examination passive movement tests which must be assessed. These are listed below (Table 10.10).

Proving unaffected

It is sometimes necessary to examine the elbow joint solely to prove that it is not causing a patient's symptoms. Under these circumstances only three passive movement tests need be performed. They should be performed as grade IV+ movements (Table 10.11).

Treatment

When pain is felt by the patient to be in a vague area around the elbow joint it is very difficult to determine which of the three joints is the primary one at fault. During examination, the accessory movements performed at the limit of the various ranges of each joint may provide the answer.

In many chronic or minor disorders, elbow extension or extension in conjunction with abduction or adduction will provide the most comparable sign. Therefore these are the most commonly used techniques in treatment. However, if an accessory

Table 10.10 Mandatory passive movement tests, when chronic symptoms occupy any part of the area from mid-humerus to mid-radius/ulna

Supine: Flexion & extension, plus in abd. & add.
Supination & pronation plus (↓) & (↓) and plus compr.
Longitudinal caudad (humeral line) in 90° Elb. F.
Olecranon movements
Functional test, grip (small & large) in F, E, Sup, Pron.
Isometric tests

Test movements begin as IV− with observation for pain response. If pain free, adequate over-pressure is applied until pain is provoked or the movement is judged 'clear'.

When a positive pain response is provoked, that test movement may need to be differentiated to determine the specific joint at fault, and/or other test movements may need to be tested so as to either exclude or incriminate other joints as contributing to the symptoms.

If all test movements appear 'clear' at first examination, they should be repeated more strongly. If still 'clear', they may prove positive when repeated at the next consultation.

Table 10.11 Proving that the elbow is, in fact, UNAFFECTED

Supine: E/Abd – Add and 'scouring'
Sup. & Pron. with IV+ OP
Olecranon tests

movement at the limit of a physiological range is a good 'comparable sign', then it would be the first technique used.

The elbow, whether being treated for pain or stiffness, is a joint which is extremely easily overtreated at any one session. Therefore, if the physiological movement of extension is used to treat pain, it is vital that the patient's arm be completely relaxed during treatment, and the technique should be completely free of even the most minor feeling of discomfort.

The technique shown in Figure 10.64 is commonly the best position in which to use grades II and III− extension. This is because the joint is completely surrounded and supported by both hands while the forearm and hand can be comfortably surrounded and supported by the physiotherapist's forearm and trunk.

If the patient's symptoms are comparatively mild, and gentle grade IV extension movements are contemplated as treatment techniques, initially the movements should be slower than those usually used, and the amount of pain provoked by the treatment should be minimal. If this care is not taken there will almost certainly be an exacerbation of the patient's pain.

Tennis elbow

If the term tennis elbow is used accurately, passive movements of the joint will be full range and painless. Under these circumstances passive movement techniques have no place in treatment. (In the author's opinion, Mill's manipulation, when used effectively, producing a good result, it does so because it manipulates the joint and not because it has stretched the tenomuscular junction.)

The term tennis elbow in the majority of cases is used loosely and careful examination will reveal that there is a joint component to the symptoms as well as the tenomuscular component. When minor joint signs are present they should be used as the passive movement treatment techniques. Initially, the joint signs alone should be treated until a clear picture of the pattern of progress can be predicted. It may then be necessary to treat the tenomuscular component while continuing with the joint treatment. However, on many occasions, the tenomuscular component recovers spontaneously when joint movement recovers.

All tennis elbows that have become chronic will have a joint component as part of the comparable joint signs.

Joint stiffness

The long-held view, that stretching the elbow is likely to cause a myositis ossificans, is taking a long time to die. When a patient has a stiff and painful joint the physiotherapist should treat the pain first so that she has a clear picture of its behaviour and irritability. Once this is known and treatment is directed towards stretching the elbow in any direction provided progression of the strength of the technique used does not unfavourably alter the pattern of the pain, the stretching techniques are completely safe. As has been indicated earlier the stretching techniques would consist of three elements:

1. A physiological movement is selected and grade IV or IV− stretching can be applied provided pain is minimal.
2. The joint is now supported at the limit of the physiological range being stretched and accessory movements (for example Figure 10.73) are performed as grade IV movements.
3. Either interspersed between the physiological movements and the accessory movements, or at

Table 10.12 Composite elbow – objective examination

HIGHLIGHT MAIN FINDINGS WITH ASTERISKS AS YOU GO

Observation

*Functional demonstration/tests
1. *Their* demonstration of *their* functional movements affected by *their* disorder.
2. Differentiation of *their* demonstrated functional movement(s).

Brief appraisal
Active movements (move to PAIN or move to LIMIT)
F, E, (as applicable bouncing F and E in full pronation and supination)
Sup, Pron (as applicable performed in F and E)

Isometric tests
Other structures in 'plan'
Thoracic outlet & ULTT.
Entrapment neuropathy.

Passive movements
As applicable
F, E Sup and Pron as IV− to IV+ to III++
Differentiating as required
1. F and E as IV+ at limit of range
   (a) F/Ab, F/Ad, E/Ab, E/Ad. Ab and Ad in the first 5° of F and full E.
   (b) (↔) (in line with humerus) ceph and caud.
       (i) on radius (radiohumeral (R/H) joint or superior radioulnar (R/U) joint add superior R/U compression to differentiate between R/H and superior R/U.
       (ii) on ulna (humeroulnar joint).
   (c) (↔) (in line with radius) ceph and caud.
       (i) on radius (R/H or superior R/U joint) add superior R/U compression to differentiate between R/H and superior R/U.
       (ii) on ulna (humeroulnar joint).
2. Sup and Pron as IV+ at limit of range.
   (a) (↓) (↑) on head of radius (superior R/U or R/H joint) add compression of superior R/U joint to differentiate between radiohumeral and superior R/U joint.
   (b) (↓) (↑) on ulna (humeroulnar joint).
3. Other differentiating tests:
   (a) (↓)(↖)(↗)(↓)(↖)(↗) on head of radius in different positions of elbow F and E.
   (b) (→) (←) on olecranon and coronoid.
4. Combined movements.
5. Canal's Slump tests.
6. Differentiation tests.
7. ULTT.
Note range, pain, resistance, spasm and behaviour

Palpation
+When 'comparable signs' ill defined reassess 'injuring movement'.

Check case records etc.

Instructions to patient
1. Warning of possible exacerbation.
2. Request to record details.
3. Instruction re 'joint care' if required.

the completion of the treatment session, grade II+ (or III− if not painful) are used through as large a range as is possible to minimize treatment soreness.

Chronic minor joint pain

When a patient has pain in the elbow which is minor and the condition has existed without change for a long time, the techniques used will be the 'comparable signs' found at examination. After the first examination and treatment, if the disorder is found to be not irritable, then subsequent treatments must be performed as grade IV or IV+ movements interspersed with grade III and III+ movements.

If the patient has a seemingly full range of movement and the comparable signs are found to be very close to the limit of the range then the two most commonly used techniques are (1) extension/ adduction as a scouring series of movements, and

(2) extension/abduction in the same manner. These techniques, when tried at the right time on the right patient/disorder, are dramatic in their relief of pain.

Composite elbow examination

Movements of each of the three (humeroulnar, radiohumeral, radioulnar) joints which combine to form the elbow do not occur in isolation. It is therefore difficult at times to determine whether pain felt on stretching supination, for example, is in fact arising from the superior radioulnar joint. This is because if supination is stretched, the humeroulnar joint undergoes a degree of torsion and the head of the radius spins and slides under the capitulum. Table 10.12 lists the test movements performed, and shows how this example of supination can be performed in ways to differentiate between the different components of the movement.

Inferior radioulnar joint

Pain from this joint is always felt locally and deep. Any referred pain is usually felt from the joint spreading upwards towards the elbow. The site of symptoms is quite different from those arising from the carpal-tunnel or the tendon sheaths[6].

The passive movements that can be produced at the inferior radioulnar joint are supination, pronation, posteroanterior (PA) and anteroposterior (AP) movements of the ulna on the radius. The last two movements can be produced with the inferior radioulnar joint positioned anywhere from the limit of pronation to the limit of supination. The largest amplitude of the movement is when the inferior radioulnar joint is positioned midway between full pronation and supination. The PA and AP movements are referred to as movements of *the ulna on the radius* because it is easier to stabilize the comparatively large distal end of the radius and produce the movement by pushing the distal end of the ulna.

The next movement possible at the radioulnar joint, either actively (with hand movements) or passively, is described as being longitudinal movement of *the radius on the ulna* either cephalad or caudad. The reasons for presenting the movement as being that of the radius on the ulna are: first, the ulna is relatively more stable at the elbow and second, one of the best ways of producing this movement is to carry out ulnar deviation of the hand, which pulls the radius in a caudad direction. Cephalad longitudinal movement of the radius on the ulna is produced by radial deviation of the wrist.

One last movement that can be produced passively at the inferior radioulnar joint consists of compression (where the radius and ulna are squeezed together), and distraction (when the distal ends of the radius and ulna are separated).

Examination

During the examination of the inferior radioulnar joint when the forearm is supinated or pronated strongly and the patient feels pain in the vicinity of the inferior radioulnar joint it is commonly erroneously assumed that the pain is arising from that joint. When it is realized that supination and pronation can also be produced at the wrist joint it is easy to see how this error is made. The differentiation examination procedure is described fully elsewhere in this chapter.

Functional demonstration/test

These should be sought first and analysed. For example, turning on a tap may be the function that provokes the pain. The question is, at what stage does it hurt? The answer is, what movement of the ulna (for example) in this position increases the provocation?

Brief appraisal

These tests consist of asking the patient to rotate his forearm and hand through a large-amplitude, firstly striking the limit of supination four or five times and then repeating the technique for pronation. The speed with which he can do this will guide the examiner as to how firmly or gently the tests will need to be performed.

Another quick test is to ask the patient to squeeze the therapist's hand and report any pain response.

Special tests

There are two important special tests for the inferior radioulnar joint. The first is performed when the inferior radioulnar joint is stretched to the limit of, say, supination. While the joint is held in this position an extra anteroposterior movement should be exerted against the anterior surface of the ulna and after assessing pain with this movement a posteroanterior movement should be applied from the posterior surface of the ulna. The same anteroposterior and posteroanterior movements should be performed with the ulna moving on the radius at the limit of pronation.

The second special test is to compress strongly the radius against the ulna and at the same time rock the radius and ulna back and forth against each other. This technique is shown in Figure 10.78.

Table 10.13 lists the full passive movement examination.

Techniques
Posteroanterior and anteroposterior movements***
Starting position

The physiotherapist stands by the patient's right side, just beyond his flexed elbow, facing his left shoulder. She holds his forearm, midway between supination and pronation, between the thumb and index finger of each hand. The distal end of his radius is held in her left hand between the thumb on the posterior surface and the flexed index finger on the anterior surface. If all her fingers are flexed they can be used to add lateral support to the index finger

---

6. Corrigan, B. and Maitland, G. D. *Practical Orthopaedic Medicine*, Butterworths, London, p. 93 (1983)

Table 10.13 Inferior radioulnar joint – objective examination

---

The routine examination of this joint must also include examination of the wrist, as supination and pronation also occur as accessory movements of the wrist joint.

HIGHLIGHT MAIN FINDINGS WITH ASTERISKS AS YOU GO

Observation

*Functional demonstration/tests

1. *Their* demonstration of *their* functional movements affected by *their* disorder.
2. Differentiation of *their* demonstrated functional movement(s).

Brief appraisal
Active movements (move to PAIN or move to LIMIT)
Routinely
Wrist, Ab, Ad (F and E).
Supination, pronation.
Note range, pain.

Isometric tests

Other structures in 'plan'
Thoracic outlet & ULTT.
Entrapment neuropathy.
Tendon sheaths.

Passive movements

Physiological movements
Routinely
Sup and Pron.
Note range, pain, resistance, spasm and behaviour.

Accessory movements
As applicable

1. (↓) (↑).
   (a) in neutral (also (↕).
   (b) at limit of pronation.
   (c) at limit of supination.

2. Sup/Pron with compression.

3. Sup and Pron differentiating for wrist.

   Note range, pain, resistance, spasm and behaviour.
   As applicable

4. Canal's Slump tests.

5. Differentiation tests.

6. ULTT.

Palpation
+When 'comparable signs' ill defined reassess 'injuring movement'.

Check case records etc.

Instructions to patient

1. Warning of possible exacerbation.
2. Request to record details.
3. Instruction re 'joint care' if required.

---

which makes the main point of contact. With her right hand she holds the distal end of his ulna with an identical grip (Figure 10.83).

Method

A posteroanterior movement of the radius on the ulna is produced by pressure against the anterior surface of the ulna with the therapist's right index finger and an equal and opposite pressure against the posterior surface of the head of the radius with her left thumb. Obviously, an anteroposterior movement of the head of the radius on the ulna would be produced by an opposite action.

If either of these movements needs to be performed strongly at the limit of its range, the therapist should grasp the radius and ulna more firmly between the thenar eminences, rather than just the thumb, and the respective fingers. The oscillation is then produced by a pushing and pulling action of the arms.

Compression**
Starting position

The physiotherapist kneels by the patient's right side beyond his flexed elbow and grasps his right hand in her two hands. Her thumb and thenar eminence, pointing towards his fingers, cover the posterior surface of the wrist, meeting in the mid line. Her fingers reach around to meet anteriorly in the mid line. The heel of her left hand cups around the lateral surface of the distal end of his radius while the heel of her right hand cups around his ulna. Both arms are directed opposite to each other at right angles to his forearm (Figure 10.84).

Method

Supination and pronation are produced by a twisting in opposite directions of the heels of the therapist's cupped hands pivoting around her stationary fingers and thumbs. Pronation of the patient's forearm is produced by pronation of her left forearm and supination of her right forearm so that the heels of her hands move away from each other. Supination is produced by supination of her left forearm combined with pronation of her right. A back and forth rocking movement between supination and pronation is continued while the compression is maintained between her two arms.

Longitudinal movement cephalad*
Starting position and method

The technique is almost identical with that shown in Figure 10.82 but emphasis must be placed on the exact position of the patient's hand and the direction

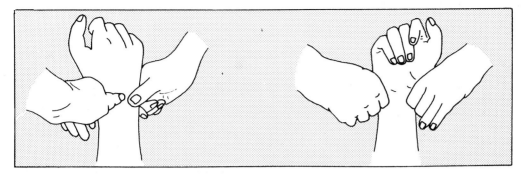

Figure 10.83 Inferior radioulnar joint; posteroanterior and anteroposterior movements

of the pressure applied by the therapist's hand. The patient's hand must be tilted towards radial deviation (abduction) and the therapist should apply her main contact through the base of the patient's

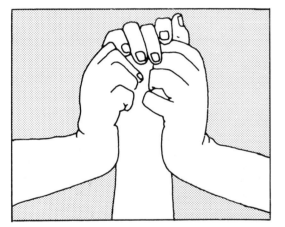

Figure 10.84 Inferior radioulnar joint; compression

thenar eminence so that the pressure is in a straight line in line with the shaft of the radius.

Longitudinal movement caudad*

Starting position and method

This is identical with that shown in Figure 10.81 but with one special qualification. The therapist must grasp around the patient's hand immediately adjacent to the base of the first metacarpal and the pisiform bone. During the movement longitudinally the patient's wrist should be deviated towards the ulnar side (adduction).

It is important to realize that during radial deviation of the hand there is a cephalad longitudinal movement of the radius in relation to the ulna. Similarly, during ulnar deviation of the wrist there is a caudad longitudinal movement of the radius in relation to the ulna.

Wrist joint

It is impossible to be too fussy when endeavouring to determine the precise site of the patient's pain (assuming his disorder is painful).

It is advisable when learning movements and techniques, to practise using an articulated set of bones.

The passive movements of the wrist (that is, the radiocarpal joint) are flexion, extension, radial and ulnar deviation, supination and pronation, medial and lateral transverse movements, posteroanterior and anteroposterior movements, longitudinal movement cephalad and caudad.

Treatment of an individual joint is often possible by general movements which affect them all. However, during examination and treatment it is necessary to differentiate between the joints.

Examination

The wrist joint is not as simple to examine accurately as one may at first think. This is why it is useful, when practising, to have an articulated skeletal hand alongside. The wrist joint's movements are intimately related to the inferior radioulnar joint and the intercarpal joints; Table 10.14 outlines the wrist joint and Table 10.18 outlines examination for all the associated joints.

Functional demonstration/tests

These can be extremely helpful in identifying a single joint, or dominant joint situation.

Brief appraisal

To discern the extent and strength that will be required of examination movements, three passive movements should be carried out. These movements are performed by moving the radiocarpal joint slowly to the limit of each range and then gently applying over-pressure. If the range is good and pain is minimal the strength of the over-pressure should be increased. If the movement is still comparatively pain-free then a full-range amplitude movement (grade III+) should be carried out.

The method described above should be applied to the four movements in turn: first to flexion and extension as depicted in Figures 10.85 and 10.86; second to radial and ulnar deviation as shown in Figure 10.89; and third to supination and pronation as shown in Figures 10.90 and 10.91. Supination and pronation as occurring at the wrist joint are not described separately in this chapter. However, these

---

Table 10.14 Wrist joint – objective examination

The routine examination of this joint must include inferior R/U joint and intercarpal joints.

HIGHLIGHT MAIN FINDINGS WITH ASTERISKS AS YOU GO

Observation

*Functional demonstration/tests

1. *Their* demonstration of *their* functional movements affected by *their* disorder.
2. Differentiation of *their* demonstrated functional movement(s).

Brief appraisal
Active movements (move to PAIN or move to LIMIT)
Routinely
F, E, Ab, Ad, Sup, Pron.
Note range, pain, (repeated and rapid).
Clenching fist.

Isometric tests

Other structures in 'plan'
As applicable Full active resisted movement through range for 'sheaths'.
Thoracic outlet.
Entrapment neuropathy.

Passive movements
Physiological movements
Routinely
F, E, radial and ulnar deviation, Sup and Pron.
Note range, pain, resistance, spasm and behaviour. All without and with compression as applicable.
Accessory movements
Routinely ($\updownarrow$), ($\updownarrow$), ($\leftrightarrow$), ($\leftrightarrow$), ($\leftrightarrow$) *ceph and caud*
As applicable

1. F and E differentiating.
2. Sup and Pron differentiating.
3. Meniscus.
4. Pisiform.
5. Wrist ($\updownarrow$), ($\updownarrow$), ($\leftrightarrow$), ($\leftarrow$) in supination neutral and pronation and in varying positions of flexion and extension.
6. Canal's Slump tests.
7. Differentiation tests.
8. ULTT.
Note range, pain, resistance, spasm and behaviour

Palpation
Include tendon sheaths and 'anatomical snuff box' as applicable
+When 'comparable signs' ill defined reassess 'injuring movement'.

Check case records etc.

Instructions to patient

1. Warning of possible exacerbation.
2. Request to record details.
3. Instruction re 'joint care' if required.

movements are very important to the normal function of the wrist, and the techniques used to differentiate between supination pain or pronation pain arising from the inferior radioulnar joint and that from the wrist joint are described on page 33. The fourth movement requiring over-pressure is AP/PA, and the fifth is distraction.

Special tests

In the section of Table 10.14 labelled 'Accessory movements – as applicable' reference is made to 'differentiating' for flexion, extension, supination and pronation. In relation to testing flexion and extension, it is necessary to know whether pain felt on flexion or extension of the hand is coming from the radiocarpal joint or the intercarpal joints. It *is* possible to differentiate between the two. In the description of radiocarpal flexion (see page 196) emphasis is placed on grasping the proximal row of the patient's carpus. Pain felt with localized movement of the radiocarpal joint is then compared with the pain felt when the whole hand is flexed.

Interestingly Mennell[7] shows radiographs of wrist flexion and extension which, he states, verify the fact that extension occurs mainly at the mid-carpal joint whereas flexion occurs at the radiocarpal joint. *Grays Anatomy* (35th edition)[8] states the opposite; 'When the wrist is flexed, both the radiocarpal and the midcarpal joints are implicated but the range of movement is greater at the latter. In extension the reverse is the case and most of the movement takes place at the radiocarpal joint.' Their statement is also substantiated by radiological evidence.

As for the Concept aspect of this book, it does not matter which is correct. The thing that does matter is that the therapist must be able to identify, when testing either flexion (or extension), which bone is flexing on which other bone(s) that reproduces the pain.

Techniques

Flexion (general) **

Starting position

The physiotherapist stands by the patient's right side beyond his flexed elbow and grasps around the medial border of his right hand with her right hand, placing her thumb against the dorsum of his metacarpals and her fingers in his palm. With her left hand immediately proximal to his carpus, she stabilizes his forearm midway between supination and pronation (Figure 10.85).

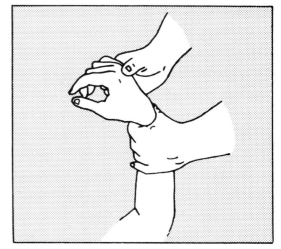

Figure 10.85 Wrist joint; flexion (general)

Method

Starting from a position midway between flexion and extension she flexes his wrist to the limit of the range with her right thumb and returns it to the starting position with her fingers. It is her index finger, positioned near his metacarpophalangeal joints, that controls most of the returning movement.

Extension (general) **

The starting position is identical with that described above for flexion, and the method consists in extending the patient's wrist from the mid position to the fully extended position with her fingers, and returning it to the starting position with her thumb (Figure 10.86).

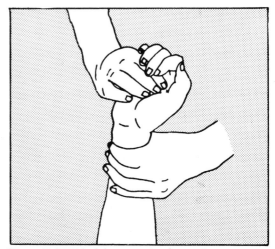

Figure 10.86 Wrist joint; extension (general)

7. Mennell, J. M. *Joint Pain,* Churchill Livingstone, London, pp. 46–48 (1964)
8. *Gray's Anatomy,* 35th edn. Churchill Livingstone, Edinburgh, p. 438 (1973)

Radiocarpal flexion***

To exclude intercarpal (and carpometacarpal) movement from radiocarpal flexion and extension, the technique comprises holding the proximal row of the carpus and not the distal row or the metacarpals. Grades II and III are the movements most commonly employed but grade IV has its place also.

Starting position

The physiotherapist stands by the patient's right hip facing his right shoulder and holds his supinated and extended arm at the wrist with both hands. His forearm is supinated for convenience but should not be held at the limit of the range. She holds with both thumbs pointing proximally on the anterior surface of the proximal row of the carpus and her fingers across the back of the carpus. The flexed index fingers form the main point of contact against the proximal row of the carpus posteriorly. The index fingers and thumbs grasp immediately opposite each other, mainly the scaphoid and lunate bones but also the triquetrum. When the grip is held firmly, the thumb contact is through the base of the terminal phalanx rather than the tip (Figure 10.87).

Method

From a position midway between flexion and extension, the patient's wrist is moved downward towards the floor while the carpus, held firmly between the physiotherapist's index fingers and thumbs, is flexed on the radius and ulna. While performing this movement the carpus must be held firmly.

Radiocarpal extension***

This movement is identical with that described for radiocarpal flexion except that the patient's forearm is partially pronated and the physiotherapist's thumbs hold the posterior surface of the proximal row of the carpal bones while her fingers hold the proximal row of the carpal bones anteriorly. The extension movement is produced through a very firm localized grasp with fingers and thumbs while lowering the wrist towards the floor as the wrist is extended. The oscillation is produced by returning the patient's arm to the starting position while at the same time returning the extended radiocarpal joint to the mid position (Figure 10.88).

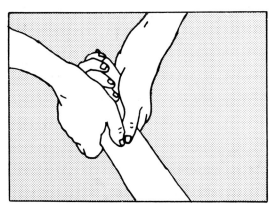

Figure 10.87 Wrist joint; radiocarpal flexion

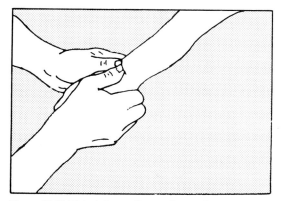

Figure 10.88 Wrist joint; radiocarpal extension

The grasp of the proximal row of the carpus must be very precise. When using this method of producing localized flexion the source of joint pain can be determined very accurately if the therapist grasps only the scaphoid or only the lunate, so that the fulcrum of the flexion (or extension) is even more localized. The precision of this test can be carried even further by grasping only the scaphoid while producing the flexion (or extension) and varying the point of contact between the scaphoid and the radius with the wrist in varying degrees of ulnar deviation or radial deviation. The same principle applies if the therapist holds only the lunate between her fingers and thumbs.

As described in detail for radiocarpal flexion, the extension movement can be similarly localized more precisely by performing the extension grasping only the scaphoid or the lunate. Similarly, the movement can be further refined by holding the wrist in varying degrees of radial and ulnar deviation.

See mid-carpal flexion and extension on page 201.

Ulnar deviation**

Starting position

The physiotherapist stands by the patient's right shoulder, facing his feet. With her left hand she grasps his forearm distally so that her index finger stabilizes around the styloid process of the ulna. She flexes his elbow to 90° and positions his forearm midway between supination and pronation. With her right hand she grasps the posterior surface of the metacarpals with her fingers reaching around the ulnar border of his hand and her thumb through the first interosseous space (Figure 10.89).

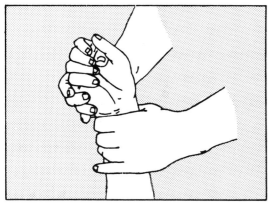

Figure 10.89 Wrist joint; ulnar deviation

Method

The oscillatory treatment movement, performed in any part of the range, is produced by supination of the therapist's right forearm, returning it to the starting position by a pronation movement.

Radial deviation**

The starting position is identical with that described for ulnar deviation with the exception that now her left thumb holds around the styloid process of the radius. The only difference in the method is that the movement is one of radial deviation produced by pronation of the therapist's right forearm.

Radiocarpal supination***

Starting position

The physiotherapist stands by the patient's flexed and supinated right forearm. She holds his forearm adjacent to the wrist with her left hand so that her thumb hooks around the lateral border of the distal end of the radius to reach the posterior surface of the radius. Her index finger makes firm contact against the anterior surface of the distal end of the ulna. With her right hand she holds across the posterior surface of the proximal row of his carpus so that her thumb hooks around the scaphoid to hold it firmly anteriorly, while her index finger lies across the proximal row of the carpal bones posteriorly making the firmest contact against the triquetrum (Figure 10.90).

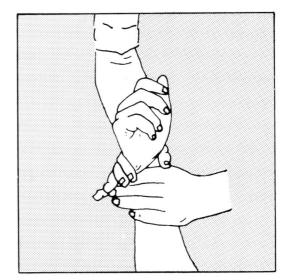

Figure 10.90 Wrist joint; radiocarpal supination

Method

Further supination of the inferior radioulnar joint is prevented by the therapist's left hand while the added supination of the radiocarpal joint is produced by her right arm acting through her wrist and hand. The tip of her right thumb and the distal end of the proximal phalanx of her index finger are the points through which all of the pressure is transmitted to the carpus while her left thumb and index finger provide counterpressure.

Although radiocarpal supination has been described with the forearm loosely supinated, it can be performed with the forearm anywhere between full supination and full pronation.

Radiocarpal pronation***

Starting position

The physiotherapist stands by the patient's right hip, facing his shoulder. With his elbow flexed to a right angle she holds the distal end of his forearm in her right hand with her thumb hooked posteriorly around his ulna and the base of her index finger against the anterior surface of the radius. With her left hand she grasps around the carpus, her thumb holding around the triquetral bone anteriorly and her index finger pressed firmly against the posterior surface of the scaphoid (Figure 10.91).

Method

The movement is produced by the physiotherapist's left hand against the carpus while her right hand stabilizes the patient's forearm by applying an equal and opposite counterpressure.

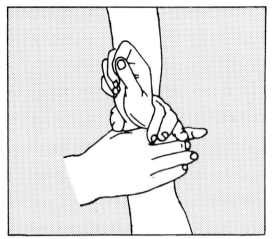

Figure 10.91 Wrist joint; radiocarpal pronation

Posteroanterior movement***

Posteroanterior movement of the carpus on the radius is mainly used in the treatment of stiff joints rather than extremely painful joints. Therefore, grades III and IV are the movements most commonly used.

Starting position

The physiotherapist stands by the patient's right hip, facing his head, and holds his forearm midway between supination and pronation. She holds the posterior surface of his hand in her left hand and the anterior surface of his distal forearm in her right hand which is fully supinated and extended at the wrist and pointing proximally. The heel of her left hand should lie over the carpus, her fingers grasping around his thumb and her thumb grasping around the ulnar border of his hand. The heel of her right

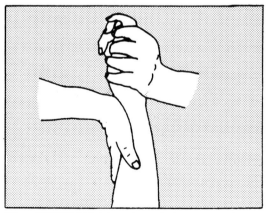

Figure 10.92 Wrist joint; posteroanterior movement

hand is placed level with the distal end of his radius and ulna while her fingers grasp around his forearm. She should crouch over his arm to direct her forearms opposite each other (Figure 10.92).

Method

If a grade III movement is employed the oscillation starts from the neutral position and is taken to the limit of the range by an equal and opposite movement of the forearm. It is important to keep the patient's hand straight to prevent any flexion or extension of his wrist. Grade IV movements are performed through a much smaller amplitude at the limit of the range.

Anteroposterior movement***

Starting position

The physiotherapist stands between the patient's right side and his elbow and faces away from him. His elbow is flexed and supported midway between supination and pronation. She grasps his palm from in front with her right hand, her thumb holding around the ulnar border of his hand and her fingers around the radial border. His thumb lies between her ring and middle fingers. The heel of her hand forms the main point of contact against his carpus anteriorly. She places the base of her left thumb opposite the distal border of the radius posteriorly and grasps around his radius with her fingers (Figure 10.93). This technique and the posteroanterior movement can also be performed using the edge of the couch as a fulcrum.

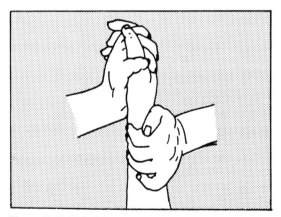

Figure 10.93 Wrist joint; anteroposterior movement

Method

The method for this technique resembles that described above for posteroanterior movement.

Lateral transverse movement***

Starting position

The patient lies supine with his arm abducted. His wrist lies at the edge of the couch with his hand beyond it and his thumb pointing towards the floor. With her right hand the physiotherapist holds firmly around the distal end of his radius and ulna, immediately around the styloid processes. Her knuckles, between the patient's distal forearm and the surface of the couch, stabilize his wrist, but it may be necessary for her to rest her forearm across his forearm or elbow to stabilize the arm.

With her left hand she grasps around the posterior surface of his hand so that her thumb and index finger grasp the carpus around the triquetral bone and the pisiform adjacent to the ulnar styloid process (Figure 10.94).

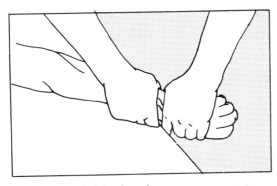

Figure 10.94 Wrist joint; lateral transverse movement

Method

Movement of the patient's hand towards the floor is produced through the therapist's left arm and shoulder. Proper movement can only be gained if the therapist's left hand moves as a single unit with the patient's hand.

The movement can be performed as an oscillatory grade IV to IV+ or as a large amplitude grade III.

Four variations can be made with the technique. These changes would be indicated when any one of them more exactly reproduces the patient's symptoms. The variations are as follows:

1. The patient's hand can be positioned in any degree of ulnar or radial deviation and held in this position while the transverse movement is produced.

2. The direction of the lateral transverse movement can be inclined posteriorly or anteriorly, where, although the available range is smaller, it may more accurately produce the comparable pain.
3. The wrist may be positioned to any degree of supination or pronation prior to applying the transverse movement.
4. The transverse movement may be performed with a degree of compression of the radiocarpal joint surfaces, or the joint surfaces may be distracted during transverse movement.

Medial transverse movement***

Starting position

The patient lies supine and abducts his arm so that his wrist is at the edge of the table. The physiotherapist grasps above and below the wrist as in the previous technique but this time the patient's thumb is pointing towards the ceiling (Figure 10.95) instead of towards the floor.

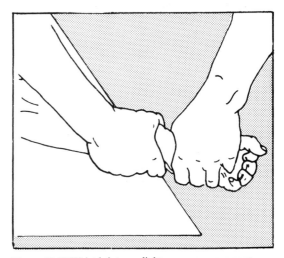

Figure 10.95 Wrist joint; medial transverse movement

Method

The technique is identical with that described for the previous movement and the emphasis is on the fact that the patient's hand and the therapist's hand move as a single unit.

The variations listed above in numbers 1–4 apply in exactly the same manner in this technique.

Intercarpal joint movement
Examination

Decisive pinpointing of the precise site of dominant symptoms offers the best of foundations on which to base the remaining examination. Pain arising from any of the intercarpal joints is always felt locally though it may radiate around the central point of the disordered joint.

The bones, joints and movements of the carpus are complex (Figure 10.90) yet it is surprising how, with skill, it is possible to assess the range of movement and the pain response to that movement between each of the bones. Therefore, if the treatment is localized to the particularly restricted and painful movement, the result will be achieved much more quickly than if general hand and wrist movements are used. As was shown and explained in Chapter 4 (Figures 4.7–4.12), the tests are intricate and require care and skill.

Functional demonstration/test

If the patient has such a function to demonstrate, it should be analysed as a first step.

Brief appraisal

There are no specific brief tests for the carpus other than to ask the patient to flick his hand into full flexion, full extension, full radial and ulnar deviation, and full supination and pronation. It is also useful to ask him to make a fist while the physiotherapist assesses movement and strength.

Special tests

The first of two special tests is to hold one carpal bone between the fingers and thumb of one hand while the fingers and thumb of the other hand hold and move the adjacent carpal bone to assess whether anteroposterior and posteroanterior movement have a full and painless range.

The second of the special tests consists of the posteroanteriorly directed pressures (which may be varied with a caudad, cephalad, medial and lateral inclination) on each of the two bones forming the joint and then over the joint space (see pages 44 and 45).

Table 10.15 lists the examination by passive movements.

When considering the carpus it must not be forgotten that the pisiform, which articulates with the triquetrum and has the ulnar nerve immediately adjacent to its radial surface, is also capable of movements which should be tested.

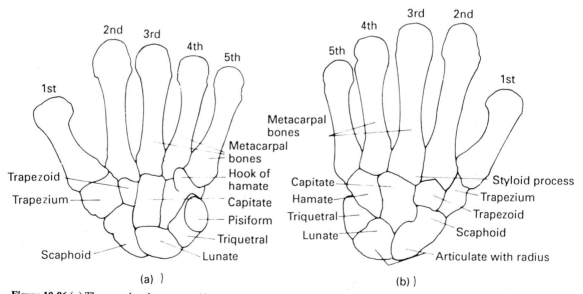

(a))   (b))

Figure 10.96 (*a*) The carpal and metacarpal bones of the left hand. Palmar aspect. (*b*) The carpal and metacarpal bones of the left hand. Dorsal aspect (Reproduced from *Gray's Anatomy* (1973), 35th edn, Edinburgh: Churchill Livingstone, pp. 336–337, by courtesy of publishers.)

Table 10.15 Intercarpal joint – objective examination

The routine examination of these joints must also include examination of the wrist joint, carpometacarpal (C/MC) joints and pisiform movements*.

HIGHLIGHT MAIN FINDINGS WITH ASTERISKS AS YOU GO

Observation

*Functional demonstration/tests

1. *Their* demonstration of *their* functional movements affected by *their* disorder.
2. Differentiation of *their* demonstrated functional movement(s).

Brief appraisal
Active movements (move to PAIN or move to LIMIT)

Isometric tests

Other structures in 'plan'
Add full active resisted movement through range for 'sheaths'
Thoracic outlet & ULTT.
Entrapment neuropathy.

Passive movements
Physiological movements
Routinely
1. Wrist F, E, Ab, Ad, Sup, Pro.
2. Mid carpal F and E.
3. Differentiating F and E.
4. Individual carpometacarpal (C/MC) F and E.

Note range, pain, resistance, spasm and behaviour.

Accessory movements
As applicable
1. (↓) and (↑) (varying angles and points of contact)
   (↕) (i.e. gliding of each carpal bone on adjacent carpal bone).
2. HF and HE of carpus.
*3. Pisiform, without compression and with compression, (←→), (←→), (←→) ceph and caud.
   Distraction.
4. C/MC joints:
   (a) (↓) and (↑) (varying angle and points of contact), (↕).
   (b) (←→), (←→) of metacarpals on carpus, with and without abduction and adduction.
   (c) (↺) and (↻) metacarpals.

Note range, pain, resistance, spasm and behaviour.

5. Canal's Slump tests.
6. Differentiation tests.
7. ULTT.

Palpation
Include tendon sheaths
When 'comparable signs' ill defined reassess 'injuring movement'.

Check case records etc.

Instructions to patient
1. Warning of possible exacerbation.
2. Request to record details.
3. Instruction re 'joint care' if required.

Techniques
Mid carpal flexion***
Starting position

The physiotherapist's grip position is critical for a flexion movement to be produced at the mid carpal row. With the patient lying supine she places the tips of her thumbs over the anterior surface of the *distal* carpal row. Her index fingers, pointing towards each other and reinforced by the middle fingers, overly the posterior surface of the *proximal* carpal row (Figure 10.97).

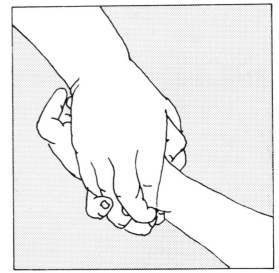

Figure 10.97 Mid-carpal joint; flexion

Method

Flexion is produced by a tilting action flexing his *hand* pivoting through the thumb tips to the *distal* row anteriorly, and being countered by a postero-anterior stabilizing pressure against the *proximal* row posteriorly. If performed correctly, there is no radiocarpal movement or carpometacarpal movement.

Mid-carpal extension***
Starting position

As above, the physiotherapist's grip is critical if the mid-carpal extension is to be effectively localized and comfortable. On the posterior aspect of the patient's hand she must place the *proximal end* of the distal phalanx of each thumb immediately over the *distal margin* of the *proximal row* of the carpal bones. Her reinforced index fingers lie firmly against the anterior surface of the distal row of the carpal bones (Figure 10.98).

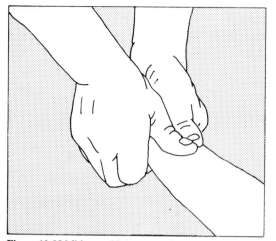

Figure 10.98 Mid-carpal joint; extension

Method

The tilting action is produced through the index fingers against distal carpal row, with the base of the thumbs preventing movement of the proximal row. Thus there is no extension at the wrist or the carpometacarpal joints.

Intercarpal horizontal extension**

Starting position

The physiotherapist stands by the patient's right side, beyond his flexed and supinated forearm, facing his head. She holds his right hand from the back with the tips of the pads of her thumbs against the centre of the carpus posteriorly and her index and middle fingers around the pisiform medially and the carpometacarpal joint of the thumb laterally (Figure 10.99).

Method

The oscillatory movement is produced by thumb pressure against the centre of the carpus posteriorly and pulling against the medial and lateral margins of the carpus with her fingers. This action is produced by extension of the therapist's wrists which is facilitated by pushing the patient's hand away from her.

The movement as described so far is a general one affecting the full length and breadth of the carpus. For examination purposes it may be found that the general horizontal extension is pain-free. When this is so, the tips of the thumbs should localize the fulcrum of the movement by limiting their point of contact to each carpal bone in both the proximal and distal rows.

With experience and practice, it is possible to determine that an individual carpal bone cannot be moved anteriorly as far as its normal range or that it may be hypermobile. By altering the fulcrum of the horizontal extension to each of the bones, one will, when pushed anteriorly, reproduce the patient's pain. It may well be that this joint sign is the main 'comparable' sign. When this is so, it may well be the technique used as treatment. It should also be pointed out that this localization of the movement will divulge whether it is a hypermobile or a hypomobile joint causing the pain.

Variations

The posteroanteriorly directed pressures should be inclined medially, laterally, cephalad, caudad, and also diagonally. These variations can be in any direction. They have been described on pages 43–45.

Intercarpal horizontal flexion**

The intercarpal horizontal flexion movement is not as useful as extension because the movement is less commonly restricted or painful.

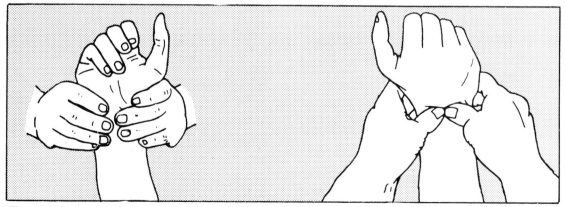

Figure 10.99 Intercarpal horizontal extension

Starting position

The physiotherapist stands by the patient's right elbow, facing across his body, and supports his supinated and flexed forearm by grasping the back of his hand in her right hand with her fingers pointing distally.

The main contact with her right hand is at the medial and lateral margins of the carpus. She places her left thumb tip against the palmar surface of the carpus to apply a direct anteroposterior pressure. This fulcrum provided by her left thumb would first be used on the proximal row and then the distal row of the carpus. She then directs both forearms opposite each other (Figure 10.100).

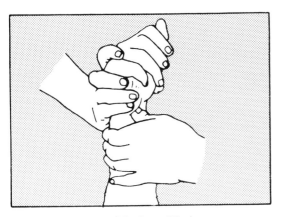

Figure 10.100 Intercarpal horizontal flexion

Method

The oscillation is produced by opposite pressure though the forearms. The right hand produces a cupping action of the patient's hand around the pivot formed by the therapist's left thumb.

Variations

The same variations in regard to the point of contact as described for intercarpal horizontal extension (see page 202) should be used. This also applies to the direction of the thumb pressure, referred to as posteroanterior, which should also be varied in inclination as described on page 44.

Posteroanterior intercarpal movement***

Localized intercarpal movements are extremely effective as treatment techniques when the movement is painful.

Starting position

The patient lies with his pronated hand resting on the couch. The physiotherapist stands by his right side, beyond his hand, and places the maximum breadth of her thumb tips, adjacent to each other, on the appropriate carpal bone or their intercarpal joint. She spreads her fingers over the adjacent area of the hand for stability (Figure 10.101). She then directs her arms and thumbs either immediately posteroanteriorly or combined with any of the inclinations described in detail on page 44.

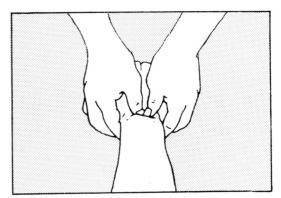

Figure 10.101 Posteroanterior intercarpal movement

Method

Posteroanterior mobilizing is produced by pressure from the therapist's arms transmitted through the spring-like action of the thumbs against the carpal bone or intercarpal joint.

Anteroposterior intercarpal movement*

Anteroposterior movement is similarly produced, but the thumb contact is against the palmar surface of the patient's supinated hand although the individual carpal bones are much harder to find anteriorly being padded so much more (Figure 10.102).

Both anteroposterior and posteroanterior pressures can be used in conjunction with horizontal flexion or extension emphasizing the movement of a particular intercarpal joint.

Longitudinal movement caudad*

The distraction technique has been described earlier (see page 193) but when it is used to treat the carpus, the physiotherapist must ensure that her grasp surrounds the metacarpals and not the carpus. Also, the movement can be emphasized more to the medial, central or lateral, mid-carpal joints by distracting the medial, central or lateral aspects of the mid-carpal joint.

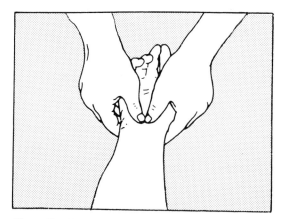

Figure 10.102 Anteroposterior intercarpal movement

Longitudinal movement cephalad*

The compression technique has been described (Figure 10.82), but with the patient's wrist in extension. To meet the present aim the therapist should grasp more distally and hold firmly around the medial four metacarpals. The compression is then transferred through his intercarpal joints. Though the technique is depicted in a neutral wrist position (Figure 10.103) the patient's wrist may be positioned anywhere between flexion and extension, radial and ulnar deviation. Also, as has been described above, each of the patient's fingers may be used so as to localize the compression to different intercarpal joints.

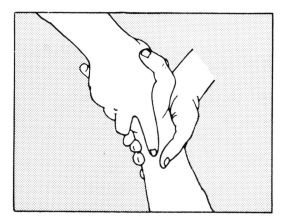

Figure 10.103 Intercarpal longitudinal movement

This technique is not used alone but has considerable application in treatment when used as a 'combined movement' in conjunction with other intercarpal movements. For example, if pain arises from the joint between the capitate and lunate, the only 'comparable sign' may be a rocking anteroposterior to posteroanterior movement directed against the joint line while compression is added in a cephalad direction through the third metacarpal bone. This example is only one of innumerable variations where the direction of pressure through different angles against different points on the carpus may be used as test movements and treatment movements.

Pisiform movement

Movement between the pisiform and the triquetral bone can be limited, thickened or inflamed, resulting in symptoms. It can irritate the ulnar nerve which is adjacent to its lateral surface. The movement can be mobilized just as can any moving part.

Starting position

With the patient lying supine, his arm outstretched and the back of his hand resting on the treatment couch, the physiotherapist maintains stability of the hand and forearm while directing pressure against the different surfaces of the pisiform to make it move on the triquetral bone. To make the mobilizing techniques comfortable she should use as much of the pad of her thumb as possible, though not at the expense of localizing the contact point, so that the direction of movement can be finely varied from one direction to another.

Method

Movement of the pisiform is produced through the thumb by pressure from the therapist's arm. The movement is an oscillatory one and in treatment usually needs to be a grade IV or III− type movement (Figure 10.104).

Variations

It is quite usual to vary the direction of the pressure against the pisiform, moving it in any direction that may either stretch into the limitation of movement, or reproduce the patient's symptoms. Previously, variations have been described for the different directions of movement. However, in relation to the pisiform it is necessary to remember that the different directions of movement can also be combined with compression of the pisiform against the triquetral bone. Coincidentally, distraction of the pisiform can be produced by gripping the medial and lateral sides of the pisiform and lifting it from the triquetrum by squeezing the fingers towards the central point beneath the pisiform.

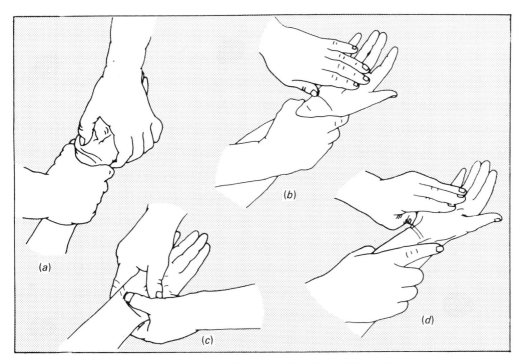

Figure 10.104 Pisiform movement (*a*) cephalad; (*b*) caudad; (*c*) medially; (*d*) laterally

Treatment

It is common with falls on the outstretched hand, which result in fractures of the radius and ulna, for the hand also to be sprained or strained. During examination, therefore, movements of the intercarpal joints should be included. Pain found on movement of any intercarpal joint or joints should be part of follow-up treatment when the arm is taken out of plaster. General movements of the wrist and hand should be used both as grade IV− and as grade II, II+ or III. Where abnormal or painful movement can be localized to one joint, the technique used should be localized to that joint rather than performed as a general movement of all carpal bones.

Carpal tunnel syndrome

This syndrome can sometimes be relieved by direct anteroposterior pressure, where the pressure reproduces the patient's symptoms. Also, the technique (Figure 10.104) can be used to stretch the flexor retinaculum. While the fingers of each hand separate the pisiform and the hook of the hamate away from the trapezium and scaphoid, the thumb tips on the posterior surface of the carpus form a fulcrum for the movement. If the patient's symptoms can be reproduced by localizing the pressure to one bone on the posterior surface of the carpus, then this bone should be used as the fulcrum point for the treatment technique. To determine whether this reproduction of symptoms is possible, the tips of the thumbs should be used on the capitate and the lunate first as the fulcrum for the horizontal extension movement. Pressure should then be applied in turn through the trapezoid, the hamate, the triquetrum and the scaphoid. The pressure can be inclined in any direction in an effort to find the exact movement for the treatment (Figure 10.105).

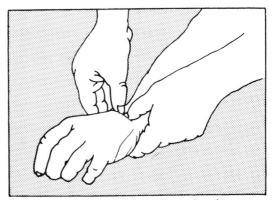

Figure 10.105 Treatment for carpal tunnel syndrome

Carpometacarpal joints

The description is here confined to the fingers; the thumb is described separately with the remainder of its movements (see pages 218–220).

These joints do not cause as much trouble as do the intercarpal joints but they are often injured when a person attempts to protect themselves when falling by trying to take the weight through the outstretched arm and hand.

Examination (and treatment) movements are similar to those used in the intercarpal joints (varying the points of contact and the inclinations of the pressures) and in the metacarpophalangeal joints (including rotation, abduction and adduction).

The examination movements are listed in Table 10.16.

Extension***

Starting position

The supine position for the patient is still the position of choice because better relaxation is possible than if he sits. If the lateral carpometacarpal joints are to be mobilized, the physiotherapist stands by his slightly flexed right forearm facing across his body. She holds his partially pronated hand in her hands, grasping from the lateral side, the relevant carpal bone in her left hand and the relevant metacarpal in her right. Her right hand grasps through the first interosseous space and the tip of her right thumb is placed against the base of the metacarpal posteriorly (Figure 10.106(a)).

When mobilizing the carpometacarpal joint of the little finger she maintains the same grip with her left hand except that she places the pad of her thumb over the patient's hamate. With her right hand she holds around the ulnar border (medial side) of the patient's right hand to grasp the fifth metacarpal, her flexed index finger supporting it distally and anteriorly, and her thumb contacting the base posteriorly (Figure 10.106(b)).

Method

Grades III and IV are the movements most commonly used with this technique. The movement is produced by the therapist moving the patient's hand away from her and applying pressure through her thumbs while applying a pulling counterpressure with her fingers to assist the extension. This movement can be performed either in large-amplitude (grade III) or small-amplitude oscillations into resistance (grade IV).

Table 10.16 Carpometacarpal joints – objective examination

The routine examination of these joints must also include examination of the intercarpal joints, and proximal and distal intermetacarpal joints and spaces.

HIGHLIGHT MAIN FINDINGS WITH ASTERISKS AS YOU GO

Observation

*Functional demonstration/tests

1. *Their* demonstration of *their* functional movements affected by *their* disorder.
2. Differentiation of *their* demonstrated functional movement(s).

Brief appraisal
Active movements (move to PAIN or move to LIMIT)

Isometric tests

Other structures in 'plan'
Full range active/resisted wrist and finger F for sheaths
Thoracic outlet & ULTT.
Entrapment neuropathy.

Passive movements
Physiological movements
Routinely
Individual C/MC F and E.
HF and HE of carpus ⎫
HF and HE of metacarpals ⎬ and differentiating
Note range, pain, resistance, spasm and behaviour.

Accessory movements
Routinely

1. (↓) and (↑) (varying angles medial, lateral ceph. and caud.).
2. (→) and (←).
3. Abduction and adduction.
4. Combining (2) and (3).
5. (↻) and (↺) of metacarpals.

All without and with compression.
Note range, pain, resistance, spasm and behaviour.

As applicable

1. Canal's Slump tests.
2. Differentiation tests.
3. ULTT.

Palpation
Include tendon sheaths
When 'comparable signs' ill defined reassess 'injuring movement'.

Check case records etc.

Instructions to patient

1. Warning of possible exacerbation.
2. Request to record details.
3. Instruction re 'joint care' if required.

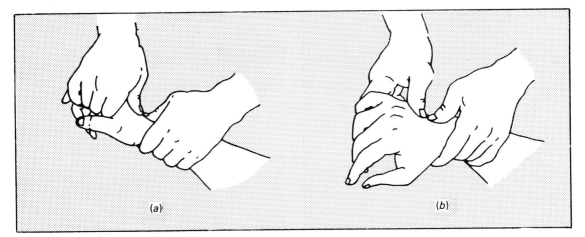

Figures 10.106 Carpometacarpal extension (*a*) of index finger; (*b*) of little finger

Flexion***

Starting position

The physiotherapist stands by the patient's upper arm, facing his feet, and holds his supinated hand in her hands. She holds around the medial border of his wrist with her left hand, placing the tip of her thumb in his palm over the appropriate carpal bone. If the carpometacarpal joint of the index finger is to be mobilized she holds the second metacarpal, through the first interosseous space, in her right hand. She places the tip of her thumb against the base of the metacarpal anteriorly and her flexed index finger against the posterior surface of the metacarpal distally (Figure 10.107).

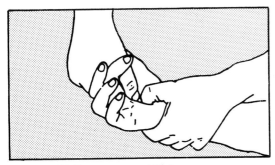

Figure 10.107 Carpometacarpal flexion

Method

The therapist produces the movement by pushing the patient's hand away from her at the same time as adducting her glenohumeral joints and extending her elbows to transmit pressure through her thumbs to his palm.

The movement of flexion can be produced by the movement of both hands as described above, or it may be produced by stabilizing the carpus with the left hand and flexing the metacarpal with the right hand.

Accessory movements***

The grip for each carpometacarpal joint has been described and related to the movements of flexion and extension.

Other movements can be produced at this joint by inclining the direction of pressure techniques against the base of the metacarpal bone or the related carpal bone. The direction of this pressure may be inclined medially or laterally, cephalad or caudad.

Combined movements

If the tip of the right thumb can be wedged between adjacent metacarpal bones, a transverse pressure can be exerted on the metacarpal bone through the tip of the thumb in conjunction with flexion, extension or rotation. Although very little movement can be felt, comparison with the other hand makes it possible to assess range. Also, it may reproduce the patient's symptoms and this may guide the physiotherapist to use this direction of movement as the treatment movement.

Rotation

Rotation of the carpometacarpal joint can be obtained by flexing to 90° the relevant metacarpophalangeal joint and then rotating the metacarpal by swinging the flexed finger medially and laterally.

Anteroposterior and posteroanterior

The base of the metacarpal can also be made to move anteroposteriorly and posteroanteriorly in relation to the adjacent carpal bone with which it articulates.

Compression

The carpometacarpal joint may also be distracted or compressed, and while in this position the other movements described above may be incorporated. When the carpometacarpal joint causes pain, the test movements performed while the joint is compressed are most likely to reproduce a 'comparable sign'.

Combined movements

The transverse movement, the rotary movements and the anteroposterior and posteroanterior movements can also be performed in conjunction with different positions of flexion, extension, radial and ulnar deviation.

Treatment

The techniques used in the treatment of the carpometacarpal joints are similar to those described for the intercarpal joints. That is, by varying the angles of movement of the carpometacarpal joints, if one is found to be more restricted than the comparable joint of the other hand and this restricted movement reproduces the patient's symptoms then grade IV type movements should be used to increase the range. Any treatment soreness produced by this technique would be relieved by continuing the same movement but producing a grade III− type technique.

To increase mobility, the restricted physiological movement is used as a grade IV movement. This is followed by performing all of the accessory movements at the limit of the physiological range being treated.

Intermetacarpal movement

The main movements between the metacarpals consist firstly of cupping and flattening the palm (which are perhaps better thought of as horizontal flexion and horizontal extension, respectively), and secondly the parallel anteroposterior and posteroanterior movements of one metacarpal relative to its neighbouring metacarpal. Though the movements are similar they are not identical.

Examination

The localized techniques described are the only special tests for this area.

The movements do not usually become disturbed unless caused by trauma.

The examination is given in Table 10.17.

Techniques

General horizontal flexion*

Starting position

When the horizontal flexion movement is performed as a general movement for the whole row of metacarpals, the physiotherapist places the pad of her left thumb pointing distally in his palm over the distal end of the third metacarpal, while cupping her right hand across the dorsum of all the metacarpals distally. Her right thumb presses against the posterior surface of the second metacarpal and her fingers, particularly her index fingers, press against the posterior surface of the fifth metacarpal (Figure 10.108).

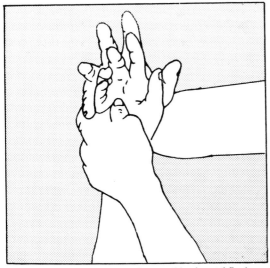

Figure 10.108 Intermetacarpal general horizontal flexion

Table 10.17 Intermetacarpal movement – objective examination

HIGHLIGHT MAIN FINDINGS WITH ASTERISKS AS YOU GO

Observation

*Functional demonstration/tests

1. *Their* demonstration of *their* functional movements affected by *their* disorder.
2. Differentiation of *their* demonstrated functional movement(s).

Brief appraisal

Active movements (move to PAIN or move to LIMIT)

Other structures in 'plan'

Full active resisted movement through range for 'sheaths'.
Thoracic outlet & ULTT.
Entrapment neuropathy.

Isometric tests

Passive movements

Physiological movements

Routinely

HF and HE of metacarpals (on bases and heads)

Note range, pain, resistance, spasm and behaviour

As applicable

1. Canal's Slump tests.
2. Differentiation tests.
3. ULTT.

Accessory movements

Routinely

1. (↓) and (↑) of each metacarpal in relation to its neighbours (bases and heads)
2. Individual HF and HE (bases or heads)

Note range, pain, resistance, spasm and behaviour.

Palpation

Include tendon sheaths.
When 'comparable signs' ill defined reassess 'injuring movement'.

Check case records etc.

Instructions to patient

1. Warning of possible exacerbation.
2. Request to record details.
3. Instruction re 'joint care' if required.

The peak of the movement can be changed by placing the left thumb against the fourth metacarpal.

Method

Small- or large-amplitude oscillations are produced by moving the hands in opposite directions.

The same movement can be localized to two adjacent metacarpals but the technique differs slightly.

Localized horizontal flexion**

Starting position

The physiotherapist stands facing the back of the patient's supinated and flexed forearm and grasps his hand with her two hands. She does this by holding the fifth metacarpal posteriorly with her right thumb posteriorly, and anteriorly with the tips of her index and middle fingers. With her left hand she holds the adjacent fourth metacarpal between the pads of her index and middle fingers anteriorly and the pad of her thumb posteriorly (Figure 10.109).

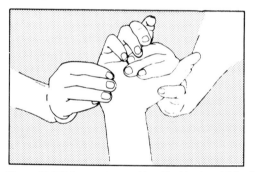

Figure 10.109 Intermetacarpal localized horizontal flexion

Method

While her left hand stabilizes the fourth metacarpal she moves the fifth with her right hand in a circular direction around it. When the second metacarpal is mobilized on the third, the physiotherapist's left hand performs the movement, whereas when the fourth and fifth metacarpals are mobilized her left hand holds the fourth metacarpal while her right hand moves the fifth metacarpal around the fourth. Mobilizing the third on the fourth the therapist's left hand does the moving and the right hand does the stabilizing. When the fourth is mobilized on the third, the reverse is the case.

General horizontal extension*

Starting position

The physiotherapist stands beyond the patient's flexed and supinated forearm facing the back of his hand which she holds in her two hands. She places the pads of her thumbs against the distal end of the posterior surface of the third metacarpal. With her fingers she holds around the medial and lateral margins of his hand to reach the anterior surface of the second and fifth metacarpals distally (Figure 10.110).

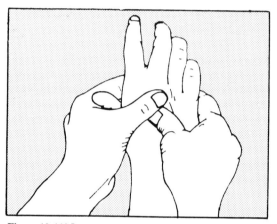

Figure 10.110 Intermetacarpal general horizontal extension

Method

The extension movement is performed by a pulling action with the fingers of both hands pivoting the patient's metacarpals around the thumbs on the third metacarpal while at the same time pushing his hand away. This can be done as a large-amplitude grade III movement or as a small movement at the limit of the range (grade IV).

Localized horizontal extension**

This movement can also be localized to two adjacent metacarpals and is performed with the same grasp as that described for localized metacarpal horizontal flexion (Figure 10.109), except that the 'method' is one of pivoting towards extension around the stabilized adjacent metacarpal (Figure 10.111).

Posteroanterior and anteroposterior movement***

The starting position is the same as that described for localized metacarpal horizontal flexion and extension (Figures 10.109 and 10.111) and the method is similar except that instead of one metacarpal pivoting **around** its neighbour they traverse **parallel** lines moving in opposite directions. One metacarpal moves anteroposteriorly or posteroanteriorly in relation to the stabilized neighbouring metacarpal.

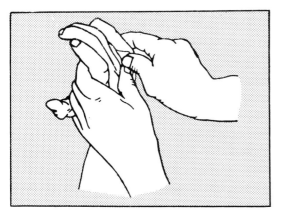

Figure 10.111 Intermetacarpal localized horizontal extension

Compression (transversely)

Starting position

The patient's hand should be grasped in a 'hand-shake' position, that is, right hand to right hand and left to left. The physiotherapist should grip around the heads of the metacarpals and her other hand should stabilize the head of the metacarpals in a straight line from the radial to the ulnar side.

Method

The therapist alternately squeezes and relaxes her grasp of the heads of the metacarpals, assessing for pain. She then compares the findings with those for the other hand.

Table 10.18 Composite wrist/hand – objective examination

HIGHLIGHT MAIN FINDINGS WITH ASTERISKS AS YOU GO

Observation

*Functional demonstration/tests

1. *Their* demonstration of *their* functional movements affected by *their* disorder.
2. Differentiation of *their* demonstrated functional movement(s).

Brief appraisal
Active movements (move to PAIN or move to LIMIT)
Clench fist and test grip
F, E, Ab and Ad of wrist
Sup and Pron

Isometric tests

Other structures in 'plan'

Passive tests
As required
Whole hand

1. F and E.
2. Radial and ulnar deviation.
3. Supination and pronation.
4. (↔) ceph and caud.
5. HF and HE.
6. Pisiform.
7. (↕), (↕), (↔), (↔), in different positions of wrist
   Sup, Pron, F and E.
8. Sheaths.
9. Tendon length and function.
10. Meniscus.

Differentiating as required

1. F and E:
   (a) Radiocarpal.
   (b) Midcarpal.
   (c) Carpometacarpal.

2. Radial and ulnar deviation.
   (a) Radiocarpal.
   (b) Midcarpal.
   (c) Carpometacarpal.

3. Supination and pronation.
   (a) Radiocarpal.
   (b) Inferior R/U joint.

4. (↔) caud and ceph.
   (a) Radiocarpal.
   (b) Intercarpal.
   (c) Carpometacarpal.

5. HF and HE.
   (a) Intercarpal.
   (b) Carpometacarpal.
   (c) Intermetacarpal.

Other test movements
(↕), (↘), (↗), (↕), (↗), (↘), (↕), (from inferior R/U to heads of metacarpals).
Canal's Slump tests.
ULTT.

Note range, pain, resistance, spasm and behaviour

Palpation

+When 'comparable signs' ill defined reassess 'injuring movement'.

Check case records etc.

Instructions to patient

1. Warning of possible exacerbation.
2. Request to record details.
3. Instruction re 'joint care' if required.

Composite examination forearm to palm

Table 10.18 is a guide to a composite examination of the joints from the inferior radioulnar joint to the intermetacarpal area. The differentiating of supination and pronation refers to holding the patient's hand and forearm fully supinated to reproduce his pain. While maintaining this position and degree of pain, the physiotherapist pronates the inferior radioulnar joint. If the patient's pain decreases, the source of the pain is the inferior radioulnar joint. If the pain increases, the supinated wrist is the source.

Chronic/minor wrist/hand symptoms

When chronic symptoms occupy any part of the area from the lower third of the forearm to the mid-metacarpal area (excluding the thumb) only selected movements need examining. However, these movements should be tested initially at a grade IV− strength. If this does not provoke a 'comparable' symptomatic response; the strength of the over-pressure should be increased until it (the test movement) can be judged to be 'clear'. Table 10.19 lists the movements to be examined.

Table 10.19 Chronic/minor wrist/hand symptoms

Supine: Flexion & extension
Supination & pronation (through metacarpals)
Radial & ulnar deviation
AP & PA movement
HF & HE
Longitudinal caudad & cephalad

Proving the area unaffected

When the joints from the inferior radioulnar joint to the intermetacarpal need to be quickly examined to prove that they are *not* contributing to the patient's disorder, the examination movements to be examined are listed in Table 10.20.

These movements should be tested by starting with grade IV− movements and then gradually increasing until IV+ and III+ grades can be performed painlessly.

Table 10.20 Proving the area unaffected

F & E (fingers to wrist)
Sup and Pro
Wrist deviation
(←→) ceph, caud.

Treatment

Movements between the metacarpals are rarely a source of pain unless the hand has been subjected to some trauma. When pain and stiffness are present, grade IV and IV+ type movements should be used, and used quite strongly.

It is more common for pain to arise from the intermetacarpal synovial joints at their bases. When this is the case the site of pain will be over the joint and the positive comparable joint signs will be among the test movements listed in Table 10.16.

Metacarpophalangeal and interphalangeal joints
Examination

As the techniques used for the metacarpophalangeal and interphalangeal joints of the fingers and the thumb are identical, description of the metacarpophalangeal joint of the index finger will suffice. When passive movement is used in the treatment of stiff fingers, mobilization is given in many directions, and movement in one direction may be coupled with movement in other directions. For example, while the metacarpophalangeal joint of the index finger is being flexed, anteroposterior or posteroanterior mobilizing pressures may be applied to the joint. Compression may also be added to these movements. Although each movement will be described separately it must be remembered that they can be used in combination.

The only quick appraisal tests are opening widely the hand and then forming a fist. Getting the patient to squeeze the physiotherapist's hand is also informative.

Table 10.21 lists the examination for the metacarpophalangeal and interphalangeal joints.

Techniques

Flexion*

Starting position

The physiotherapist holds the proximal phalanx of the patient's index finger in her right hand between her thumb and index finger, both of which are directed proximally. With her left hand she stabilizes his hand, particularly around the second metacarpal, between her finger and the thumb. The joint is then flexed to the comfortable limit of the range (Figure 10.112).

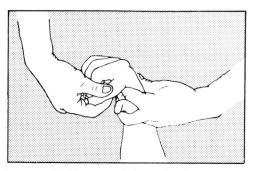

Figure 10.112 Metacarpophalangeal flexion

Method

If grade IV movements are required, a small amplitude oscillation is performed with the therapist's right hand while she stabilizes the metacarpal

Table 10.21 Metacarpophalangeal and interphalangeal joints – objective examination

HIGHLIGHT MAIN FINDINGS WITH ASTERISKS AS YOU GO
Observation
***Functional demonstration/tests**
1. *Their* demonstration of *their* functional movements affected by *their* disorder.
2. Differentiation of *their* demonstrated functional movement(s).
Brief appraisal
Active movements (move to PAIN or move to LIMIT) *Routinely*
F, E, spreading; fist/grip. Note range and pain, repeated and rapid.
Isometric tests
Other structures in 'plan' *As applicable* Full active resisted movement through range for 'sheaths' Joint restriction cf. muscle/tendon restriction Thoracic outlet Entrapment neuropathy
Passive movements *Physiological movement routinely* F, E. Note range, pain, resistance, spasm and behaviour. *As applicable* Joint restriction cf. muscle/tendon restricted. *Accessory movements Routinely*
1. (↔) ceph and caud, Ab, Ad (↔), (↔), (◯), (◯)
2. The above in different positions of other physiological ranges
As applicable
1. Same movements under compression.
2. Ab, with (↔) and (↔).
3. Ad with (↔) and (↔).
4. Canal's Slump tests.
5. Differentiation tests.
6. ULTT. Note range, pain, resistance, spasm and behaviour
Palpation Include tendon sheaths +When 'comparable signs' ill defined reassess 'injuring movement'.
Check case records etc.
Instructions to patient
1. Warning of possible exacerbation.
2. Request to record details.
3. Instruction re 'joint care' if required.

with her left. Any grade of movement can be performed with this grasp but grade I movements are rarely required.

Extension*

Starting position

This technique is the same as that described for flexion except that the metacarpophalangeal joint is comfortably extended.

Method

The oscillatory movement can be produced by the combined action of extending the proximal phalanx on the metacarpal and the metacarpal on the phalanx. The movement can also be produced by stabilizing the metacarpal and moving the proximal phalanx into extension. Small or large oscillations can readily be produced.

Abduction**

Starting position

The physiotherapist holds the posterior surface of the patient's right hand with her right hand and his index finger with her left hand. She holds the posterior surface of his hand from the radial side and places her thumb, pointing distally, against the lateral surface of the second metacarpal distally, while her fingers grasp the ulnar border of his hand. The pad of her left thumb, pointing proximally, stretches along the lateral surface of the proximal phalanx to its base (Figure 10.113).

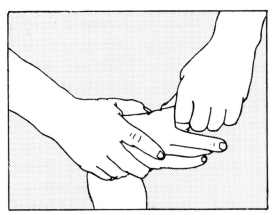

Figure 10.113 Metacarpophalangeal abduction

Method

The oscillatory abduction produced by movement of the therapist's two hands combines abduction with pushing the patient's hand away. Moving his hand

away as the joint is abducted makes the mobilization easier to perform. As with other techniques small or large-amplitudes in any part of the range can easily be performed.

Adduction**

Starting position

It is not as easy to hold the metacarpal during this technique as it is during abduction. The physiotherapist holds the posterior surface of the patient's hand around its radial border with her left hand, wedging as much of the tip of her thumb as she can into the second interosseous space against the ulnar surface of the distal end of the second metacarpal. She reaches with the fingers of her left hand both around his thumb and through the first interosseous space to stabilize his hand. With her right hand she grips his index finger with the pad of her right thumb, pointing proximally, against the medial surface of the proximal phalanx (Figure 10.114).

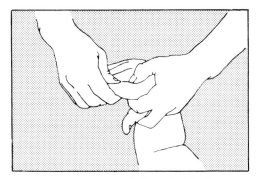

Figure 10.114 Metacarpophalangeal adduction

Method

The adduction movement is produced by the therapist's arm acting through both hands while pushing the patient's hand away from her.

Medial rotation**

Starting position

The physiotherapist stabilizes the patient's second metacarpal with her left hand by holding it firmly between her fingers anteriorly and her thumb posteriorly while she holds his slightly flexed index finger in her right hand. The metacarpophalangeal joint is flexed approximately 10° and the proximal interphalangeal joint 80°. She places the tip of her right thumb against the medial aspect of the proximal interphalangeal joint and the tips of her index and middle fingers against the lateral surface

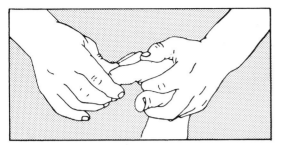

Figure 10.115 Metacarpophalangeal medial rotation

of the middle and distal phalanges (Figure 10.115). The maximum range of medial rotation is obtained when the metacarpophalangeal joint is positioned in a few degrees of flexion which places it midway between its limits of flexion and extension. This is not necessarily the position in which the rotation is performed in treatment but it is the position of greatest range in a normal joint. The degree of flexion and extension in which the medial rotation is used in treatment is usually either the most restricted range of medial rotation or the most painful.

Method

The movement is produced entirely by the therapist's right hand while her left hand stabilizes his hand. She pivots the distal phalanx around her thumb tip, causing the proximal phalanx to medially rotate.

Lateral rotation**

Starting position

The physiotherapist holds across the posterior surface of the patient's hand with her left hand threading her fingers around the lateral border, her index finger passing through the first interosseous space to reach the palm and her remaining fingers grasping around the thenar eminence.

She holds his flexed finger in her right hand with her thumb against the lateral surface of the proximal interphalangeal joint and her index finger against the medial surface of the distal interphalangeal joint (Figure 10.116).

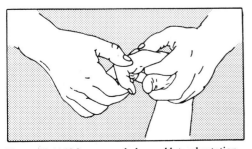

Figure 10.116 Metacarpophalangeal lateral rotation

Method

The therapist produces the rotation by movement of her left hand and forearm while her right hand stabilizes the patient's hand.

Longitudinal movement caudad**

Starting position

The physiotherapist grasps firmly around the lateral border of the patient's right hand with her left hand and holds his index finger in her right hand. His second metacarpal, held in her left hand, is grasped between her flexed index finger threaded through the first interosseous space and her thumb so that the proximal interphalangeal joint of her index finger is against the anterior surface of the distal end of the metacarpal and her thumb is held firmly against the shaft posteriorly. With her right hand she grasps his index finger in a similar fashion, her fully flexed index finger holding the proximal phalanx anteriorly while her thumb grasps along the shaft posteriorly. His metacarpophalangeal joint is then positioned midway between its other ranges to permit maximum caudad movements; this usually requires a slight degree of flexion (Figure 10.117).

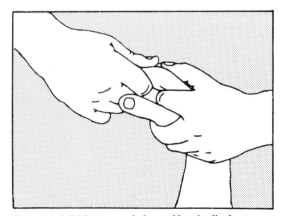

Figure 10.117 Metacarpophalangeal longitudinal movement caudad

Method

While holding the metacarpophalangeal joint in a small degree of flexion the therapist produces distraction by pulling her hands away from each other. The selected position of metacarpophalangeal flexion is maintained during the mobilization by firm pressure against the anterior surface of the patient's metacarpal and phalanx adjacent to the joint with her index fingers at their proximal interphalangeal joints.

Longitudinal movement cephalad*

Starting position

As described for distraction the physiotherapist holds the patient's second metacarpal firmly between her fully flexed index finger and thumb. She holds his index finger similarly except that she holds all of his index finger, slightly flexed at each interphalangeal joint, between her fingers and palm (Figure 10.118).

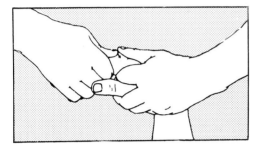

Figure 10.118 Metacarpophalangeal longitudinal movement cephalad

Method

The movement is applied by a squeezing together of the therapist's hands. During this movement it is essential to hold the metacarpal and the index finger firmly.

When the joint is the source of pain and, on examination, both active and passive physiological movements are painless, the passive movements should be repeated while the joint surfaces are compressed. One or more of these movements are commonly found to be painful. The painful movement can then be used in treatment, by making the use of the compression as described above.

Posteroanterior movement***

Starting position

The patient's second metacarpal is held firmly in the physiotherapist's left hand with her fully flexed index finger anteriorly and her thumb posteriorly. Her thumb contacts the posterior surface proximal to the joint while the proximal interphalangeal joint of her index finger contacts the anterior surface. This positioning is necessary to counter the posteroanterior pressure against the head of the phalanx. She grasps the proximal phalanx of his index finger in her right hand with her fingers hooking around the anterior surface and the tip of her thumb against the head of the proximal phalanx posteriorly (Figure 10.119).

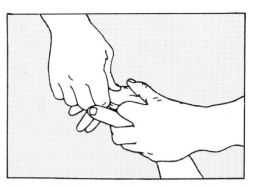

Figure 10.119 Posteroanterior metacarpophalangeal movement

Method

The posteroanterior movement is produced by pressure acting through the tip of her right thumb against the posterior surface of the head of the proximal phalanx immediately adjacent to the metacarpophalangeal joint. The movement, which can be performed in any degree of metacarpophalangeal flexion or extension, must not be produced by the flexors of the right thumb.

Anteroposterior movement***

Starting position

The physiotherapist grasps the patient's second metacarpal between her fully flexed left index finger anteriorly and the tip of her thumb which contacts the posterior surface of the metacarpal distally. She holds the proximal phalanx of his index finger between her fully flexed right finger and thumb, with her proximal interphalangeal joint against the anterior surface of the base of the proximal phalanx adjacent to the joint and her right thumb against the posterior surface of the phalanx more distally (Figure 10.120).

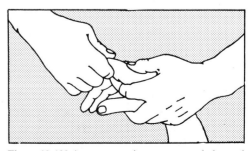

Figure 10.120 Anteroposterior metacarpophalangeal movement

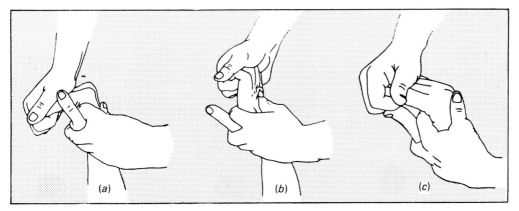

Figures 10.121 General movements metacarpophalangeal and interphalangeal joints. (*a*) and (*b*) flexion/extension; (*c*) circumduction

Method

The oscillation is produced by an anteroposterior pressure against the head of the proximal phalanx anteriorly. This movement may be performed in any degree of metacarpophalangeal flexion or extension.

When general mobilizing of all fingers in every direction is used as a general loosening procedure the following techniques may be used. These techniques are less specific but they have the effect of making the joints feel freer and more comfortable.

General flexion, extension, circumduction

Starting position**

The physiotherapist holds across the back of the patient's right hand from the medial side with her left hand. She grasps through his first interosseous space with her fingers to reach his palm and holds across the back of his hand with her thenar eminence and thumb. With her right hand she holds his four fingers, also from the medial side, between her fingers anteriorly and her thenar eminence posteriorly. With this grasp she can perform flexion, extension or circumduction.

Method

1. From a position of say 60° of metacarpophalangeal flexion and almost full interphalangeal extension the therapist can extend the metacarpophalangeal joints while at the same time flexing the interphalangeal joints. This movement can be performed as a grade II movement (Figure 10.121(a) and (b)). The reverse move-

ment is then performed to reach the starting position.
2. With the middle and distal phalanges held firmly in her right hand she can carry out circumduction of the metacarpophalangeal joints by a circling action with her right hand. During all of these movements she must hold his metacarpals very firmly between the fingers and thumb of her left hand (Figure 10.121(c)).

Treatment

The metacarpal and interphalangeal joints are so shaped that as the joint is flexed the distal joint surface 'slides' anteriorly on the proximal joint surface. It would seem therefore, at least theoretically, that if one of these joints is painlessly stiff in flexion then to stretch the joint structures by using grade IV flexion movements, pressure should be applied to the posterior surface of the base of the distal bone at the same time, to encourage that forward movement of the base on the head.

When flexion is painful as well as restricted then during the use of flexion as a stretching technique the base of the distal bone forming the joint should be moved anteroposteriorly as well as posteroanteriorly.

It is uncommon for a patient to have pain arising from one of these joints without some degree of stiffness. Under these circumstances all of the accessory movements (rotation, transverse movement both medially and laterally, anteroposterior and posteroanterior movements, longitudinal movement caudad, abduction and adduction) should be utilized at the limit of the range. Following these stretching techniques the loosening movements shown in Figure 10.121 should be carried out.

Thumb movements

Movements of the thumb are identical with those of the fingers even though the planes of the thumb movements do not coincide with those of the fingers. The movement of opposition is an additional thumb movement. Opposition takes place at the carpometacarpal joint and in terms of passive movement it is a combination of flexion, abduction, and rotation. Because the carpometacarpal joint lies in a different plane its movements will be described.

Examination

Brief appraisal

Varying angles of posteroanterior pressure on the trapezium, trapezoid, base of first metacarpal and the joint line combined with extension are quick to perform and are usually very informative. Table 10.22 outlines the examination.

Techniques

Carpometacarpal flexion**

Starting position

The physiotherapist stabilizes the patient's wrist in her left hand with her fingers across the anterior surface and her thumb posteriorly. She must make sure that her index finger crosses in front of his trapezium to stabilize it during thumb flexion while not obstructing metacarpal movement. She grasps his thumb in her right hand with her thumb across the posterior surface of the metacarpal and her index finger across the anterior surface (Figure 10.122).

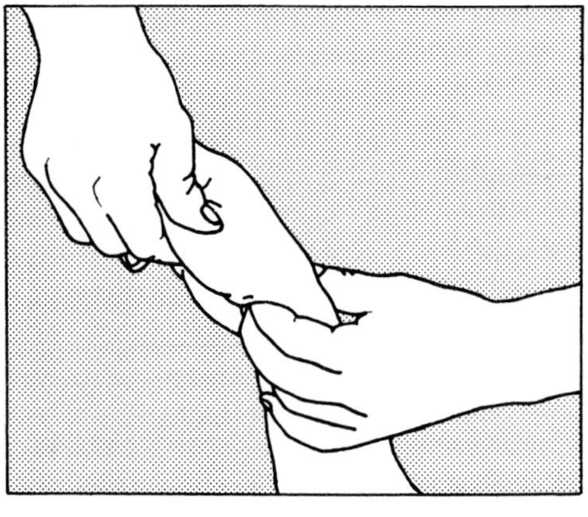

Figure 10.122 Carpometacarpal flexion

Table 10.22 Carpometacarpal joint of thumb – objective examination

HIGHLIGHT MAIN FINDINGS WITH ASTERISKS AS YOU GO

The routine examination of this joint must include the adjacent intercarpal joints and wrist.

Observation

***Functional demonstration/tests**

1. *Their* demonstration of *their* functional movements affected by *their* disorder.

2. Differentiation of *their* demonstrated functional movement(s).

Brief appraisal
Active movements (move to PAIN or move to LIMIT)
Add active movements of thumb including gripping and fist.

Isometric tests

Other structures in 'plan'
Full active resisted movement through range for 'sheaths'
Joint restriction cf. muscle/tendon restriction
Entrapment neuropathy

Passive movements
Physiological movement
Routinely
1. Thumb F, E, Ab, Ad.
2. Differentiating F, E, Ab, Ad Rotn and opposition.
3. HF and HE of carpus.

Note range, pain, resistance, spasm and behaviour.
Accessory movements
Routinely

1. (↓) and (↑) of first metacarpal on trapezium.
2. (→) and (←) against metacarpal on carpus, with and without abduction and adduction, with and without compression.
3. (↻) and (↺) of metacarpal, with and without compression.
4. (↓) adjacent intercarpal and 1st C/MC joint.

Note range, pain, resistance, spasm and behaviour
As applicable

1. Intercarpal tests.
2. C/MC (↓) with E.
3. Canal's slump tests.
4. Differentiation tests.
5. ULTT.
Note range, pain, resistance, spasm and behaviour

Palpation
Include tendon sheaths
+When 'comparable signs' ill defined reassess 'injuring movement'.

Check case records etc.

Instructions to patient

1. Warning of possible exacerbation.
2. Request to record details.
3. Instruction re 'joint care' if required.

Method

The flexion movement is produced through her right hand while her left hand stabilizes the proximal part of the joint.

Carpometacarpal extension**

Starting position

This is the same as that described above except that the tip of her left thumb is placed against the dorsal surface of the trapezium, with which the metacarpal articulates, and the trapezoid with which it has a ligamentous attachment (Figure 10.123).

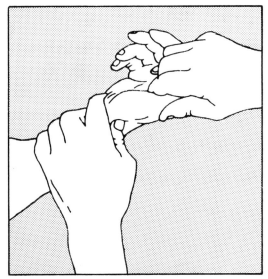

Figure 10.123 Carpometacarpal extension

Method

The extension movement is produced mainly through her contact on the anterior surface of the first metacarpal pivoting it around her right thumb while her left thumb stabilizes the proximal part of the joint. The movements of flexion and extension can be performed in various degrees of abduction or adduction but the one usually used is the one that is most restricted or most painful.

Adduction, abduction and opposition***

Adduction, abduction and opposition are performed with basically the same techniques as described above. With one hand the physiotherapist stabilizes the carpus, particularly the trapezium, while the other hand produces the movement of the metacarpal in the desired direction. During opposition, medial rotation is included as part of the oscillatory movement.

Longitudinal movement cephalad***

This is produced by the same method as has already been described for the index finger (see page 207) and is used in treatment in much the same way. It can be used in conjunction with flexion, extension, abduction, adduction or rotation as dictated by the signs found on examination.

Posteroanterior movement at the first carpometacarpal joint

Pressures in posteroanterior, anteroposterior, transverse medial and lateral directions can be exerted against the trapezium, the trapezoid or the base of the first metacarpal. Only posteroanterior movement will be described as the remainder should then be self-explanatory.

Starting position

The physiotherapist grasps the patient's thumb with her right hand and the radial border of his wrist with her left hand. She places the tips of both thumbs, tip to tip, in one of three main positions:

1. Against the posterior surface of the first metacarpal immediately adjacent to the carpometacarpal joint (Figure 10.124).
2. Against the trapezium.
3. On the joint line.

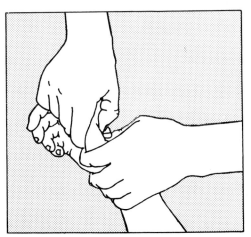

Figure 10.124 Posteroanterior movement at the first carpometacarpal joint

Method

The posteroanterior movement is produced by pressure of the thumbs against the base of the metacarpal. The pressure should arise from the therapist's arms and must not be produced by the thumb flexors.

Chronic/minor symptoms
Proving thumb unaffected

Under either of the above circumstances the most telling of the test movements listed in Table 10.23 below are:

1. A rocking flexion–extension movement of the carpometacarpal joint combined with anteroposterior and posteroanterior movements respectively but performed with strong joint surface compression.

Table 10.23 Chronic/minor base of thumb symptoms

Proving that the thumb is, in fact, unaffected
F-E, E with ( ), Rotn with compression

2. Rotary movements performed with strong compression.

Treatment

The carpometacarpal joints of the thumb are a common source of pain. It is surprising how often the physiological movements of the carpometacarpal joints of the thumb are painless both actively and passively yet when posteroanterior movement of the metacarpal on the trapezium, and/or when the joint surfaces are compressed during extension, the patient's symptoms are immediately reproduced. Use of this technique, interposing III− grades between stretching IV or IV+ grades with a controlled degree of pain, is dramatically effective.

11

Lower limb

Hip joint

The hip is much more stable than the shoulder joint. Movement at the hip cannot be produced to the same degree by thumb pressure against the head of the femur as can be produced in the glenohumeral joint. The shape of the acetabulum and the accessibility of the head of the femur make this difficult. However, small oscillatory movements of the head of the femur within the acetabulum can be produced, particularly when the leg is used as a lever.

Examination

Subjective examination

Most patients are able to point to the site of pain when it arises from the hip. The most common sites are deep in the buttock at the hip joint or in the groin. The pain, when it is over the greater trochanter, usually indicates a disorder of the bursa. It must not be forgotten that referred pain in the area of the quadriceps and knee is common with hip disorders, and it is not uncommon for the hip and quadriceps area to be asymptomatic and yet for there to be pain felt in the knee.

Objective examination

The routine passive movement 'hands-on' examination for the hip joint is given in Table 11.1.

Functional demonstration/tests

If the patient is able to demonstrate how he can provoke his symptoms, this should be analysed first.

Brief appraisal

The quickest way to make a general assessment of a patient's hip disorder is to ask him to walk forwards in his usual manner and to walk backwards; then to flex his hip and knee so as to put his foot up on a step. If those movements do not reveal any abnormality he should be asked to squat, firstly allowing him to do it as he chooses, and secondly observing any differences if he squats while on his toes or with his feet flat on the floor.

Special tests
Flexion/adduction

Flexion/adduction is as important to the hip as the quadrant movement is to the glenohumeral joint. When all other movements are pain-free, this movement can be restricted and painful when compared with the opposite hip. Used as grade III or IV it is extremely useful when treating a hip which is the source of minor symptoms. Grade II type movements can be used effectively in the treatment of osteoarthritic hips during an exacerbation.

Grade IV***
Starting position
The patient lies near the right-hand edge of the couch while the physiotherapist stands by his right thigh, facing across his body. She flexes his hip to a right angle, allowing his knee to flex comfortably. She interlocks the fingers of both hands and cups them over the top of his knee. She then adducts his hip fully until his right ilium starts to lift from the couch. To maintain balance, she places her right

Table 11.1 Hip joint – objective examination

HIGHLIGHT MAIN FINDINGS WITH ASTERISKS AS YOU GO

Observation

*Functional demonstration/tests

1. *Their* demonstration of *their* functional movements affected by *their* disorder.
2. Differentiation of *their* demonstrated functional movement(s).

Brief appraisal

Active movements (move to PAIN or move to LIMIT)
Routinely (but modified as required)

Gait
(Full rotation, and other movements, while standing on one leg)
Squatting or flexing knee to chest
Going up and down step
Lumbar spine
Hip F, E, Ab, Ad, (◯) and (◖)

Isometric test

Other structures in 'plan'

Passive movements
Physiological movements

1. F/Add (if all tests negative so far), in F/Add do (◯) and (◖) or F, E, (◯) and (◖) in F and E. Ab and Ad, in F and E.
   Add compression medially and/or cephalad where applicable
2. Tensor fascia lata.
3. Canal's Slump tests & ULTT.
4. Differentiation tests.
Note range, pain, resistance, spasm and behaviour
Accessory movements
As applicable

1. (↔) ceph and caud, (↕), (↕), (↦), (↤) and (◯◖) in various hip positions.
2. Add compression (ceph & medial) where applicable.

Note range, pain, resistance, spasm and behaviour

Palpation
(especially bursae)
+ when 'comparable signs' ill-defined reassess 'injuring movement'

Check case records etc.

Instructions to patient

1. Warning of possible exacerbation.
2. Request to record details.
3. Instruction re 'joint care' if required.

knee on the couch, level with his left knee, and leans against the lateral surface of his femur so that her chin is close to her hands. Her left thigh, pressed firmly against the edge of the couch at the level of his right hip, gives her the added control to prevent her weight falling fully against his right thigh (Figure 11.1).

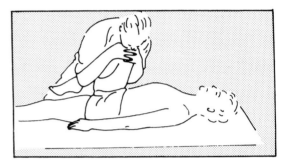

Figure 11.1 Hip joint; flexion/adduction

Method

There are three methods for testing the flexion/adduction. Though they all assess the arc of the adduction while the hip is in various angles of flexion, they assess differing pain responses by varying the method of producing the adduction:

1. From the described starting position, the therapist uses her body to adduct the patient's femur across his body. She then adducts further for two or three oscillations and then releases some of the adduction. Her next step is to flex the hip a further few degrees and repeat the adduction. This is repeated in different angles of hip flexion until the whole range is assessed. This should be the first method used[1] (see Appendix 2, S5).
2. From the same described starting position the therapist first adducts his hip to lift his right ilium off the table. She then increases his hip adduction by applying pressure through his knee downwards in line with the shaft of the femur thus pushing his right ilium down onto the table again (Figure 11.1). If the shaft of the femur has been retained in its relationship to the vertical the pelvis will have adducted under the femur at the hip (see Appendix 2, S6).

   This method of adducting the hip has the added component of driving the head of the femur posteriorly in the acetabulum. The technique can produce groin pain in a normal hip. However, if the movement is being tested on a patient complaining of groin pain, it will be reproduced earlier in the range when compared with his normal hip.

1. Maitland, G. D. *Shoulder Quadrant and Hip F/Add,* Videotape No. 6 (42 mins.). Postgraduate Study Centre Hermitage, Medizinische Abteilung, Bad Ragaz, Switzerland CH-7310 (1979)

3. To find the position of the painful limitation which requires treatment by this third method, the hip should be moved through an arc of flexion in adduction from a position of 20–30° below 90° of hip flexion to approximately 140° where the knee is pointing towards the patient's left shoulder. To test this arc of movement the therapist, starting with the patient's hip in a position of less than 90° of flexion and full adduction, applies and maintains a constant pressure through the knee along the shaft of the femur in these two directions while at the same time moving his thigh through a further 70° of flexion. At all times during the movement the femur should lie midway between medial and lateral rotation. When movement is normal the knee will follow the arc of a circle (Figure 11.2 (a)). A small abnormality will be felt as a bump on the smooth arc of this circle (Figure 11.2 (b)) and this point may be painful. The movement should always be compared with movement of the other hip.

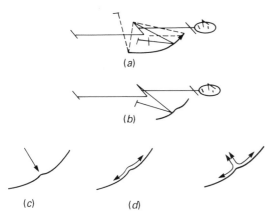

Figure 11.2 Diagrammatic representations of hip flexion/adduction

When flexion/adduction is thought to be normal on examination, both medial and lateral rotation should be added, as grade IV movements, to several over-pressure positions of flexion/adduction before judging normality. Pain response and available ranges guide the judgement.

Grade IV movements can be directed against the painful limitation in three ways. The first is simply a flexion/adduction movement directed at the limitation; this movement is depicted as a single-headed arrow in Figure 11.2 (c). The second method is to move from flexion through 10 or more degrees of extension and then to return while maintaining moderate pressure in adduction so that the movement can rub back and forth over the painful limitation. A double-headed arrow in Figure 11.2

(d) depicts this movement. The third method, perhaps the most important of all, is the small movement that nudges at either side of the limitation in back and forth oscillations in an arc, as shown in Figure 11.2 (e) by the two double-headed arrows.

Techniques

Flexion/adduction

Grade III***

Starting position

The physiotherapist rests her right knee on the couch and leans her left thigh against the edge. Having flexed the patient's hip, she holds his flexed knee with her two hands then adducts and flexes his hip to the limit of the range at the chosen point on the arc. Before commencing the oscillatory movement she alters her grip to support his knee entirely with her left hand, leaving her right hand free to support his right foot and thus prevent flapping. In this position she maintains the mid-rotation movement (Figure 11.3).

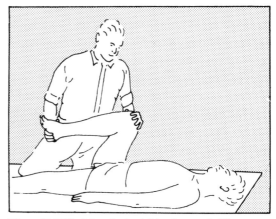

Figure 11.3 Hip joint; flexion/adduction, grade III

Method

The large-amplitude oscillation of approximately 30° (or even up to more than 90°) directed towards the limitation must traverse a straight line and the amplitude of foot movement must equal that of his knee. With her body positioned to form the stop at the outer limit of the movement, she swings his knee away from her to the limit of the flexion/adduction range where his pelvis begins to lift from the couch. These large-amplitude oscillations are difficult to perform smoothly without hip rotation. They are, however, extremely valuable in the treatment of the through-range moderately painful hip.

Grade II***

Starting position

The physiotherapist stands at the level of the patient's right thigh, facing his left shoulder. After flexing his right hip and knee she positions her body as a stop at the lateral extent of the flexion/adduction movement. She holds his knee in her left hand and his foot in her right and faces in the direction of the flexion/adduction movement. She stands further away from the patient for this grade than for grade III (Figure 11.4).

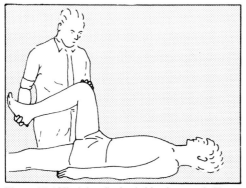

Figure 11.4 Hip joint; flexion/adduction, grade II

Method

The large-amplitude movement, which does not reach the limit of the range, is performed by a back and forth movement of the therapist's arms. The depth of range into which this is taken is governed by the onset of pain and whether this pain increases with further movement. This technique, in its various grades, is among the most useful of all hip mobilizations.

Neither flexion nor adduction will be described as separate techniques because they are simply variations of the foregoing, and also because they are not usually restricted when flexion/adduction is free.

Medial rotation***

This movement, which is frequently restricted and painful, may be more restricted in hip flexion than in extension or vice versa, and such variations should be sought during examination. When movement is very painful, and grade I or II movements are required for treatment, they should be performed in the position as near to midway between the limits of available pain-free physiological flexion and extension as comfort will permit. This is the position where movement is freest and in which a patient relaxes best.

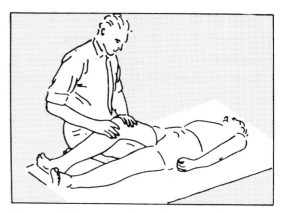

Figure 11.5 Hip joint; medial rotation, grades I and II

Although the technique shown in Figure 11.5 is titled 'rotation', it is related to shaft rotation and not rotation that is 'spin' of the hip joint[2]. In fact, when the femur rotates, the movement of the head of the femur in the acetabulum is a combination of 'slide' and 'roll' combined with a small degree of abduction and adduction. The abduction and adduction occur because when the physiotherapist rolls the patients' knee away from her, the posterior aspect of the patient's knee does not slide on the therapist's thigh but adducts slightly. Similarly, as she pulls the knee back towards her, the knee moves laterally, that is, it abducts.

When grades III and IV are required, the movement should be performed in the degree of flexion or extension where the painful limitation exists or, if general mobilization is required, it should be performed in both flexion and extension.

Grades I and II***

Starting position

The patient lies near the right-hand edge of the couch. The physiotherapist stands at the level of his right knee. With her right knee on the couch she positions her thigh carefully to support his thigh and calf to give him a comfortable and small degree of hip and knee flexion while his heel rests on the couch. She holds around his knee with both hands (Figure 11.5).

Method

She imparts small rotary movements to the femur by light pressures against the lateral surface of his knee. For grade I movement very little movement should be performed whereas when grade II is required a large-amplitude of medial rotation is performed.

2. Williams, P. L. and Warwick, R. *Gray's Anatomy,* 36th edn., Churchill Livingstone, Edinburgh, p. 437 (1980)

Alternative method for grade I***

Starting position

The patient lies on his left side with pillows between his legs so as to support his hip in a neutral and pain-free position. The physiotherapist leans across his hip, positioning it in her left axilla and with her left hand she holds around and under his knee so as to stabilize it and to feel hip rotation. With her right hand she holds under his right ankle and foot to stabilize the foot.

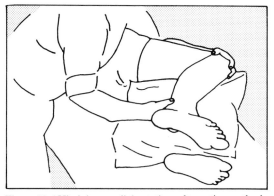

Figure 11.6 Hip joint; medial rotation, alternative method for grade I

Method

While the therapist holds around the knee with her left hand, maintaining a constant position of abduction/adduction and flexion/extension, she produces very small oscillatory movements by raising and lowering the patient's foot with her right hand.

Throughout the technique the patient should be questioned, to determine whether any pain or *even discomfort* is felt in the hip.

In extension supine (grades III and IV)*

Starting position

The patient lies supine near the right-hand edge of the couch on a slight angle to bring his left foot near the edge of the couch and leave his right knee free of the edge. The physiotherapist, kneeling by his right thigh, facing his left knee, supports under his knee with her left forearm, and holds his right foot with her right hand. While stabilizing his knee with her left forearm, she medially rotates his hip by raising his heel laterally (Figure 11.7).

Method

The therapist produces grade IV movements by moving the patient's right foot laterally to the limit of the range while maintaining an equal and

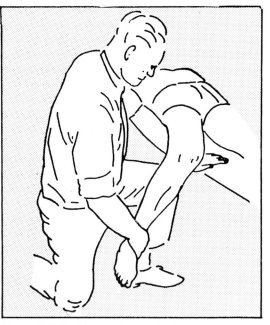

Figure 11.7 Hip joint; medial rotation in extension supine, grades III and IV

opposite counterpressure against the lateral side of his knee with her left forearm. Oscillatory rotation is controlled by her right hand. The pressure with her left arm should be quite firm; in fact this hand feels the tension of the movement even more than does her right hand.

When grade III movements are required, a large-amplitude oscillation is produced by lowering the patient's right foot which releases the pressure against her left arm. While raising and lowering his foot she must exercise care maintaining the patient's thigh in a constant position so that only medial rotation is produced.

In extension prone (grades III and IV)**

Starting position

The patient lies prone and flexes his knee to a right angle. The physiotherapist, standing by his right knee and facing his hip, rests her left knee on the couch, her thigh forming a comfortable stop for his leg at the limit of medial rotation of his hip. She holds his heel in her right hand and his forefoot in her left, medially rotating his hip and adjusting her left leg to the height required to prevent medial rotation (Figure 11.8).

Method

The therapist produces medial rotation of the patient's hip by drawing his foot towards her until it reaches her thigh. The foot and leg are then

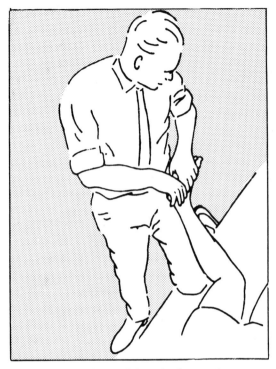

Figure 11.8 Hip joint; medial rotation in extension prone, grades III and IV

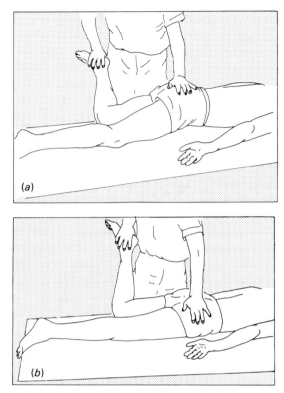

Figure 11.9 Hip joint; medial rotation: (*a*) right ilium raised; (*b*) right ilium posteroanterior pressure downwards

repeatedly oscillated back and forth by her arms. A better action is usually obtained if, while she draws his foot towards her, she inverts his foot a little. She may need to position her right hand against the lateral side of his thigh during the medial rotation to prevent hip abduction. Treatment movements from II+ to IV− can be given with complete control in this position.

As with nearly all passive movement treatment techniques, the movement of the joint may be produced from either of the bones forming the joint. For example, a grade IV medial rotation of the hip joint may be produced from a starting position similar to that shown in Figure 11.8 (but sufficiently rotated for the patient's left ilium to be raised a few centimetres off the table). By stabilizing the patient's lower leg, the therapist can produce medial rotation of his right hip by oscillatory pressures on his left buttock moving his left ilium towards the table (Figure 11.9).

In flexion (grades III and IV)**

Starting position

The patient lies supine near the right-hand edge of the couch and the physiotherapist stands by his right hip, facing his left knee. She flexes his hip and knee

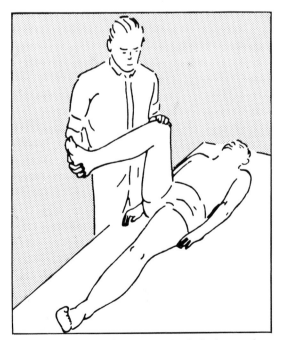

Figure 11.10 Hip joint; medial rotation in flexion, grades III and IV

to a right angle, supporting his knee with her left hand and his right heel with her right hand. She medially rotates his hip, preventing abduction by pressure against the lateral surface of his knee with her left hand (Figure 11.10).

Method

Medial rotation is produced by her right hand moving his foot in an arc around his knee while maintaining a constant knee position with her left hand.

Lateral rotation

Lateral rotation is required less often. When necessary, it is usually performed with the hip in flexion. When the joint is painful, requiring grade I or II movements, the technique is identical with that described for medial rotation except for the direction of the movement (see Figure 11.5). An alternative position for grade I is for the technique to be performed in exactly the same way as described for medial rotation with the patient lying on his left side and having pillows between his legs. The one difference is that the therapist's right hand produces the lateral rotation as very small oscillatory movements by gently pushing the patient's foot into the pillows and then returning it to its starting position. The position is as in Figure 11.6 but with the difference that the therapist's right hand holds around the foot and ankle. Grades III and IV are similar to those performed for medial rotation except that in extension the technique cannot easily be performed with the patient supine because the edge of the treatment couch hinders movement of the leg.

In flexion supine*

Starting position

The physiotherapist stands by the patient's right hip, facing his left knee, and flexes his hip and knee to a right angle. She holds his knee in her left hand and his foot in her right hand. Stabilizing his knee with her left hand, she laterally rotates his hip until the limit of the range is reached, at the same time adjusting the position of her body to face his left shoulder (Figure 11.11).

Method

Grade III or IV oscillatory movements are produced by moving the patient's foot back and forth in an arc around his knee. The therapist's left hand and trunk maintain the position of his knee, the centre of the arc of movement. If the hip is flexed a few degrees during the medial rotation phase of the oscillation and then extended back through those few degrees during lateral rotation, the technique is sometimes

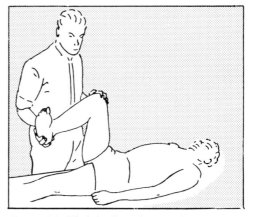

Figure 11.11 Hip joint; lateral rotation in 90° flexion supine

easier. This action lessens the amount of work for the right hand.

Starting position

The patient lies prone and the physiotherapist stands by his left knee, facing his right hip. She flexes his right knee to a right angle, holds his right forefoot with her right hand and his heel with her left hand. With her right knee on the couch, she positions her thigh to provide the stop at the limit of his lateral rotation. She then laterally rotates his hip by lowering his foot towards her until the limit of the range is reached (Figure 11.12).

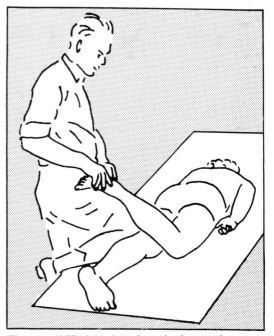

Figure 11.12 Hip joint; lateral rotation in extension prone

In extension prone

Method

The therapist performs the oscillatory rotation by a back and forth action with her arms. The technique is improved if the movement of the lateral rotation is combined with some eversion of his foot.

Lateral movement**

This movement is depicted with the hip positioned in almost 90° of flexion. It must be realized, however, that exactly the same lateral movement of the hip can be produced in any degree of hip flexion or extension, in different angles of abduction or adduction, and with varying degrees of rotation.

Starting position

The patient lies on his back and flexes his hip and knees to the chosen angle. The physiotherapist stands alongside the patient's hip, pressing her upper sternum against his knee while interlocking her fingers and holding around the medial surface of his thigh as near as is practicable to the hip joint. Her arms and chest also stabilize his lower leg (Figure 11.13).

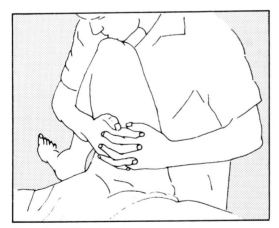

Figure 11.13 Hip joint; lateral movement

Method

Considerable movement can be produced by this technique. It can be used solely as a lateral displacement of the head of the femur in the acetabulum. To achieve this movement the physiotherapist should ensure that the angle of the hip abduction or adduction does not alter as the proximal end of the femur is moved laterally. This may require considerable movement of the patient's knee position to avoid the tendency of his pelvis to roll as the hands pull the head of the femur laterally. Again, it is not the therapist's hands that produce the lateral oscillatory movement. This time the patient's whole limb and the therapist's hands, arms and thorax move as one solid entity while she rocks back and forth on her feet. By this method she can produce any movement between grade I and IV.

Alternatively, while producing the lateral movement of the hip joint, the therapist may:

1. Stabilize the patient's knee, preventing its lateral movement, so that the lateral movement of the hip is combined with a small degree of horizontal adduction of the hip.
2. While stabilizing the patient's limb and applying lateral movement to the hip, lean backwards, carrying the patient's hip into a small degree of horizontal abduction.

If the technique is to be used as an accessory movement at the limit of another range of movement as part of the treatment to restore range, then before applying lateral movement she should position the hip at the limit of the range she aims to improve (i.e. the limit of flexion, extension, abduction, adduction, medial rotation or lateral rotation) before taking up any remaining slack in the direction of lateral movement. She should then use the oscillatory lateral movement as a grade IV or IV+ movement. Also, under circumstances where improvement in range is the goal, the lateral movement asserted by the therapist's hands may be performed simultaneously with movement in the direction of the chosen upper range. For example if the aim is to improve medial rotation the starting position is adopted where the hip is flexed to a neutral convenient position and medially rotated to the limit of the range. To perform the technique the therapist twists her trunk to face towards his feet while producing the lateral movement. Again it is emphasized that the patient's whole limb and the therapist's hands, arms and trunk move as one entity as movement is produced by the rocking action on her feet.

Straps or belts are used by some therapists to produce this movement. This has the one disadvantage which is that the therapist does not have the feedback information of the quality and range of the movement which is available and can be assessed when the movement is performed through the therapist's hands. This principle applies to all belt or strap techniques described by other authors. Nevertheless, a small therapist treating a heavy patient requiring strong grade IV movements is well justified using such equipment.

When extremely gentle and very finely controlled lateral movement is needed a different starting position must be used.

Grade I**

Starting position

The patient lies on his side and pillows are placed between his comfortably flexed legs. The physiotherapist stands behind the patient and grasps around his thigh anteriorly and superiorly (Figure 11.14).

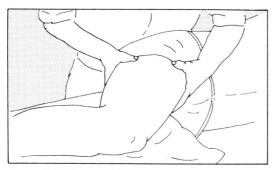

Figure 11.14 Hip joint; lateral movement, grade I

Method

The therapist very gently oscillates a lateral hip movement. She should endeavour, with the whole palmar surfaces of her fingers, to feel the femur and control the tiny movements. It is also necessary repeatedly to determine by questioning if the movement is free of any symptoms.

Longitudinal movement caudad***

Longitudinal movement is most useful when hip movements are very painful. The amount of movement possible is very small but when the patient has considerable pain and it is performed in a comfortable position for the patient this movement is soothing.

Starting position

The physiotherapist supports under the patient's slightly flexed hip and knee with her right leg. Depending upon the amount of hip flexion which is comfortable for the patient, she either kneels on her right shin and places her right thigh diagonally under his knee, or she sits on the edge of the couch and places her right leg fully flexed at the knee and laterally rotated at the hip, under his thigh. She then encircles the distal end of his femur with her hands (Figure 11.15).

Method

Oscillatory longitudinal movements are produced by pulling gently on the femur. This technique can be

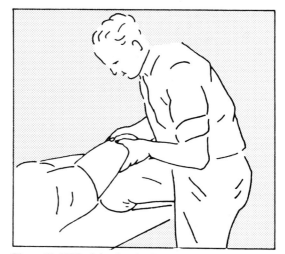

Figure 11.15 Hip joint; longitudinal movement caudad

assisted by a rolling or sliding movement of the therapist's support under the patient's thigh in the direction of the treatment movement. When the joint is very painful, movements should be performed so gently that there is no discomfort. This technique can be performed in varying degrees of hip flexion.

Alternative method for grade I

Starting position

The patient lies on his left side with the pillows between his legs. His hips are positioned in mid flexion/extension and his knee comfortably flexed. The physiotherapist, standing behind the patient, places her thumbs on the greater trochanter, her fingers spread widely to help stabilize the thumb position, and her forearms directed in line with the patient's femur (Figure 11.16).

Method

Extremely gentle comfortable longitudinal movements can be produced at the hip joint by this

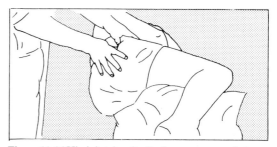

Figure 11.16 Hip joint; longitudinal movement caudad, alternative method for grade I

method. It is important that the thumbs should not be the prime movers in producing the oscillatory movement but should act as spring-like contact points, feeling the movement that is taking place. The therapist's arms and body gently rock back and forth in line with the femur to produce the hip movement.

Alternative method for grade I or II**

Starting position

The patient lies on his left side with pillows between his legs to limit adduction of the right hip. The patient's hips and knees are flexed for comfort and for positioning the hip in a neutral position.

The therapist leans across the patient, cradling his pelvis with her left axilla. She then grasps the lower end of the femur with both hands (Figure 11.17).

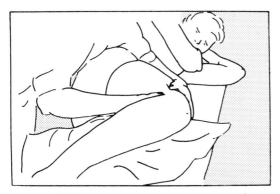

Figure 11.17 Hip joint; longitudinal movement caudad, alternative method for grade I or II

Method

The therapist stabilizes the pelvis in her left axilla to prevent it moving while the technique is being performed. The longitudinal movement is produced through her hands, which clasp the distal end of the femur. The movement should be produced by her arms; she cannot use her body because she would then lose control of the patient's pelvis position.

In flexion

Longitudinal movement of the hip is an accessory movement which can be used with the femur in many different positions. The two following techniques show longitudinal movement being applied to the hip while it is in flexion. The first is neither adducted nor abducted during the technique and the second, while still in flexion, is also in some degree of abduction.

Starting position (in flexion)

The patient's hip is flexed to 90° and his knee is fully flexed. The physiotherapist, with the fingers of both hands interlocked, grasps around the anterior surface of his thigh as far proximally as she can reach. She stabilizes the hip and knee angle by cradling his knee between her head and shoulder (Figure 11.18).

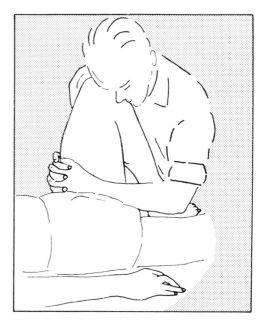

Figure 11.18 Hip joint; longitudinal movement caudad in flexion

Method (in flexion)

The therapist's grasp of the patient's leg is such that, as she rocks back and forth on her feet, her whole trunk and the patient's leg rock in the same direction.

Starting position (in flexion/abduction)

The starting position for this technique is identical with that described for the preceding technique except that the patient's femur is abducted to any chosen range (Figure 11.19).

Method (in flexion/abduction)

The method used for producing this longitudinal movement is identical with that described for the preceding technique. The patient's leg and the therapist's trunk and arms move as a single unit as she rocks back and forth on her feet.

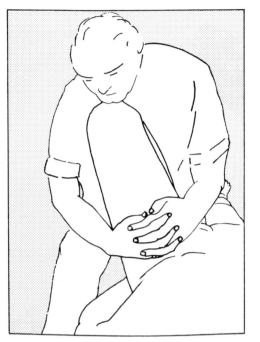

Figure 11.19 Hip joint; longitudinal movement caudad in flexion/abduction

Compression***

The hip has two directions for compression. The first is with the compression in line with the shaft of the femur as it would be in the standing position. This is called 'longitudinal movement cephalad'. The second is a medially directed pressure against the greater trochanter compressing the articular surface of the head of the femur into the laterally facing surface of the acetabulum.

Longitudinal movement cephalad***

The compression technique can be used on its own or in conjunction with rotation in the gentle grades, or with flexion and extension when these movements are performed between full extension and 20° of flexion. It is best suited to the patient who has pain on weight bearing. It therefore serves its best purpose in grades III and IV.

Starting position

The physiotherapist supports the patient's leg in a slight degree of hip and knee flexion in the same way as described above for longitudinal movement caudad. She holds his leg with her right hand cupped over the tibial tubercle while supporting under his knee with her left hand (Figure 11.20).

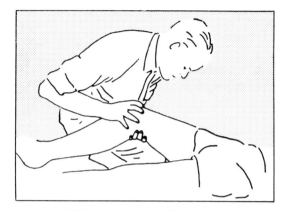

Figure 11.20 Hip joint; longitudinal movement cephalad

Method

The oscillatory movement, pushing the head of the femur into the acetabulum, is performed by the physiotherapist's right hand thrusting against the front of the tibia in the line of the femur. The return oscillation is governed almost entirely by her left hand. As with the caudad technique the movement can be performed in varying degrees of hip flexion. If strong techniques are used there will be considerable pelvic movement. The strength of technique initially is varied either to produce slight pain or to reach a point just short of this.

Alternative technique***

While compression is sustained in the position described above, other movements can be added. For example, Figure 11.21 shows a rotary movement being produced: a medial/lateral movement of the patient's lower leg and foot while compression is maintained along the shaft of the femur though his knee.

Compression medially***

This technique has an important role in treatment and is often linked with a patient having chronic hip symptoms which nearly always prevent him lying on the side of his painful hip.

Starting position

The patient lies on his right side (this being the pain-free side in these circumstances) and the physiotherapist leans across the patient from in front placing the cupped heel of her left hand over his left greater trochanter. She positions her left shoulder directly above her left hand and supports his (left) lower leg along the maximum distance medially (Figure 11.22).

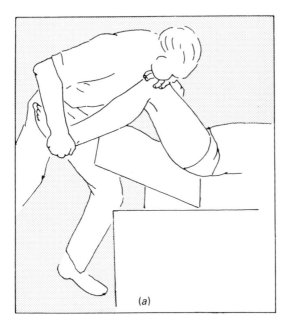

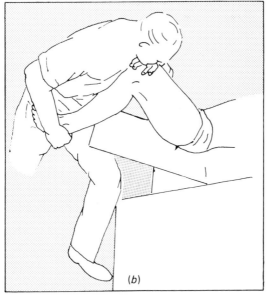

Figure 11.21 Hip joint; rotation added to longitudinal cephalad compression: (*a*) towards medial rotation; (*b*) towards lateral rotation

Method

Six techniques for using compression will be described:

1. A sustained squeezing together of the head of the femur medially into the laterally facing articular surface of the acetabulum is sustained while, with her left shoulder she squashes the head of the femur towards the floor in an oscillatory over-pressure fashion. The length of time spent sustaining the compression is estimated in comparison with the length of time the patient is able to lie on his disordered hip before becoming aware of symptoms (Figure 11.22 (a)).

The technique can be performed with the patient lying on his painful hip, the medial compression being produced by the therapist transmitting pressure through his pelvis (lateral iliac crest and greater trochanter) to squash the opposite trochanter into the table.

2. While the compression medially is sustained (or oscillated if required) she uses her body and right arm to pivot around his left hip to produce extension (Figure 11.22 (b)).

3. To produce hip flexion with the compression medially she pivots in the opposite direction (Figure 11.22 (c)).

4. Abduction is produced by the therapist laterally flexing her trunk to the left (Figure 11.22 (d)).

5. For lateral rotation she curves her body forwards and over his left hip which results in his foot being lowered towards the floor while his knee is retained in the mid-flexion/extension, abduction/adduction ranges (Figure 11.22 (e)).

6. The reverse action of the therapist's body produces medial rotation (Figure 11.22 (f)).

Posteroanterior movement**

Very little posteroanterior movement of the head of the femur takes place in the acetabulum. However, this technique can be used to good effect for the very painful joint. It can also be used as an accessory movement at the limit of a physiological range when the aim of treatment is to increase the range of movement of the hip joint.

When used for treating pain, pillows are used between the patient's leg and the thigh is positioned midway between the limit of its ranges. Usually this means that the hip is flexed, the correct range being that which is pain-free. Very gentle oscillatory movements that are painless should be produced by pressures transmitted through her thumb.

When the movements are being used to increase the range of movement in any particular direction, flexion for example, the hip is flexed to the limit of its range and the therapist's hands rather than her thumbs are used to produce the posteroanterior movement.

Starting position

The patient lies on his left side with pillows between his legs and feet. The physiotherapist stands behind him and places the pads of both thumbs, pointing

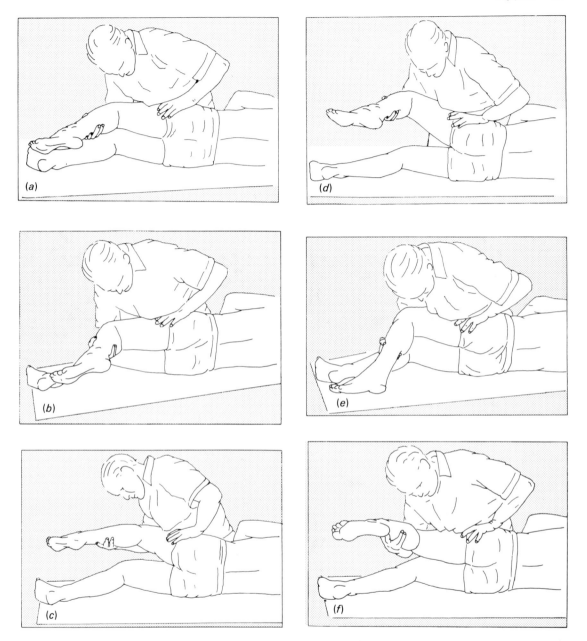

Figure 11.22 Hip joint; compression medially: (*a*) in neutral; (*b*) in extension; (*c*) in flexion; (*d*) in abduction; (*e*) in lateral rotation; and (*f*) in medial rotation

towards each other, against the posterior surface of the greater trochanter (Figure 11.23). This is the starting position for grades I and II.

If the technique is being used as a stretching technique, the patient's hip is flexed as far as possible and the physiotherapist applies the oscillatory grade IV movement, using the heel of her hand.

Method

When painless grade I movements are used for treating pain, soft gentle small oscillatory movements are produced by the physiotherapist's body and arms through the thumbs stabilized against the trochanter. As with other techniques that make use

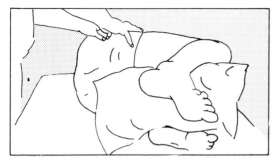

Figure 11.23 Hip joint; posteroanterior movement

of the physiotherapist's thumbs, the movement should not be produced by the thumb's intrinsic muscles. Throughout the technique the patient is asked if he can feel any pain or discomfort.

When the technique is used for stretching hip flexion the physiotherapist may need to use one hand against the femur while the other hand maintains hip flexion and/or stabilizes the pelvis by pressure anteroposteriorly against the right antero-superior iliac spine.

Anteroposterior movement

Starting position

The patient lies on his left side with pillows between his legs and thighs as described above. The pillows must support between his feet also to avoid unwanted lateral rotation. The physiotherapist stands in front of the patient and places her thumbs on the anterior surface of the greater trochánter. She should endeavour to use a large surface area of the pads of the thumbs so as to make the technique as comfortable as possible. Spreading her fingers will help to stabilize her thumbs, which should be in direct bone-to-bone contact with the trochanter (Figure 11.24).

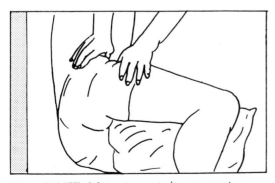

Figure 11.24 Hip joint; anteroposterior movement

Method

As described above the oscillatory movement is produced by the therapist's body and arms and not by intrinsic thumb muscles.

Although the movement has been described as, and titled, anteroposterior movement, the actual direction of the pressure against the anterior surface of the greater trochanter may be varied through an arc of approximately 30°. If the technique is performed well it is surprising how much movement can be produced and felt.

Abduction

Abduction can be performed in three main ways. The first two are abduction in flexion and abduction in extension; the third is a combined extension/abduction movement which is the opposite from flexion/adduction described on page 222.

In flexion*

It is simpler if abduction in flexion is performed in a position of approximately 60° flexion with the patient's foot resting on the couch even though a degree of lateral rotation occurs with the abduction. Grades II and IV are the most frequently used treatment movements in this position. When the joint is very painful, grade I movements are used in a position of approximately 20° hip flexion (see Figure 11.15). When grade IV movements are used, as in Figure 11.25, both legs should be flexed so that the painless hip can be abducted fully to stabilize the pelvis during the mobilization of the painful stiff hip.

Starting position

The physiotherapist stands by the flexed hip and knee of the patient, whose foot rests on the couch level with his left knee. She rests her right lower leg across his foot to stabilize it. She supports his knee with her left hand over the femur and her right hand over the tibia. Before performing the mobilization, she abducts his knee to the limit of the range which she intends using for treatment and stands close to his leg to form a stop, preventing further abduction (Figure 11.25).

Method

The oscillation is performed in small or large-amplitudes by the action of her hands on his knee. His pelvis must be watched carefully to see that the hip movement is not taken beyond the point at which it begins to move.

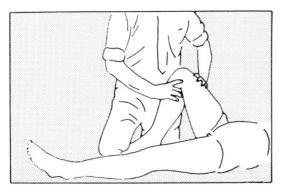

Figure 11.25 Hip joint; abduction in flexion

In extension**

The patient lies with both legs abducted comfortably. The physiotherapist, standing by his right lower leg, facing his hip, places her right knee immediately adjacent to his right leg. Sitting back on her right heel she supports under his right knee with her left hand and under his ankle with her right hand (Figure 11.26).

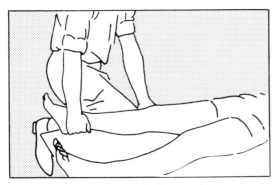

Figure 11.26 Hip joint; abduction in extension

Method

The oscillation, usually not exceeding an amplitude of 10–15°, is performed by the therapist's arms while the patient's leg is supported just free of the couch. Her right leg forms the stop at the limit of the abduction range. If more hip extension is required, a folded blanket or pillow can be placed under the patient's buttocks.

Extension/abduction**

The main use for extension/abduction is to treat pain rather than to restore range by stretching. It is therefore used mainly as a grade II movement.

Starting position

The physiotherapist stands in a similar position to that described for flexion/adduction as a grade II movement (see page 224). The difference is that she moves backward to lower the patient's leg in extension/abduction to the limit of the treatment range.

Method

The mobilization is performed through an amplitude of 20–40° of hip movement by the therapist's arms while at the same time she carefully maintains the hip in a mid-rotation position.

Extension**

Extension is best performed with the patient supine because movement at the hip can be performed in any part of the range whether it is limited or not. If there is a limitation of extension, the physiotherapist supports under the patient's knee with her right thigh in much the same way as has been described for longitudinal movement (see Figure 11.15). The technique described here will be for a grade II movement.

Starting position

The patient lies near the right-hand edge of the couch and the physiotherapist stands by his right lower leg facing his left knee. She holds laterally around and under his knee with her left hand and under his heel from the medial side with her right hand (Figure 11.27).

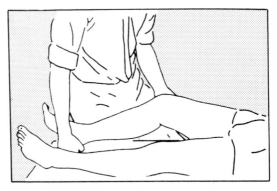

Figure 11.27 Hip joint; extension

Method

The therapist with her left hand raises his knee 6 or 8 in. (15–20 cm) from the couch and with her right hand keeps his heel off the couch and approximates it 3 or 4 in. (7.5–10 cm) towards his right buttock.

She then carries his heel away from his buttock and allows his knee to lower to the limit of the extension. His heel is kept off the couch throughout the movement.

As has been mentioned, if the extension is limited she will support under his knee with her thigh to provide a stop at the limit of the movement. If a greater range of extension is required, a pillow can be placed under his buttocks. His left hip and knee may be flexed for comfort.

Chronic/minor hip symptoms

Proving the joint is unaffected

The movements required in both of these circumstances are the same. They are:

1. In standing:
   (a) F/E.
   (b) Abd/Add.
   (c) Med/Lat Rotn.
   (d) squatting on heels.
2. In supine: Medial rotation and lateral rotation in different positions of F and of F/add: (and in E/abd and E/ad).

Treatment

The majority of patients referred for physiotherapy to the hip have, on examination of hip movements, a combination of stiffness and pain. It then becomes a question of priorities: should the physiotherapist initially treat pain or restriction of movement? It is usually wiser to treat pain for at least the first one or two sessions. If treating pain does not effect improvement, the stiffness can be treated and the only loss to the patient will have been time. However, if the choice is made to treat the stiffness first and it causes a marked exacerbation then although it will not harm the joint disorder it does produce unnecessary discomfort for the patient, and it shows that the wrong approach was used at the current phase of the disorder.

The rotary technique shown in Figure 11.5 is very useful for the treatment of hip pain. Earlier in this book emphasis was placed on using accessory joint movements in a neutral position when techniques are directed towards treating the pain. Although this rotary technique is not an accessory movement, it is of particular value in the treatment of pain when a patient has a diagnosis of osteoarthritis of the hip. It is also most useful as a very large-amplitude grade III movement to relieve soreness when this soreness is produced by strong stretching techniques.

Another technique of great value is flexion/adduction. The technique, in its different grades, has been described in detail in this chapter. If a patient has minimal pain, or intermittent pain

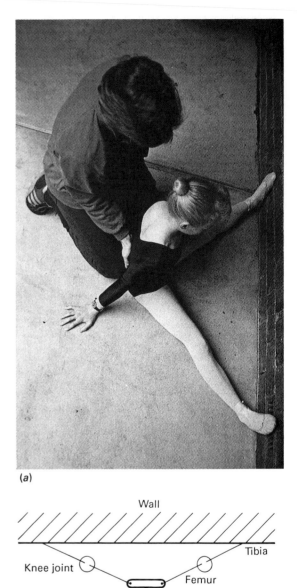

(a)

(b)

Figure 11.28 (*a*) and (*b*) Hip joint; the patient's 'functional demonstration/test' position: the position she adopted to demonstrate reproduction of her medial knee pain in both knees which she felt during training. (*c*) and (*d*) Hip joint; pelvis stabilized and one single movement used to increase

provoked by sudden unexpected movements, then flexion/adduction performed as a grade IV movement readily relieves this pain. This treatment technique would be performed as shown in Figure 11.2 (c–e). It is often important to add lateral

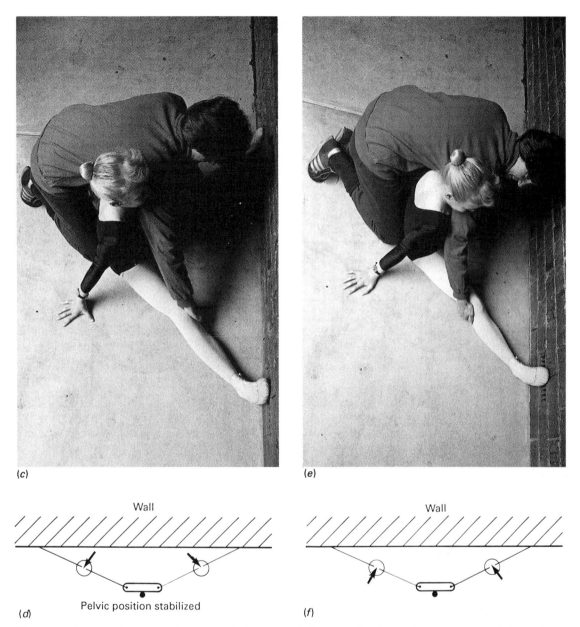

(c)

(e)

Wall

Pelvic position stabilized

(d)

Wall

(f)

hip stress and decrease knee stress simultaneously. The arrows indicate the direction in which pressure was applied to the knees. This pressure in fact decreased knee stress and increased hip stress. Because the 'differential test' reproduced her knee pains, the fault must have been in the hips and not the knees. (e) and (f) Hip joint; pressure directed medially at the knees increases the stress at the knees and decreases the stress at the hips when performed in the patient's 'functional demonstration/test' provoking position

lateral rotation to the technique. Obviously, the technique will cause discomfort or pain but this pain is readily relieved by performing the technique as shown in Figure 11.2 (c) as a very gentle but large-amplitude grade III movement.

When the hip joint is stiff, restricting functional activities, the same pattern of treatment is used as has been described in Chapter 7. That is, the particular movement that is restricted is performed as a gentle grade IV oscillatory movement for one minute or so, and is followed by grade III accessory movements at the limit of the restricted range.

This routine is repeated three or four times. Any treatment soreness is then easily relieved by performing a large painless grade III movement in the direction of the stiff movement being stretched.

Example

The following 'patient history and treatment' story exemplifies four areas of the 'Concept':

1. Hypermobility.
2. Local knee pain arising from a pain-free hip.
3. Making use of a movement or position which the patient can perform to knowingly provoke his/her symptoms.
4. Use 'differentiation tests' to determine the source of the symptoms which the patient can provoke.

A young girl, who had great promise as a ballerina, was referred for treatment because of pain she was experiencing in both knees following intensive ballet practice sessions.

She could provoke her pain in both knees by attempting to do the 'splits' with feet against a wall in the sitting position, and trying to get her symphysis pubis as close to the wall as possible (Figure 11.28 (a)).

Most therapists would consider that this knee pain would be coming from the knees as they were being stressed in this position. The concept says 'prove it' by differentiation tests IN THIS DEMONS-TRATED PROVOKING POSITION because knee pain *can* be referred from a painless hip. This was done as seen in Figure 11.28 (c).

Her knee pain was increased during the tests (Figures 11.28 (b) and (d)).

If the stressing of the knees is increased by the therapist reversing the direction her pressure on the girl's knees (which would simultaneously decrease the stress placed on her hips by the provoking position) her knee pain would decrease or disappear (Figure 11.28 (e) and (f)).

Passive examination of her knees proved them to be normal.

As would be expected of a ballerina, her range of hip movement in this direction was abnormally great. As this hypermobile range was not adequate for the work she was doing, it was necessary to use strong passive stretching techniques to increase this range with the expectation that when she had the range she needed, the pain would go. This in fact occurred and she was able to sit on the floor with her pelvis and trunk vertical while both legs were abducted fully to form a straight line in the coronal plane with both thighs on the floor; she lost all of her knee pain.

Knee

The techniques will be divided into those applied to the tibiofemoral joint, the patellofemoral articulation and the superior tibiofibular joint.

Tibiofemoral joint

The tibiofemoral joint has physiological movements of flexion and extension and a small range of rotation. It also has accessory movements of abduction, adduction, rotation, posteroanterior and anteroposterior movements, medial and lateral movements, and longitudinal movement cephalad and caudad.

Examination
Functional demonstration/tests

A position or movement by which the patient can provoke his disorder is analysed first.

Brief appraisal

A variety of tests can be used to assess the severity of a patient's knee disorder, and a particular sequence of tests is suggested below. If test 2 reveals obvious pain then there is no need to proceed with tests 3 and 4. However, if test 2 does not give the information being sought then tests 3 and 4 can be usefully used. The range of knee movement may be measured and the degree and site of pain provoked by these tests can be recorded and used as asterisked signs against which progress can be measured. The tests are as follows:

1. The patient, sufficiently undressed, should be (a) asked to balance on the one bad leg and then (b) asked to walk forward away from the examiner and to return while she assesses any abnormality or asymmetry in his gait.

    If the gait seems normal and symmetrical then the patient should be asked to walk backwards away from, and towards, the therapist. This often reveals asymmetry in gait not seen when walking forward.
2. Stepping up and down a small step with the work being done by the bad leg.
3. The patient should be asked to squat, using his hands to maintain balance if necessary. He should not be told to squat in any particular manner. The examiner observes the spontaneous method he uses. It is his knee for which the quick tests are being used so it matters little whether he squats with his feet flat or on his toes.

    If he is able to do so, he should be asked to bounce in the full squat position, vigorously enough and with feet far enough apart, to bounce his buttocks downwards so that, if possible, his ischial tuberosities will pass his heels. The physiotherapist should make an assessment of any pain or discomfort; this is particularly important when the patient is able to bounce symmetrically. If the knee is normal the feeling in the joint which the patient experiences should be the same in both knees.

If the patient is only able to squat symmetrically a small distance and then continue to bend further by tilting towards the good side, the range of knee flexion on that side moves further while the painful side does not increase its range. Accordingly the physiotherapist should assess the range of knee flexion of the disordered knee together with the site and severity of pain.

4. It is useful to compare the range of knee flexion found in test (2) above with that which the patient can perform in the non-weight-bearing position lying supine.
5. Another useful test of knee flexion is to ask the patient to adopt the position where he is kneeling with his weight forwards on his hands. He should then be asked to sit back gradually until he reaches the limit of his range. If his range is normal he should be able to sit at least on his heels or even past his heels.

Tests (3) and (4) above are not strictly 'quick tests'. All of the information which the 'quick test' will give will be disclosed by tests (1) and (2). However, if test (2) reveals a marked limitation due either to joint stiffness or pain then tests (3) and (4) follow logically so that the pattern of knee flexion is more clearly shown. It will be revealed more clearly because the test movements are done with the patient's full control and there will be no body-weight transmitted through the joint.

Special tests

As has been mentioned in relation to other joints, the knee can be responsible for minor symptoms yet have a full painless range of flexion and extension. However, if grade IV extension/abduction, extension/adduction, flexion/abduction and flexion/adduction are not examined, the joint may be considered to be normal because important physical joint signs and reproduction of pain will have been missed. The two extension movements are the main test and extension/abduction is the most common to elicit joint signs. These four movements are described under the heading 'Techniques'.

Palpable swelling is a common finding in knee disorders but it is important to realize that such increase in synovial fluid can be localized to, or greater at, one area of the whole synovial pouch. In

Table 11.2 Tibiofemoral joint – objective examination

The routine examination of the tibiofemoral joint must also include examination of the patellofemoral (P/F) joint, the superior tibiofibular joint (and the hip).

HIGHLIGHT MAIN FINDINGS WITH ASTERISKS AS YOU GO

Observation
In standing from anterior, posterior and especially laterally.

*Functional demonstration/tests

1. *Their* demonstration of *their* functional movements affected by *their* disorder.
2. Differentiation of *their* demonstrated functional movement(s).

Brief appraisal
Active movements (move to PAIN or move to LIMIT)
(Balance on toes for coordination)
Routinely (but modified as required)

Gait

As applicable

Squatting to onset of pain
Lumbar spine
F and E in standing
Specific movements that aggravate
The injuring movement
Movements under load
Knee extension lag
Speed of test movements

Isometric test

Other structures in 'plan'
Entrapment neuropathy, LLTT

Passive movements
Physiological movements
Routinely

F, E, (◯), (◯) in F and E
Note range, pain, resistance, spasm and behaviour
Test hip (especially F/Ad) Pat/Fem and Sup. Tib/Fib to exclude
Accessory movements
Routinely

Ab, Ad, in various positions of F/E
(↓), (↓), (→), (→) in various positions of F/E

As applicable
(↓), (↓), (→), (→), (◯), (◯) with compression
E/Ab, E/Ad, F/Ab/, F/Ad
Note range, pain, resistance, spasm and behaviour

Palpation
+ when 'comparable signs' ill-defined reassess 'injuring movement'

Check case records etc.

Instructions to patient

1. Warning of possible exacerbation.
2. Request to record details.
3. Instruction re 'joint care' if required.

other words, the increased fluid does not necessarily spread evenly within the joint. The localization indicates the site of the disorder, for example, superomedial patellofemoral articulation.

Table 11.2 below lists the full passive movement tests of the tibiofemoral joint.

Techniques

Extension/abduction***

Grade III

Starting position

The physiotherapist stands by the patient's right ankle, facing his left hip. She rests her right knee and lower leg on the couch at right angles to his leg and supports his right heel across her thigh adjacent to her anterior superior iliac spine. Her right hand supports his knee by being placed around the medial aspect of the joint line so that her fingers reach the medial condyle of the tibia posteromedially and her thenar eminence covers it anteromedially. The heel of her left hand may be placed in one of three positions: cupped over the lateral epicondyle of the femur, on the lateral condyle of the tibia, or directly over the joint line. As with her right hand, the fingers of her left hand reach posteriorly while the thenar eminence is positioned slightly anteriorly. It is necessary for her left forearm to be almost at right angles to the shaft of the femur and tibia so that the abduction component can be produced (Figure 11.29).

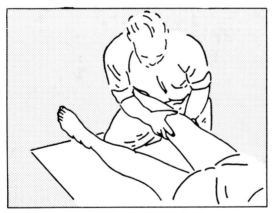

Figure 11.29 Tibiofemoral extension/abduction

Method

If a grade III movement is required, the patient's knee is raised and lowered through a distance of approximately 5 or 6 in. (13–15 cm) by the therapist's hands. A constant pressure is maintained

against the lateral surface of his knee by the heel of her left hand, placed in one of the three positions described above. Each of the three positions will produce a slightly different movement of the tibiofemoral joint. When the heel of her left hand is against the femur and a strong abducting pressure is applied, the femur will tend to move slightly medially on the tibia while abduction during extension is taking place at the joint. However, when the heel of her hand is placed against the tibia, the tibia will tend to move medially on the femur during the extension/abduction. When the heel of the physiotherapist's hand is on the joint line there will be no medial movement of the femur on the tibia or tibia on the femur, so that the movement produced at the tibiofemoral joint will be simply extension/abduction. The stronger the abduction pressure required, the more she needs to crouch to bring her left shoulder close to his knee.

She must not support his lower leg above his ankle and she must firmly hold his foot against the iliac crest with her right elbow. This hold of his ankle enables the addition of longitudinal movement to the extension/abduction whenever it is required, as well as providing a counterpressure for the abduction pressure applied to the knee.

Grade IV**

If grade IV+ movements are required, it is more economical for the therapist to stand by the patient's right knee, holding from the lateral side under his heel with her right hand while her left hand is placed anterolaterally over the joint line of his knee. She is then in the best position to control firm small-amplitude movements while varying the pressure of abduction or extension that she wishes to emphasize (Figure 11.30).

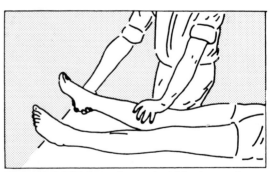

Figure 11.30 Tibiofemoral extension/abduction, grade IV+

Extension/adduction***

The technique for extension/adduction is essentially the same as the technique described for grade III and IV+ extension/abduction, with the obvious difference that this time it is the therapist's right forearm which should be at right angles to the femur and tibia so as to exert the adduction component. As described above for extension/abduction, the heel of her right hand can be placed over the medial epicondyle of the femur, the medial condyle of the tibia or the joint line. Also, as mentioned above, the three different positions of the heel of the therapist's right hand produce three slightly different movements at the tibiofemoral joint.

Extension**

Extension is performed with the therapist's left hand (as shown in Figure 11.30) in one of two positions:

1. The cupped hand is placed on the anterior surface of the femur immediately adjacent to the superior border of the patella. The extension produced in this position is identical with that produced with the *active* movement: that is, the articular surface of the tibia moves (slides) anteriorly on the articular surface of the femur. This positioning of the therapist's left hand is the one used in the treatment of a painless knee disorder when the aim is to restore the last few degrees of knee extension (convex/concave principle).
2. This second position has the cupped left hand placed over the anterior surface of the *tibia* immediately superior to its tuberosity. The extension movement now goes against the physiological active movement rule of concave (tibia) and convex (femur) rule.

An example of this concept's rule

Other manipulative therapist authors argue the axiom that all examination and treatment passive movements must be performed in the directions (slide, role, spin) in which they occur actively.

This is anathema to the concept propounded in this book; in fact the concept says the opposite, on the basis of the very positive importance of the 'PAIN provoked with movement' principle. The 'comparable' – 'appropriate' pain response is nearly always found with the unphysiological movement rather than the physiological movement.

Sometimes the grade II+ or III− movements of extension are performed more effectively if the physiotherapist stabilizes the patient's knee and produces extension by lifting his foot, rather than by using the technique described above which stabilizes the foot and lowers the knee. This may be because the techniques have slightly different tibiofemoral relationships and the patient may find it easier to relax with one than with the other.

Starting position

The physiotherapist stands by the patient's right thigh and kneels on her left shin to support under the lower end of his femur with her left thigh. When his knee is flexed and his foot supported on the couch, she moves her left thigh to his calf also. With both hands she holds distally around his lower leg from behind. Her left elbow should be by the inside of the patient's knee so that the axis of her left arm will coincide with the axis of his knee movement (Figure 11.31).

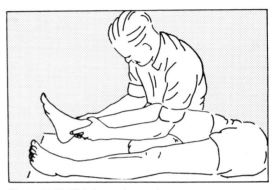

Figure 11.31 Tibiofemoral extension

Method

This position is used for grade III movements and the amplitude is usually 25–30°. The therapist raises and lowers his leg through the arc of movement with her arms. An abduction or adduction component can be added to this movement if desired but the technique is less effective than that described previously (see page 240) where the three hand positions can be used.

Flexion/abduction***
Starting position

The physiotherapist, standing beside the patient's right knee, flexes his hip to a right angle and fully flexes his knee. She supports his knee in her left hand and grasps anteriorly around his ankle with her right hand so that with her fingers pushing laterally against the medial surface of his calcaneum posteriorly and her thumb hooked around his lateral malleolus she can fully medially rotate his tibia (Figure 11.32).

Method

This technique utilizes small- or large-amplitude oscillations as diagonal movements into flexion/abduction while strongly maintaining the rotation. His heel should be lateral to his ischial tuberosity. If

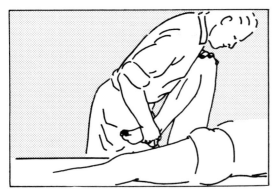

Figure 11.32 Tibiofemoral flexion/abduction

the tibial rotation is lost the diagonal component of the movement will include medial rotation of the hip rather than the small abduction movement of the knee that can be produced. The physiotherapist needs to keep close to the patient's lower leg to enable her to control the pressure against the ankle.

Flexion/adduction***

Flexion/adduction is identical with that described above except that strong lateral rotation of the tibia is maintained throughout the diagonal movement of flexion/adduction. The starting position for the therapist's right hand must be changed so that her fingers hook around the patient's medial malleolus while her thumb and the metacarpophalangeal joint of the index finger apply pressure in a posterior direction on the anterior surface of the tibia. Because of the adduction component, the patient's heel is directed medial to his ischial tuberosity (see Figure 11.33).

Abduction and adduction**

The maximum amplitude of movement that can be produced in this direction is obtained when the knee is held approximately 10° short of full extension.

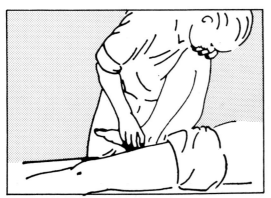

Figure 11.33 Tibiofemoral flexion/adduction

Starting position

When this technique is used as a form of treatment, the position adopted is identical with that described for extension/abduction. The therapist maintains 10° flexion by her finger support under the patient's knee (see Figure 11.29).

Method

Abduction movement is produced by the pressure of her left hand against the lateral surface of his knee. Adduction is produced by pressure against the medial side of his knee with her right hand.

Anteroposterior movement

The anteroposterior movement is very useful in the treatment of extremely painful knees when it is applied as a grade I movement with the knee supported on a soft pillow in a few degrees of flexion. In less painful conditions it can be used as a grade III or IV movement in any position of knee flexion/extension, abduction/adduction or rotation. Anteroposterior movement has its greatest range in position of knee flexion varying from 10° to 70°.

Grade I***

Starting position

The patient lies with a soft pillow placed under his knee, supporting the femur more than the tibia, in not more than 10° of knee flexion. The physiotherapist stands by his right lower leg, facing his knee, and places the pads of her thumbs against the anterior surface of the tibia either side of the tibial tubercle. Her fingers rest against the adjacent

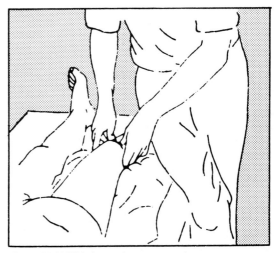

Figure 11.34 Tibiofemoral anteroposterior movement, grade I

surfaces of the tibia and fibula. She should position the metacarpophalangeal joints of her thumbs almost vertically above the pads so that the pressure will be directed through these joints (Figure 11.34).

Method

Small oscillatory movements are produced by the therapist's arms acting through her thumbs. These finely controlled movements should not be performed by the flexor muscles of the thumbs.

In flexion (grade IV)***
Starting position

The patient lies with his foot resting on the couch so that his knee is flexed approximately 70°. The physiotherapist stands by his right ankle and rests her right lower leg across his foot to stabilize the position. She positions the heel of her right hand over the anterior surface of the tibia immediately adjacent to the joint line and spreads her fingers over the front of his knee. Her left hand is placed behind his knee with her palm over the upper calf (Figure 11.35).

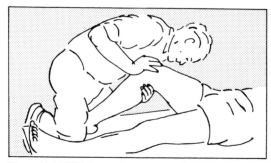

Figure 11.35 Tibiofemoral anteroposterior movement, grade IV

Method

Anteroposterior mobilizing is produced by pressure of the heel of the therapist's right hand against the upper end of the tibia. Her left hand acts as a support and produces the return movement when a large-amplitude is required.

Posteroanterior movement**

Posteroanterior movement in grades I and IV have the same application in treatment as the anteroposterior movements and the techniques are essentially the same as those described above.

Grade I
Starting position

For grade I movements the patient's knee is supported as shown in Figure 11.36).

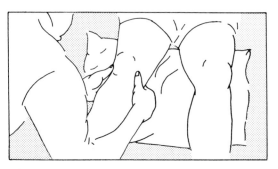

Figure 11.36 Tibiofemoral posteroanterior movement, grade I

Method

The posteroanterior movement is produced by the therapist's pressure transmitted through her fingers against the posterior surface of the tibia proximally.

Grade IV
Starting position

For grade IV movements with the patient lying prone the physiotherapist rests her right tibia on the couch with her knee fully flexed while supporting the patient's distal shin across her upper thigh.

There are two methods by which the movement can be produced. The therapist can place the pads of her two thumbs on the posterior surfaces of the medial and lateral condyles of the tibia, using as much as possible of the pads of her thumbs, as bone-to-bone contact may be uncomfortable (Figure 11.37). Alternatively, she can support the patient's

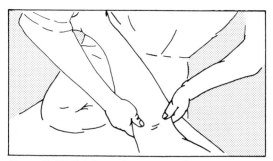

Figure 11.37 Tibiofemoral posteroanterior movement, grade IV

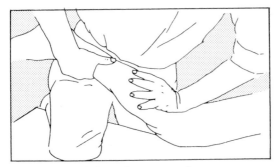

Figure 11.38 Tibiofemoral posteroanterior movement, grade IV alternative position

left shin in her right hand while the heel of her left hand is placed on the posterior surface of the tibia as far proximally as possible. The fingers of her left hand lie over the gastrocnemius (Figure 11.38).

Method

The grade IV oscillatory movements of the head of the tibia on the femur with the knee in some flexion, if performed by the thumbs, are produced by arm movement. In no circumstances should the oscillation be produced by the intrinsic thumb muscles because if this is done, the technique causes discomfort to the patient and the therapist is unable to appreciate the extent and feel of the movement.

When the heel of the therapist's left hand is used to produce the movement the pressure against the tibia originates from the therapist's trunk and arm movement.

With this particular technique the movement can be performed in three slightly different ways, producing three distinctly different movements at the tibiofemoral joint:

1. As the head of the tibia is moved forwards the therapist can, with her right hand, carry the distal end of the tibia an equal distance so that the whole lower leg moves through a full parallel line.
2. As the pressure is exerted posteroanteriorly through her left hand the physiotherapist can slightly lift the patient's distal tibia so that, combined with the posteroanterior movement, there will be a degree of knee flexion taking place.
3. As the posteroanterior movement at the head of the tibia is taking place the therapist, with her right hand, can lower the distal end of the patient's tibia so that there is a degree of tibiofemoral extension as the posteroanterior movement is taking place.

Lateral movement**

Both lateral movement and medial movement (description of which follows this technique) are accessory movements and can be tested in various angles of knee flexion/extension. In the text that follows the knee is supported in a position of 90° of flexion. The movement is described as movement of the tibia on the femur.

Starting position

With the patient lying supine, his hip and knee flexed and his foot resting on the table, the physiotherapist stands level with his foot and faces towards his head. She places the heel of her right hand on the medial condyle of the tibia and the heel of her left hand on the lateral epicondylar area of the femur. She then leans forwards and extends her wrists so that both forearms are directed parallel to each other. Her right forearm will be positioned on a slightly lower plane than her left forearm (Figure 11.39).

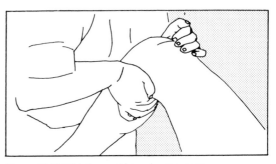

Figure 11.39 Tibiofemoral lateral movement

Method

The technique is merely one of pushing the arms towards each other, but it is necessary to have the pressure along the line of each forearm directed correctly such that if the patient's knee were not there the physiotherapist's right arm would pass parallel to but below her left arm.

Medial movement**
Starting position

The difference in position between medial movement and lateral movement is that the physiotherapist changes her contact points around the patient's knee. For medial movement she places the heel of her right hand on the medial epicondylar area of the patient's femur and the heel of her left hand against the lateral condyle of his tibia (Figure 11.40).

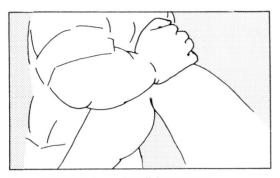

Figure 11.40 Tibiofemoral medial movement

Method

The method for this technique is identical with that described for lateral movement, with the forearms being parallel, but this time the therapist's left forearm is below her right forearm.

Medial rotation***

When used in the treatment of extremely painful joints this technique can be very effective. Medial rotation of the tibia on the femur as a grade I movement can be produced either by anteroposterior pressure against the anterior surface of the medial tibial condyle or by posteroanterior pressure against the posterior surface of the lateral condyle, or by a combination of both. In the case of the first, the starting position and method are the same as described for anteroposterior movement (see page 243) except that the thumbs are placed anteriorly on the medial condyle. If the movement is produced by posteroanterior pressure against the lateral condyle the technique is the same as mentioned above for posteroanterior pressure except that the pressure is applied only to the lateral condyle (see Figure 11.36).

Grade IV in flexion is the next most useful technique for medial rotation. It can be performed with the patient supine or prone.

In flexion supine***

Starting position

The physiotherapist stands by the patient's right hip, facing his feet, flexes his right hip and knee to a right angle and holds the knee between her left arm and her side. With her left hand pronated she holds his forefoot from the lateral side and with her right hand holds posteriorly and medially around his heel (Figure 11.41).

Method

The medial rotation movement is produced by a pulling action of both hands while she stabilizes his

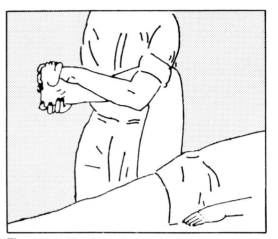

Figure 11.41 Tibiofemoral medial rotation supine

knee against her body. Large-amplitude movements involving 30° of movement can easily be performed. Small oscillatory grade IV stretching movements can also be performed easily in this position.

It should be appreciated that the technique also includes foot and ankle movement while producing rotation of the knee.

In flexion prone***

Starting position

The patient lies prone near the edge of the couch and the physiotherapist stands by his right thigh, facing his feet. She flexes his knee to a right angle and places the heel of her right hand against the medial surface of his heel and her fingers over the sole of his heel with the tips reaching the lateral surface. With her left hand she grasps the dorsum of his forefoot with the heel of her hand against the lateral border and her thumb over the sole. If strong movements are to be used she crouches over his foot to direct her forearms opposite each other (Figure 11.42).

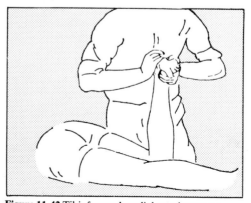

Figure 11.42 Tibiofemoral medial rotation prone

Method

Small or large amplitudes can be produced by a pulling and pushing action of both hands in opposite directions. It is essential to prevent the forefoot inverting when pressure is applied to its lateral surface by the left hand.

As with the preceding technique, movement takes place in the foot and ankle as well as the knee. This does not make it any less effective in producing knee rotation. However, if the foot or ankle is painful the knee rotation may need to be produced by grasping the malleoli.

Lateral rotation**

This movement need not be described because its technique and application are similar to medial rotation.

For grade I movements, posteroanterior pressure against the posterior surface of the lateral tibial condyle will produce medial shaft rotation of the tibia at the tibiofemoral joint with the emphasis at its lateral compartment. The axis for this rotary movement is medial to the intercondylar eminence. This axis can be brought back to the intercondylar eminence position by simultaneously using anteroposterior pressures against the anterior surface of the medial tibial condyle.

Lateral rotation can be produced by the reverse procedure as can the site of the axis of the rotation.

These movements can be performed with the patient supine or prone (Figure 11.37, prone; Figure 11.34, supine).

The stronger movements in knee flexion can be performed with the patient supine or prone as described above for medial rotation.

Longitudinal movement caudad***

This movement is used in treatment in two main ways. One method is used for very painful knees when grade I movements are given and the other method is used in conjunction with other knee movements. When combined with other movements, it may be included either to make the technique more comfortable or to provide maximum gapping of the joint surfaces. Gapping is often used in conjunction with abduction, extension and rotation.

Starting position

The patient lies near the right-hand edge of the couch with his knee support in a few degrees of flexion by a pillow. The physiotherapist, standing by his right foot, facing his knee, grasps around the head of his tibia with both hands so that her thumbs overlap to reach the opposite side of the tibial

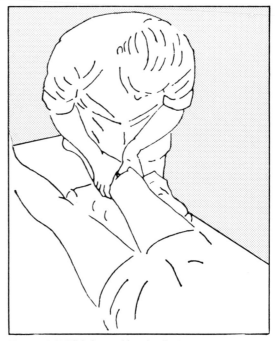

Figure 11.43 Tibiofemoral longitudinal movement caudad

tubercle. Her fingers reach around the medial and lateral borders of the tibia to the posterior surface (Figure 11.43).

Method

Tiny amplitude oscillations are produced by pulling lightly on the head of the tibia in line with the shaft of the femur.

Longitudinal movement cephalad**

Occasionally, compression of the joint surface is important when included with other accessory or physiological movements in the treatment of a painful joint. To effect improvement in such a joint, treatment may require a technique which reproduces the pain. This may require including compression of the joint surfaces while applying other movement techniques.

The starting position is the same as that described for longitudinal movement caudad but the compression is provided by the therapist's hands against the head of the tibia moving it towards the head of the femur with an oscillatory movement.

Patellofemoral articulation forms part of the knee joint but is described separately. The superior tibiofibular joint should also be examined when the site of symptoms indicates possible involvement. This, too, is described separately.

Examination sequences

Chronic/minor knee symptoms

The following tests should be performed:

1. Mandatory passive movement tests, when chronic symptoms occupy any part of the area from lower third of femur to upper third of tibia/fibula (hip excluded).
2. Supine: extension with ↕ tibia and femur (and lag).
3. Flexion.
4. Shaft rotation in 90° knee flexion.
5. Anteroposterior and posteroanterior movement in knee flexion.
6. Medial and lateral movements in 90° knee flexion.
7. Abduction and adduction in knee extension and 20° flexion.
8. Patellar/femoral movements without and with compression.

Test movements begin as IV− with observation for pain response. If pain-free, adequate over-pressure is applied until pain is provoked or the movement is judged 'clear'. If all are 'clear' the following test movements should be included:

9. Extension/adduction and extension/abduction with ↕ tibia.
10. Superior tibiofibular joint, anteroposterior and posteroanterior movement without and with compression.

When a positive pain response is provoked, that test movement may need to be differentiated to determine the specific joint at fault, and/or other test movements may need to be tested so as to either exclude or incriminate other joints as contributing to the symptoms.

If all test movements appear 'clear' at first examination, they should be repeated more strongly. If still 'clear' they may prove positive when repeated at the next consultation.

Proving unaffected

The following tests should be performed:

1. Extension with ↕ tibia, and femur, extension/abduction and extension/adduction.
2. Shaft rotation in 90° flexion.
3. Abduction and adduction.
4. Patellofemoral movements with compression.
5. Superior tibiofibular ↕ and ↕ with compression.

Treatment

Although longitudinal movement cephalad and caudad and compression are not frequently used as solo techniques in treatment, they may be used in conjunction with abduction/adduction, rotation or flexion/extension movements. An example of this, described by Cyriax[3], is the combination of longitudinal movement caudad and rotation used in attempts to reduce displaced menisci.

The techniques that can be used in the treatment of knee conditions are varied. They extend from the gentlest mobilizations using grade I anteroposterior/posteroanterior oscillatory movements for extremely painful knees to the stronger grade IV+ stretching type mobilizations or to the techniques referred to above for the reduction of internal derangements.

Treatment by knee extension

Knee conditions referred for physiotherapy frequently present with a lack of active full-range extension and even if the range passively is full it is usually painful with over-pressure. The degree of pain felt on extension will often be found to be less than the degree of pain that can be produced (with less over-pressure) when abduction is combined with the extension. The same is true of flexion compared with flexion/adduction and flexion/abduction. Extension is commonly more positive than flexion. As some people normally experience pain if over-pressure is applied to passive knee extension it is proper to compare the disordered knee with the normal knee. It is not commonly realized how much over-pressure the normal knee can accept and therefore therapists may miss an abnormality of knee movements. It is therefore necessary to emphasize that one should be prepared to carry out fairly vigorous knee extension tests provided these are done under the right circumstances and are progressed from exploratory gentle extension movements through stages of increasing pressure. Provided the movement is a slow controlled movement the patient will have both the time and the muscular ability to prevent a too strong pressure being applied. In fact, it is quite extraordinary how strong the knee flexors are even when the knee is hyperextended.

By reference to any text of anatomy or biomechanics it is understood and accepted that as the knee is actively extended, the tibia, with its concave surface, slides forwards on the convex condyles of the femur. It would seem from this that if passive stretching is being applied to improve the range of extension the physiotherapist should place one hand on the anterior distal surface of the femur pushing it towards the floor while her other hand lifts under the patient's heel. This would permit the anterior surface of the proximal end of the tibia to move

3. Cyriax, J. and Cyriax, P. *Illustrated Manual of Orthopaedic Medicine*, Butterworths, London, p. 99 (1983)

anteriorly on the femoral condyles. In the clinical situation however, as compared with the academic situation, better improvement in the range of knee extension will be obtained if the physiotherapist places her hand, not on the femur, but on the tubercle of the tibia. It is also interesting and important to note that if the technique is performed with one hand on the tibia rather than the femur the stretching technique will be more painful and therefore a more 'comparable sign'. As this pain is always a more 'comparable joint sign', it is therefore an important guide to the amount of over-pressure which should be given in the treatment and as a measure for progress.

Another interesting aspect to the use of knee extension as a treatment technique is that if the patient has pain and slight restriction on knee extension and has also some limitation of knee flexion and an active extension 'lag', then passive extension treatment techniques consistently restore the active extension to full range without giving any exercises, and also flexion, usually recover at the same time. To gain this improvement in extension lag and knee flexion it is a necessary corollary that by using the knee extension as the treatment technique (with or without adduction or abduction) the passive knee extension will increase in range and the pain will disappear.

Treatment of knee pain

When a patient has a very painful knee which is made worse with walking, or has increased pain with the first few steps following rest, the treatment techniques are directed towards treating pain. The accessory movements that can be used include oscillatory rotary movements, longitudinal movement cephalad and caudad, posteroanterior and anteroposterior movements, and medial and lateral transverse movements. These would be performed with the knee supported in some degree of flexion and the physiotherapist would use her thumbs to make small amplitude oscillatory movements short of causing any pain or discomfort.

Although it is not truly an accessory movement, the technique that is most successful in the treatment of this kind of disorder is rotation. The most comfortable method for this technique would be to place an easily moulded pillow under the supine patient's knee. The therapist then holds over the top of the patient's knee so that she can feel the medial and lateral coronary ligament with her middle finger and thumb, her palm being over the patella, while with her other hand she comfortably grasps around the medial and lateral malleoli. Starting from a neutral mid-position for rotation she would gently and slowly rotate the tibia through approximately 5° of medial rotation and then rotate

laterally from that position to 5° of lateral rotation from the mid-position. This rotary oscillation would be continued from side to side smoothly and slowly while at the same time feeling the proximal end of the tibia rotating back and forth under her finger and thumb. While performing the movement she should ask the patient whether he feels any sign of discomfort, rubbing or movement. Ideally, the patient should feel nothing but if the therapist has any doubts about what he might be feeling, she should perform exactly the same technique on the other knee and ask him whether the feeling in both knees with the same amplitude of movement is the same. For initial treatment to be successful there should be no difference in the feeling within both knees. If this can be achieved the technique should be performed on the painful knee for no longer than 1 minute. The patient should be warned of the possibility of exacerbation following the first treatment. At the next treatment session, if there has been any exacerbation, the amplitude should be made smaller and distraction should be added to the technique. If there has been no exacerbation then the amplitude can be increased and perhaps even taken into a small degree of discomfort. From this point on, the treatment can be progressed.

Knee flexion

When, due to trauma, knee flexion is markedly limited though not very painful, and knee extension is full range and painless with strong over-pressure, then the principles of treatment are applied as outlined in Chapter 7. That is, knee flexion is the technique used as a sustained stretching small amplitude movement the limit of the range interspersed with grade IV accessory movements at the limit of the flexion range. If the caudad movement of the patella is restricted, it should be mobilized

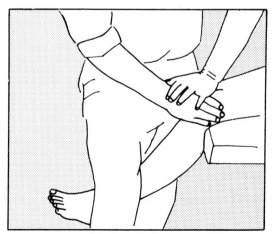

Figure 11.44 Stretching knee flexion

also. The technique involves holding the patient's knee at the limit of flexion, and even stretched further, by the physiotherapist's legs. This leaves her two hands free to stabilize the patella with one hand while applying very strong oscillatory movements against the superior border of the patella, attempting to move it distally as strongly as possible (Figure 11.44).

Instability

Instability is discussed under the headings of 'straight non-rotary (medial, lateral, anterior or posterior), and rotary (anteromedial, anterolateral, posterolateral and combined) instabilities' by Corrigan[4]. It is important to remember the difference between stable-instability and unstable-instability (see page 63). Restoring a full pain-free range of extension with anteroposterior movement combined with abduction and adduction will clear the pain-inhibition of the stable-instability and thereby restore stability.

The Apley's test and McMurray's test are well-known important differentiation tests, as is reduction of torn meniscus causing a 'locked-knee'[5,6].

The technique consists in holding the patient's knee at the limit of flexion, and even stretched further, by the physiotherapist's legs. This leaves her two hands free to stabilize the patella with one hand while applying very strong stretching oscillatory movements against the superior border of the patella, attempting to move it distally as strongly as possible.

4. Corrigan, B. and Maitland, G. D. *Practical Orthopaedic Medicine,* Butterworths, London, p. 140 (1983)
5. Corrigan, B. and Maitland, G. D. *Practical Orthopaedic Medicine,* Butterworths, London, pp. 146–151 (1983)
6. Apley, A. G. and Solomon, L. *Apley's System of Orthopaedics and Fractures,* Butterworths, London, pp. 288–292 (1982)

Patellofemoral articulation

The four main movements of the patella are longitudinal movement cephalad and caudad, and transverse movement medially and laterally. In practice it may be necessary to combine them in pairs to produce diagonal movements cephalad or caudad to elicit pain. When these movements are full range and painless, compression of the patella against the femur should be added to the test movements to elicit the pain.

Whereas transverse movements medially or laterally are best tested or performed in treatment by thumb pressures against the medial border of the patella, longitudinal movements are more comfortably performed by hand pressures.

Two rotary movements are also important. The first, and most important of the passive rotary movements is rotated around the anatomical longitudinal axis. This movement produces contact between the medial articular facet of the patella and the medial condyle of the femur (Figure 11.45).

The second rotation is in the coronal plane around the sagittal axis (Figure 11.46).

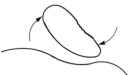

Figure 11.45 Rotation around the femoral longitudinal axis

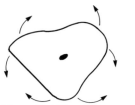

Figure 11.46 Rotation around the sagittal axis

Table 11.3 Patellofemoral articulation – objective examination

The knee movement should also be examined as part of the examination of the P/F articulation.	**Passive movements** *Physiological movements* *Routinely*
HIGHLIGHT MAIN FINDINGS WITH ASTERISKS AS YOU GO	Knee F, E Test to exclude hip *Accessory movements* *routinely*
Observation	1. Lift and compress
*Functional demonstration/tests	2. (→), (←) (and vary angles of knee F/E) ⎫ Repeat and at limit of 3. (↔) ceph and caud (add med. and lat. inclinations) ⎬ each add rotation
1. *Their* demonstration of *their* functional movements affected by *their* disorder. 2. Differentiation of *their* demonstrated functional movement(s).	4. (↻), (↺) without and with compression in neutral resting position (sagittal axis) 5. (↻), (↺) around axis of femoral shaft.
Brief appraisal **Active movements** (move to PAIN or move to LIMIT)	Note range, pain, resistance, spasm and behaviour *As applicable*
Active quick tests (as applicable, standing Knee F and E, squat)	1. Above movements with compression. 2. Above movements with knee in different angles of flexion. 3. Above movements with knee in different angles of flexion and with compression. 4. LLTT.
Routinely (but modified as required)	
Gait Sitting Knee E from F (weak, pain inhibited, painful arc) Muscle power through range Extension lag	
As applicable	**Palpation** + when 'comparable signs' ill-defined reassess 'injuring movement'
Stairs Lumbar spine	**Check case records etc.**
Isometric test (quads, holding patella caudad)	**Instructions to patient**
Other structures in 'plan' Entrapment neuropathy	1. Warning of possible exacerbation. 2. Request to record details. 3. Instruction re 'joint care' if required.

Unless the disorder is mild/chronic and is not irritable, exacerbation, even with moderately gentle techniques, is common and surprisingly easy to provoke.

Examination

Subjective examination

The site of symptoms is almost always felt at the deep surface of the patella; it can be easily identified, if care is taken examining, provided the differentiation is made between the anterior tibiofemoral area and the patellofemoral area.

Reproducing the pain when walking up and down stairs is indicative of a patellofemoral disorder, and the degree of difficulty, plus lingering or latent pain, is an important assessment of the irritability of the disorder.

Functional demonstration/tests

The demonstrations are usually knee flexion under load. Differentiation is clarified by the therapist increasing the patella compression during the demonstration.

Brief appraisal

A useful functional test for assessing range and pain is to ask the patient to squat. When the patient reaches the very beginning of pain the physiotherapist immediately estimates the angle of knee flexion then asks the patient to stand upright again. If pain is minimal, it should be determined why the patient is unable to squat fully. Perhaps he feels his knees are too weak to allow him to bend further or it may be due to pain or stiffness.

The behaviour of pain or stiffness will determine the kind of examination and treatment used. For example, if the patient is able to squat fully without any discomfort then the special tests used in examination may need to be vigorous. However, if he is able only to squat through say 40° of knee flexion, with increasing pain limiting the squat, then gentle passive patellofemoral movements should be used in examination and treatment.

It is very interesting to compare with the available range of non-weight-bearing knee flexion while the patient, while sitting with his thighs supported and his lower legs pendant, is in the supine position. Often there is quite a marked difference.

Another facet of patellofemoral movement worthy of including in examination is to ask the patient while sitting with his thighs supported and his lower legs pendant, to extend his knee into the fully hyperextended position. Frequently an arc of pain presents midway through the range. If the movement is painless, however, it is worth repeating the knee extension against the physiotherapist's resistance applied at the distal end of the tibia.

Special tests

The purpose of special tests is to move the patella through a full amplitude of movement, as in any radius of a circle, while applying a compressive force against the anterior surface of the patella, thereby rubbing the posterior surface of the patella against the femur.

Techniques

Compression**

Starting position

The patient lies supine with a pillow under his knee. This technique can be carried out in different degrees of knee flexion. The physiotherapist places one hand under the posterior surface of the femur distally, and then places the heel of her other hand over the patella. The centre of the patella should fit between the therapist's thenar and hypothenar eminences and her forearm should be directed vertically through the patient's knee (Figure 11.47).

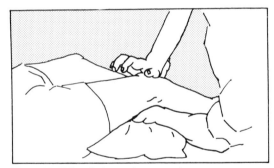

Figure 11.47 Patellofemoral compression

Method

The technique is one of gently squeezing the patella against the femur. Pressure should be applied gently and slowly against the patella, the patient being asked to report any feeling of discomfort or pain as the pressure is applied.

If no discomfort is felt, maximum pressure can be applied against the patella, and a strong small-amplitude grade IV+ movement produced.

When this technique is painless or only minimally painful, then a technique can be used where the patella is hit sharply by the heel of the therapist's hand so as to knock the patella sharply against the femur. The first session should be very short (not exceeding 20 seconds) and an assessment made on the following day to guide whether stronger techniques can be used or whether, because an exacerbation has been caused, gentler techniques are indicated.

Transverse movements medially***

Starting position

The physiotherapist stands by the patient's right knee and places the pads of her thumbs, pointing towards each other, against the lateral border of the patella. The fingers of her left and right hands point medially to rest across the distal end of the femur and proximal end of the tibia respectively. Her thumbs are hyperextended at the interphalangeal joints to bring as much of the pad as possible into contact with the lateral border of the patella (Figure 11.48).

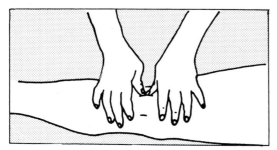

Figure 11.48 Patellofemoral articulation; transverse movement medially

Method

Oscillatory movements are imparted to the patella through the therapist's thumbs by her arms. If grade I movements are required, small-amplitude oscillations of less than a quarter of an inch (5 mm) from the normal resting position of the patella are performed. For other grades of movement the patella is displaced more medially, reaching the limit of its excursion for grade III and IV movements.

Transverse movements laterally***

These movements are merely the reverse of the above and therefore do not require description.

Longitudinal movement caudad***

Starting position

The physiotherapist stands by the patient's right knee and places the heel of her left hand near the pisiform bone, against the superior margin of the patella. With her left wrist extended she directs her forearm distally. She places her right hand pointing proximally, over the patella with her fingers and

thumb passing either side of the heel of her left hand. Her right hand serves three purposes: it provides stability for the left hand, it guides the patella during movement and it can be used to apply compression to the patella when desired (Figure 11.49). If stronger techniques are used the therapist should face the patient's feet.

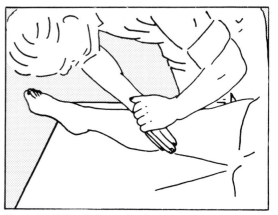

Figure 11.49 Patellofemoral articulation: longitudinal movement caudad with compression added

Method

The caudad movement of the patella is produced by the heel of the therapist's left hand while the direction of the movement is guided by her right hand. Her two hands and his patella move as a single unit. If compression is required during the movement, the patella is pressed against the femur by the therapist's right hand.

If the movement signs indicate that the movement described above should be combined with a medial inclination, she moves her point of contact against the superior border of the patella slightly laterally and alters the direction of her arms to lie in the direction of the diagonal movement (Figure 11.50).

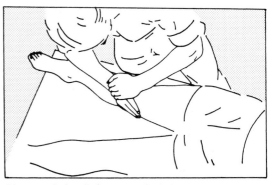

Figure 11.50 Patellofemoral articulation; longitudinal movement combined with a medial inclination and compression

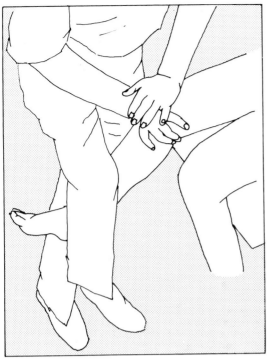

(a)

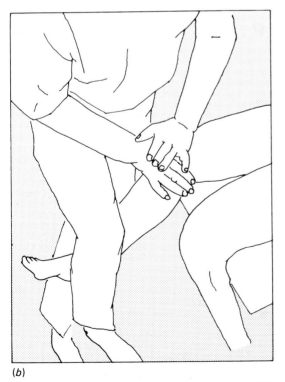

(b)

Figure 11.51 Patellofemoral movement in knee flexion: (*a*) caudad, (*b*) cephalad

Patellofemoral movement in knee flexion***

The most comparable pain response is frequently found to be a cephalad–caudad longitudinal movement with the knee in a position of flexion.

Starting position

The patient sits with his knee over the edge of the table. The physiotherapist cups her right palm over the patella and places the heel and ulnar border of her left hand against the superior margin of the patella. She stabilizes his lower leg between her lower legs (Figure 11.51).

Method

The therapist can produce movement in any direction (cephalad, caudad, angled, the two rotary directions, and even medially and laterally), and compression can be added with this same hand position. Movement is produced by arm movement acting through the hands.

Longitudinal movement cephalad***

This technique employs the same hand position over the patella as is used for the caudad technique, but the movement is produced through the ulnar border of the therapist's right hand. To guide the direction of the movement, she uses the palm of her right hand (cupped over the patella) and the cupped base of the palm of her left hand (Figure 11.52).

Distraction***

Distraction is the term used to indicate that the patella is lifted away from the femur so that there is no contact between them. This is a very gentle procedure and movements longitudinally, medially and laterally, can be performed very gently in the distracted position.

Starting position

The patient lies supine with his knee extended. The physiotherapist places both thumbs in the space between the patella and femur medially (or laterally). She then places her index fingers in the space on

the opposite side. A combination of two acts is necessary to progress to the next stage of the starting position. She should gently squeeze her fingers and thumbs together to reach under the patella, at the same time extending and radially deviating both wrists so that her fingers and thumb lift against the under-surface of the patella (Figure 11.53 (a) and (b)).

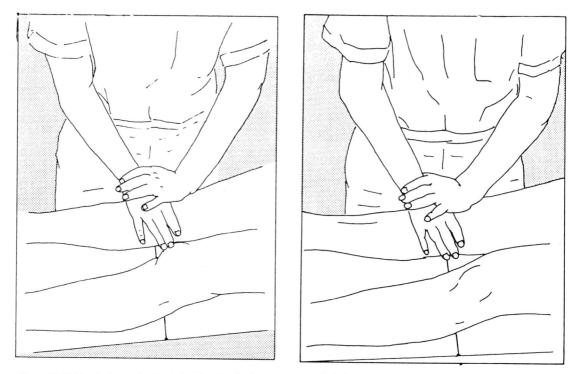

Figure 11.52 Patellofemoral articulation; longitudinal movement cephalad

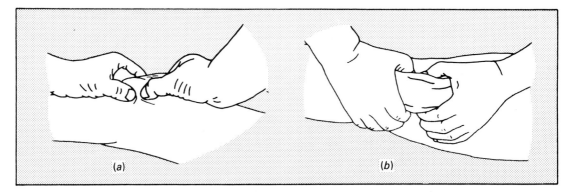

Figure 11.53 Patellofemoral distraction

Method

The technique is a very gentle slow oscillatory movement consisting in raising and lowering the patella. The patella should not be lowered to the extent where it comes into full contact with the femur. While performing the technique by repeated oscillations, care should be taken to avoid discomfort under the patella.

The above technique can be progressed by the therapist, after having lifted the patella, moving it medially, laterally, cephalad or caudad. As a modification it is also useful to produce diagonal movements as shown with the other techniques in this chapter.

Treatment

The treatment of patellofemoral disorders calls for a high degree of skill and considerable delicacy. When patellofemoral movement is painful the initial session or sessions need to be carried out extremely gently. It is far better to perform movements too gently and for too short a time than to find out at the following session that they had been performed excessively even to the smallest degree. If the physiotherapist has any doubt as to how gently she should begin, then oscillatory distraction should be her first choice. Once the effect of this has been assessed she will know how slowly to progress in small steps without causing any exacerbation.

On the other hand, there are times when maximum amplitude movements should be performed in one or more directions, at the same time maintaining a strong compressive force on the patella.

If it is found on examination that the patient is able to squat fully without pain and all examination tests have revealed only minimal signs, it may be necessary to move the patella quite forcibly while the tibiofemoral joint is flexed approximately 40° and compression applied both by the physiotherapist's hand, and secondly by resisting the patient's knee extension. This would be done with the patient in the sitting position.

Chronic/minor symptoms
Proving unaffected

Movements of the patella should be assessed with firm compression:

1. Cephalad and caudad (knee extension and half flexion).
2. Cephalad and caudad, angled.
3. Rotation (anteroposterior on medial border).

Superior tibiofibular joint

The superior tibiofibular joint is often forgotten when seeking the source of lateral leg and knee pain. Although not a frequent cause of pain, it is sufficiently common to warrant inclusion in routine examination.

Examination
Subjective examination

Symptoms are mainly felt at the joint itself although pain can be referred down the anterolateral aspect of the lower leg. With this referral, examination for entrapment of the peroneal nerve should be undertaken.

Table 11.4 Superior tibiofibular joint – objective examination

> The knee movements should also be examined as part of the examination for the superior tibiofibular (T/F) joint. Ankle joint movements should also be checked as the superior tibiofibular joint moves with full range ankle movements.
>
> HIGHLIGHT MAIN FINDINGS WITH ASTERISKS AS YOU GO
>
> **Observation**
>
> ***Functional demonstration/tests**
>
> 1. *Their* demonstration of *their* functional movements affected by *their* disorder.
> 2. Differentiation of *their* demonstrated functional movement(s).
>
> **Brief appraisal**
> **Active movements** (move to PAIN or move to LIMIT)
>
> **Isometric tests**
>
> **Other structures in 'plan'**
> Entrapment neuropathy
>
> **Passive movements**
> *Accessory movements*
> *Routinely*
> (↕), (↕), (⟷) ceph and caudad (by ankle inversion and eversion)
> (↺↻) (by ankle/leg Rotn)
> Note range, pain, resistance, spasm and behaviour
> *As applicable*
>
> 1. Repeat above, adding compression.
> 2. Repeat (↕), (↕), (⟷) ceph and caud by lying on side using hand for IV+ with compression.
> 3. LLTT.
>
> **Palpation**
> Entrapment neuropathy
> + when 'comparable signs' ill-defined reassess 'injuring movement'
>
> **Check case records etc.**
>
> **Instructions to patient**
>
> 1. Warning of possible exacerbation.
> 2. Request to record details.
> 3. Instruction re 'joint care' if required.

Objective examination

The two movements that can be tested and used in treatment are posteroanterior movement and anteroposterior movement.

When these two movements are found to be painless they should be tested while the joint is compressed.

Movements of the ankle produce movement at the superior (and inferior) tibiofibular joint – inversion and eversion of the hind-foot produce caudad and cephalad tibiofibular movement respectively. Medial and lateral rotation (especially passively) at the ankle also produces tibiofibular movement.

Vigorous posteroanterior movement and anteroposterior movement, both performed with very strong compression, are very informative.

Examination for the superior tibiofibular joint is listed below in Table 11.4.

Anteroposterior movement***

Starting position

The patient lies with his right hip and knee flexed and his foot resting on the couch. The physiotherapist sits on his foot to stabilize it and places her thumbs against the anterior border or the head of the fibula. Both thumbs point posteriorly with the pads in contact with the head of the fibula (Figure 11.54 (a)).

Method

Anteroposterior pressures are exerted against the head of the fibula through stable thumbs. It is extremely difficult to differentiate between different grades of movement but they can be varied by altering the strength of the pressures.

If the addition of compression is necessary, the heel of the left hand is placed over the head of the fibula laterally while the fingers lie over the knee. The right thumb maintains its contact against the anterior margin of the fibula. The left forearm is directed so that it can apply a medially directed pressure against the head of the fibula as well as assisting the right thumb in its anteroposterior pressure (Figure 11.54 (b)).

Posteroanterior movement***

For examination purposes posteroanterior movement can be tested with the patient supine with his knee and hip flexed as described above. A pulling pressure is then applied behind the head of the fibula. However, when this movement is used for treatment the patient should lie prone.

Starting position

The patient lies prone near the right-hand edge of the couch. The physiotherapist, standing alongside the patient's foot, places her left knee on the couch and supports his right lower leg across her thigh. This position supports the patient's knee in approximately 30° of flexion. She then places the pads of her thumbs against the posterior border of the head of his fibula, with the fingers of her left hand spreading medially across his upper calf and those of her right hand reaching anteriorly around the fibula (Figure 11.55 (a)).

Method

Posteroanterior mobilizing is performed by pressure from the therapist's arms through her thumbs against the head of the fibula. She must not produce movement with the muscles of her thumbs as this immediately becomes uncomfortable to the patient.

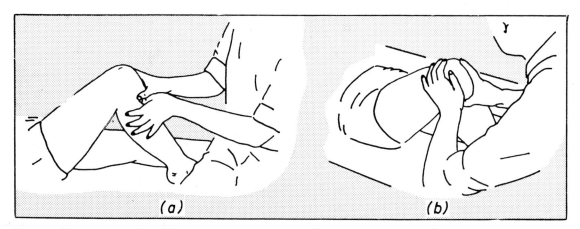

Figure 11.54 Superior tibiofibular: (*a*) anteroposterior movement; (*b*) anteroposterior movement with compression

Table 11.5 Composite knee – objective examination

HIGHLIGHT MAIN FINDINGS WITH ASTERISKS
AS YOU GO

Observation

*Functional demonstration/tests

1. *Their* demonstration of *their* functional movements affected by *their* disorder.
2. Differentiation of *their* demonstrated functional movement(s).

Brief appraisal
Active movements (move to PAIN or move to LIMIT)
As applicable

Gait: forwards, backwards, on heels (especially backwards), on toes
Squat, on toes, on feet flat, bounce
Height of step possible
On all fours sit towards heels
Sit, resist available extension
Supine, quads lag

Isometric test
Of quads in different ranges of F/E

Other structures in 'plan'
Entrapment neuropathy & LLTT

Passive movements
Tibiofemoral joint

1. E, E/Ab, E/Ad, Ab, Ad, F, F/Ab, F/Ad
2. ($\updownarrow$) and ($\updownarrow$), ($\leftrightarrow$) and ($\leftrightarrow$) in 90° knee F and E
3. ($\circlearrowright\circlearrowleft$) in various positions of knee F/E

   } Without and with compression

Differentiate medial & lateral compartments and sup. T/F joint.
Patellofemoral joint

1. ($\leftrightarrow$), ($\leftrightarrow$) in knee F and E.
2. ($\leftrightarrow$) ceph, caud, Med. and Lat. inclinations with and without compression.
3. In sitting (knee F 90°) ($\leftrightarrow$) ceph, caud, med. and lat. inclinations with and without compression.
4. ($\circlearrowright\circlearrowleft$) in sagittal and femoral axes.

Superior tibiofibular joint

1. ($\updownarrow$) ($\updownarrow$) with and without compression.
2. ($\leftrightarrow$) ceph and caud (by ankle Inv and Ev) with and without compression.

Palpation
+ when 'comparable signs' ill-defined reassess 'injuring movement'

Check case records etc.

Instructions to patient

1. Warning of possible exacerbation.
2. Request to record details.
3. Instruction re 'joint care' if required.

The movement can be performed under compression by changing the position of the therapist's right hand so that the heel of the hand is placed against the lateral surface of the head of the fibula (Figure 11.55 (b)).

Alternative method

Both anteroposterior and posteroanterior movement without compression or with (especially the latter) can be performed with the patient lying on his side. The medial aspect of his lower leg should be fully supported on the table and his ankle must be in a loose neutral mid range position.

The movement is produced through the therapist's thumbs or cupped hands, in much the same way as that shown for the inferior tibiofibular joint in Figure 11.57.

Longitudinal movement cephalad and caudad

Starting position

The patient lies prone with his knee flexed to a right angle. The physiotherapist holds the patient's foot in her hands and produces caudad longitudinal movement by strongly inverting the patient's heel. A cephalad longitudinal movement is produced by the therapist everting the patient's heel. This movement can readily be felt in the normal subject by palpating the head of the fibula with one hand while inverting and everting the model's heel with the other hand.

Treatment

Little comment need be made on treatment of superior tibiofibular joint problems. It is not very easy to determine whether the superior tibiofibular joint is responsible for a patient's symptoms and often this can only be ascertained by performing strong techniques with strong compression and comparing these on the faulty leg with symptoms felt when repeated on the good leg. When a comparable sign is found this movement should be used in treatment. Initially it should be performed firmly but not vigorously. If the test signs are obvious then the posteroanterior or anteroposterior movement should be performed without compression. It is quite common, however, for the techniques to be performed with strong compression. When this is necessary, the movements should be reasonably vigorous and may need to be repeated for four groups, each lasting approximately 1 minute.

When the superior tibiofibular joint is responsible for symptoms, it responds very readily and rapidly to passive mobilizing techniques.

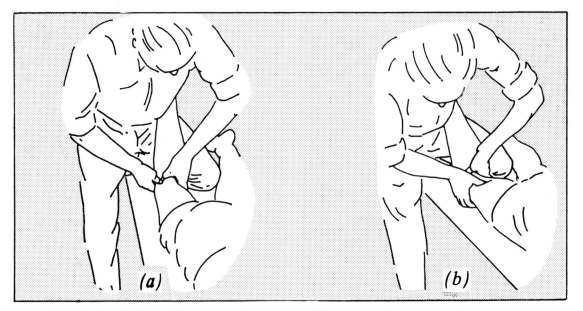

Figure 11.55 Superior tibiofibular: (*a*) posteroanterior movement; (*b*) posteroanterior movement with compression

Chronic/minor superior tibiofibular symptoms

Proving unaffected

The best technique for passive movement examination, under these circumstances, has the patient lying on his side with his medial malleolus resting on the edge of the table and his foot free beyond the edge. In this way strong ankle movements can be added to the superior tibiofibular posteroanterior and anteroposterior movements under compression:

1. ↕↕ with compression.
2. ↔ especially caudad with ankle inversion (adduction).

Composite knee joint

Having discussed in detail the examination and treatment techniques for the tibiofemoral joint, the patellofemoral joint and the superior tibiofibular joint, the examination for the three joints is brought together as the composite knee examination (Table 11.5).

To prove that all three joints are 'unaffected', the following tests are performed (Table 11.6).

Table 11.6 Composite knee unaffected

T/F, E with (↕), E/Ab, E/Add. F with OP Shaft Rotn in 90° F Ab and Ad P/F movements with compression Sup T/Fil (↕) (↕) with compression and ankle movements.

Inferior tibiofibular joint

The inferior tibiofibular joint is more often the cause of symptoms than the superior tibiofibular joint and should be routinely examined when ankle pain is present.

The movements described relate to movement of the fibula on the larger more stable tibia. The movements are anteroposterior and posteroanterior movement of the fibula on the tibia which, during examination, may require testing while the joint surfaces are compressed.

Strong rotation of the talus (produced via the foot) also produces movement at the tibiofibular joint as does compressing the talus into the mortice.

Longitudinal movement can be produced by inverting and everting the heel (see page 257). It must also be remembered that the 'close-packed' position, which spreads the inferior tibiofibular joint, is produced by anteroposterior movement of the talus (see Figure 11.71) as well as dorsiflexion. The full examination is listed in Table 11.7.

Examination

Subjective examination

The site of pain is always local though other joints may be involved in the disorder.

Objective examination

Functional demonstration/tests

Any movement which the patient can perform to demonstrate his disability should be analysed as the first part of the objective examination.

Brief appraisal

Although there are many movements the patient can be asked to do which will guide the kind of examination, there are two main tests.

The first test is to ask the patient to walk on his heels, and if he can do this, he should attempt hopping on the heel of the painful foot.

The second test is to ask the patient to squat while keeping his heels on the floor. In this position the mortice joint is jammed into the close-packed position, thus spreading the inferior tibiofibular joint apart, while the patient's bodyweight is being taken through this area.

Special tests

There are no specific 'special' tests for this joint other than the movements described in the following text.

Table 11.7 Inferior tibiofibular joint – objective examination

> Movement of the ankle joint should also be examined as part of the examination for the inferior tibiofibular joint.
>
> HIGHLIGHT MAIN FINDINGS WITH ASTERISKS AS YOU GO
>
> **Observation**
>
> ***Functional demonstration/tests**
>
> 1. *Their* demonstration of *their* functional movements affected by *their* disorder.
> 2. Differentiation of *their* demonstrated functional movement(s).
>
> **Brief appraisal**
> **Active movements** (move to PAIN or move to LIMIT)
> *Routinely (modified as required)*
> Gait, heel and toe walking towards and backwards, hopping (especially heel)
> Squatting
> DF, PF; Inv. and Ev.
> Note range and pain
>
> **Isometric tests**
>
> **Other structures in 'plan'**
> Full active resisted movement through range for 'sheaths'
> Joint restriction cf. muscle/tendon restriction
> Entrapment neuropathy
>
> **Passive movements**
> *Physiological movements*
> *Routinely*
> Ankle DF, PF, hind-foot add., abd. (↕) (↕) talus in mortice, (↻) (↺).
> Note range, pain, resistance, spasm and behaviour
>
> *As applicable*
> The injuring movement
> *Accessory movements*
> *Routinely*
> Ankle (↕), (↕), (↻), (↺), (↔) ceph and caud, Inv., Ev.
> T/F (↕), (↕), (↕), with and without compression, (↔) ceph and caud (by using ankle Inv. and Ev.) without and with compression
> Note range, pain, resistance, spasm and behaviour
>
> **Palpation**
> Palpate tendon sheaths
> + when 'comparable signs' ill-defined reassess 'injuring movement'
>
> **Check case records etc.**
>
> **Instructions to patient**
> 1. Warning of possible exacerbation.
> 2. Request to record details.
> 3. Instruction re 'joint care' if required.

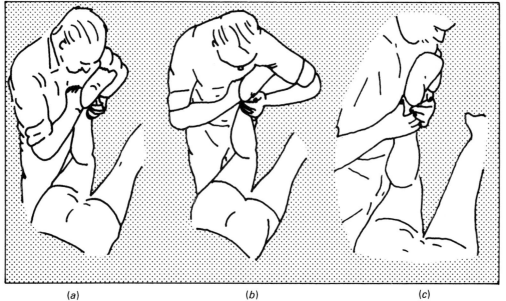

Figure 11.56 Inferior tibiofibular: (*a*) posteroanterior movement; (*b*) posteroanterior movement with compression; (*c*) grades I and II posteroanterior movement with thumb

The objective passive movement examination is given in Table 11.7.

Techniques

Posteroanterior movement***

Starting position

The patient lies prone with his right knee flexed to a right angle. The physiotherapist stands by his right knee, facing his left thigh, and places the heel of her pronated right hand against the posterior border of the lateral malleolus and the heel of her left hand against the anterior border of the medial malleolus. The fingers of her right hand are directed forward towards his toes and the fingers of her left hand towards his heel. Both forearms are directed opposite each other and parallel to the central axis of the patient's trunk (Figure 11.56 (a)).

Method

Oscillatory mobilizations, which are only possible in small amplitude, are produced by the therapist's arms exerting alternating pressure and relaxation against the malleoli.

With compression***

Compression can be applied during this movement by the therapist adjusting her position so that she faces his left hip and directs her forearms diagonally through the ankle (Figure 11.56 (b)).

Grades I and II**

If extremely gentle movements are required, she should support the distal end of the patient's tibia in her left hand as described above with the heel of her hand against the anterior surface, while the pad of her right thumb is placed behind the lateral malleolus with her fingers spreading medially for stability (Figure 11.56 (c)). The mobilization is then produced by the right arm acting through the thumb.

Alternative method

An alternative method of producing posteroanterior movement which some therapists may find easier to perform is now described. It is certainly a much easier position in which to use grades III and IV, stretching techniques, and also one in which it is easy to add the compression component.

Starting position

The patient lies on his left side and flexes his hip and knee to a right angle so that the medial surface of his lower leg and foot are lying flat on the table. The physiotherapist stands behind the patient's leg and uses two hands to apply pressure against the posterior border of the lateral malleolus. Her hands work together as a single unit, performing a very localized technique in which only her pisiform contacts the lateral malleolus posteriorly (Figure 11.57).

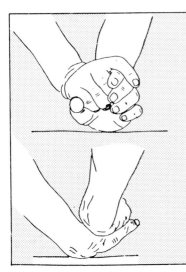

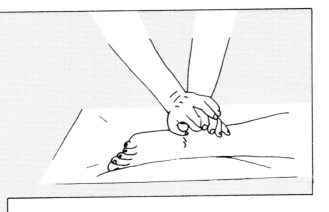

Figure 11.57 Inferior tibiofibular posteroanterior movement, alternative method

Method

The therapist uses her body to transmit the movement to the fibula while her elbows act as springs.

Anteroposterior movement**

Starting position

The patient lies prone with his knee flexed to a right angle. The physiotherapist stands by his knee, facing his left lower leg, and places the heel of her fully pronated left hand against the anterior surface of the lateral malleolus with her fingers spreading posteriorly around his ankle. She places the heel of her supinated right hand against the posterior surface of the medial malleolus with her fingers spreading anteriorly around the ankle. Her forearms are directed opposite each other parallel to the central axis of the trunk (Figure 11.58 (a)).

Method

The small-amplitude oscillatory mobilization is produced by the therapist's forearms applying equal and opposite pressures through her hands. She will have more control of the movement if she crouches over her hands.

With compression***

To apply compression during anteroposterior movement, she alters her position to face his left foot and directs her forearms diagonally across the central axis of the trunk while still maintaining them in the coronal plane (Figure 11.58 (b)).

Grade II**

If extremely gentle movements are required, the physiotherapist should support the distal end of the patient's tibia in her right hand as described above while placing the pad of her left thumb against the anterior border of the lateral malleolus. Her fingers provide stability by their position on the front of the leg. The mobilization is produced by her left arm acting through the thumb (Figure 11.58 (c)).

Alternative method

An alternative position for producing anteroposterior movement may be found easier to perform by some therapists.

Starting position

The patient lies on his left side with his hip and knee flexed so that the medial surface of his lower leg and foot rest evenly on the table.

The physiotherapist stands in front of the patient's foot and places her pisiform against the anterior border of the lateral malleolus (Figure 11.58 (d)).

Method

The therapist produces an oscillatory movement of the fibula on the tibia by rocking her body so that her trunk produces movement of her hands against the malleolus. The movement is produced by body movement and not by arm movement.

The physiotherapist can alter the direction of her arm in relation to the malleolus so that the technique is a purely anteroposterior one or she may alter it to include compression.

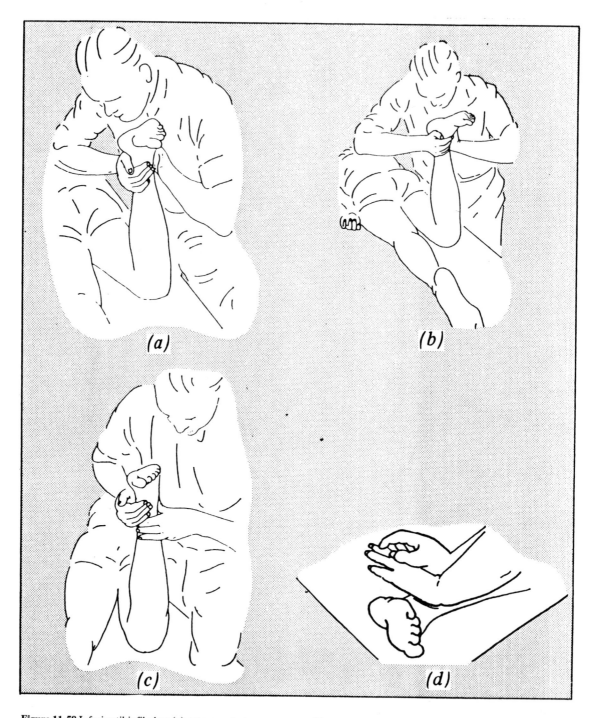

Figure 11.58 Inferior tibiofibular: (*a*) anteroposterior movement; (*b*) anteroposterior movement with compression; (*c*) grade II movement with thumbs; (*d*) alternative method, and grade IV movement with compression

In this position she is also able to direct her pressure on the lateral malleolus towards the patient's head or towards his feet so that a component of longitudinal movement, either cephalad or caudad, can also be incorporated.

Compression**
Starting position

The patient lies prone with his knee flexed to a right angle. The physiotherapist stands beyond his knee, facing his left hip. She bends slightly at the waist to position her left shoulder over his foot, placing the heel of her left and right hands over the medial and lateral malleoli respectively, with the fingers of both hands directed towards his knee. Her forearms are directed opposite each other (Figure 11.59).

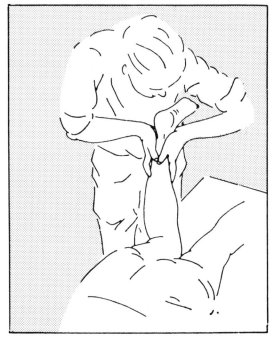

Figure 11.59 Inferior tibiofibular compression

Method

There is very little movement in this direction but a patient with symptoms arising from this joint is well aware of pain during technique. Compression is produced through the operator's forearms by alternating pressures against the malleoli.

During treatment it may be necessary for the therapist to alter the direction of her forearms slightly to permit slight anteroposterior or posteroanterior movement of the fibula in relation to the tibia.

Alternative method

The same movement can be performed with the patient lying on his side. The physiotherapist places one hand under the lateral malleolus, cupping it in her palm near the heel of her hand. With her other hand she presses through the medial malleolus, placing the thenar eminence near the heel of her hand against it (Figure 11.60).

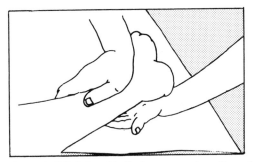

Figure 11.60 Inferior tibiofibular compression, alternative method

Inferior tibiofibular movement during ankle rotation

When the talus is rotated strongly in the mortise it spreads the inferior tibiofibular joint. Also, during medial rotation, the fibula is pulled anteriorly in relation to the tibia and during lateral rotation it moves posteriorly. The rotation can be produced by the therapist using the patient's heel and foot as a lever (Figure 11.61 (a)). The patient's report of the site of pain will indicate whether the pain is arising from the intertarsal joints, the ankle joint or the inferior tibiofibular joint.

Differentiation

The movement can also be produced by holding the talus between the index finger and thumb of both hands so that the talus can be rotated in the mortise (Figure 11.61 (b) and (c)). If pain is reproduced with this movement it is still difficult to discern whether the pain is arising from the ankle joint or the inferior tibiofibular joint.

Heel tap

This technique should be used as an examination procedure routinely when the inferior tibiofibular joint is thought to be contributing to a patient's ankle pain. It consists of hitting the sole of the patient's heel, driving the talus into the mortise and both jarring and spreading the inferior tibiofibular joint. The technique is described in full on page 272 (see Figure 11.75).

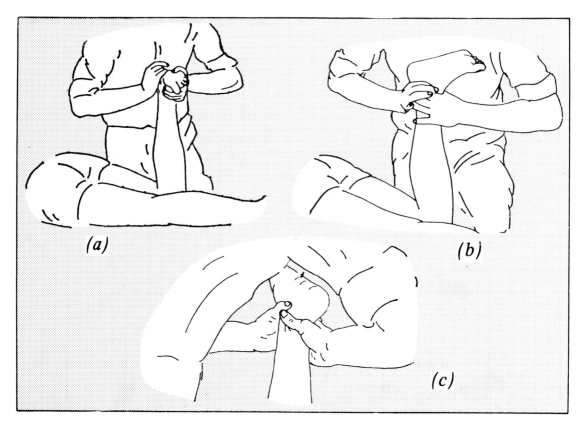

Figure 11.61 Inferior tibiofibular movement during ankle rotation: (*a*) medial rotation using foot leverage; (*b*) medial talocrural rotation; (*c*) lateral talocrural rotation

Treatment

When a patient's foot is subjected to fairly severe trauma the inferior tibiofibular joint is often affected by the strain. This fact is often overlooked because the condition of the joints below is more severe and more limiting. However, a faulty inferior tibiofibular joint can prevent normal walking and should not be omitted from the routine examination of the foot and ankle.

When the joint is found to be the source of symptoms the examination technique that reproduces the patient's symptoms, or the examination technique that discloses a loss of range, is the technique that should be used in treatment. A treatment session would involve gentle grade IV−

type movements interspersed with grade III− movements if pain is a dominant factor. If the aim of treatment is to increase range, the movement needing to be increased should be stretched as a strong IV+ movement. Following approximately 1 minute of this strongly performed technique, the joint should be held in this position of stretch, while grade IV+ accessory movements are stretched in each direction. Following the accessory movement stretches, the stretching of the stiff physiological movement should be repeated as a grade IV+ movement. The total stretching treatment will consist of alternating between stretching the physiological movement and stretching the accessory movements while the joint is held at the limit of the physiological range.

Ankle joint

When learning movements and techniques of the foot it is advisable to have an articulated set of bones available (Figures 11.62 and 63).

During examination and treatment of the ankle joint, the required movements are more easily performed by using the foot as a lever, thus incorporating intertarsal movement with talocrural movement[6]. However, mobilization techniques are most effective if they are localized to the movement of the faulty joint. During most techniques, movement can be isolated to the hind-foot (that is the calcaneus and talus) but it is sometimes difficult to differentiate completely between subtalar and ankle movement disorders.

The accessory movements that should be examined at the ankle joint are anteroposterior and posteroanterior movements of the talus, longitudinal movement cephalad and caudad of the talus within the ankle joint and rotation. The physiological movements are inversion (or adduction), eversion (or abduction), dorsiflexion and plantar flexion.

Examination

Subjective examination

An accurate determination of the site of symptoms is essential because it guides the examiner towards where the objective needs to be orientated. It is also important to know whether the patient can touch 'the' painful site(s) or whether it is too deep to reach.

The referral of symptoms in the foot, as in the hand, helps in determining whether there is tarsal tunnel involvement.

Objective examination

Functional demonstration/tests

These are usually found in movements during weight-bearing. Once in the painful position, local intertarsal (etc.) movements are used to find the painful movement of the faulty joint.

Brief appraisal

The patient should first be asked to walk forwards, away from and then towards the physiotherapist. This should be followed by walking backwards away from, then towards the physiotherapist.

If the above tests reveal no abnormality, the patient should be asked to walk on his toes and then on his heels. This should be followed by hopping on the toes of the disordered foot and then hopping on the heel.

The patient should then be asked to squat, without specific directive. If he squats fully and painlessly with his heels off the ground then he should be asked to squat again, keeping his heels on the ground as this forces greater dorsiflexion.

Careful execution of the accessory movements, noting range and pain, is important in the assessment of ankle disorders. An accessory movement that is often forgotten is that of longitudinal movement caudad (see Figure 11.76).

The full examination is listed in Table 11.8.

Techniques

Plantar flexion***

Starting position

The patient lies prone with his knee flexed to a right angle while the physiotherapist, standing by his knee, holds his calcaneus posteriorly in her right hand and anteriorly over the neck of the talus in her left hand. She places her left knee on the couch to support his right shin, a position which greatly assists relaxation. With her right hand she holds his calcaneus with her thumb around the lateral surface, her medial three fingers around the medial surface and her index finger, especially the palmar surface of the metacarpophalangeal joint, firmly contacting the sole. She places the web of the first interosseous space of her left hand over the neck of the talus adjacent to his ankle so that her thumb rests against the lateral side of his foot and her fingers against the medial malleolus. Both arms remain near her side as she stands near his foot (Figure 11.64).

Method

Plantar flexion movements of small or large-amplitude are easily controlled from this position and can be performed in any part of the range. The movements are performed by her arms.

If movement of the forefoot (that is that part of the foot distal to the navicular bone) is to be included, the therapist places her left hand more distally on the dorsum of the patient's foot. If grade III+ movements of the whole foot are required, the starting position should be altered as follows.

Grade III+***

Starting position

The patient lies prone with his feet near the end of the couch. The physiotherapist stands by his feet,

6. Maitland, G. D. *The Foot: Differentiation*, Videotape No. 25 (45 mins.). Postgraduate Study Centre Hermitage, Medizinische Abteilung, Bad Ragaz, CH7310 Switzerland (1982)

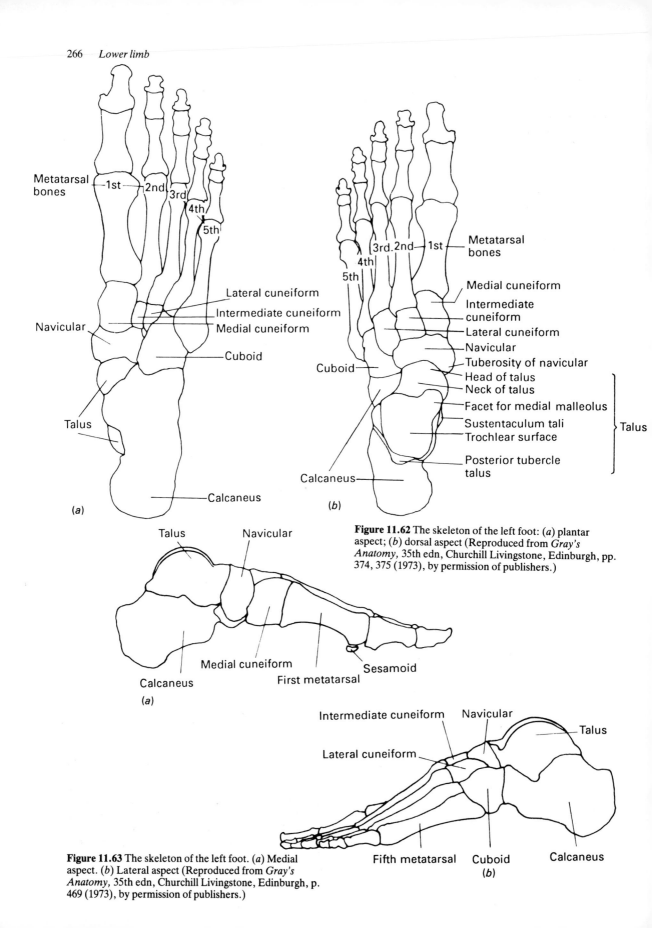

Metatarsal bones — 1st — 2nd — 3rd — 4th — 5th

Lateral cuneiform
Intermediate cuneiform
Medial cuneiform

Navicular

Cuboid

Talus

Calcaneus

(a)

Metatarsal bones — 3rd. 2nd — 1st — 4th — 5th

Medial cuneiform
Intermediate cuneiform
Lateral cuneiform
Navicular
Tuberosity of navicular
Head of talus
Neck of talus
Facet for medial malleolus
Sustentaculum tali
Trochlear surface
Posterior tubercle talus
} Talus

Cuboid

Calcaneus

(b)

Figure 11.62 The skeleton of the left foot: (*a*) plantar aspect; (*b*) dorsal aspect (Reproduced from *Gray's Anatomy,* 35th edn, Churchill Livingstone, Edinburgh, pp. 374, 375 (1973), by permission of publishers.)

Talus   Navicular

Medial cuneiform

First metatarsal

Sesamoid

Calcaneus

(a)

Intermediate cuneiform   Navicular

Lateral cuneiform

Talus

Fifth metatarsal   Cuboid   Calcaneus

(b)

Figure 11.63 The skeleton of the left foot. (*a*) Medial aspect. (*b*) Lateral aspect (Reproduced from *Gray's Anatomy,* 35th edn, Churchill Livingstone, Edinburgh, p. 469 (1973), by permission of publishers.)

Table 11.8 Ankle joint – objective examination

As hind-foot intertarsal movements must be examined as part of the examination of the ankle joint it is simpler to describe them together. The inferior tibiofibular joint should also be examined.

HIGHLIGHT MAIN FINDINGS WITH ASTERISKS AS YOU GO

Observation

*Functional demonstration/tests

1. *Their* demonstration of *their* functional movements affected by *their* disorder.
2. Differentiation of *their* demonstrated functional movement(s).

Brief appraisal
Active movements (move to PAIN or move to LIMIT)
Routinely (but modified as required)

Gait, walking forwards and backwards, towards and away from you, then similarly for walking on heels and toes, walking with feet in inversion and eversion, forwards, backwards and sideways. Heel and toe hopping
Squatting (spontaneous then flat heels) where possible
DF, PF, Inv., Ev.
Note range and pain

Isometric test

Other structures in 'plan'
Full active resisted movements through range for 'sheaths'
Joint restriction cf. muscle/tendon restriction
Entrapment neuropathy
LLTT

Passive movements
Physiological movements
Routinely

DF, PF, Inv., Ev.

As applicable

DF and PF differentiating
Inv. and Ev. differentiating
Note range, pain, resistance, spasm and behaviour

Accessory movements
Routinely

($\circlearrowright$) and ($\circlearrowleft$), ($\dagger$), ($\dagger$)
($\leftrightarrow$) ceph and caud (tibial line)
($\rightarrow$) ($\leftarrow$) subtaloid varying inclinations ($\dagger$),($\dagger$)
subtaloid
Note range, pain, resistance, spasm and behaviour
As applicable
Differentiating ($\circlearrowright$), ($\circlearrowleft$), ($\dagger$), ($\dagger$), ($\leftrightarrow$) ceph and caud
Repeat with compression.

Palpation
include tendon sheaths
+ when 'comparable signs' ill-defined reassess 'injuring movement'

Check case records etc.

Instructions to patient

1. Warning of possible exacerbation.
2. Request to record details.
3. Instruction re 'joint care' if required.

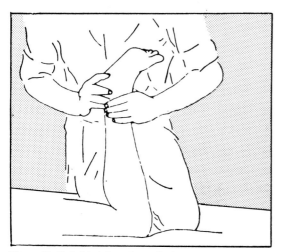

Figure 11.64 Ankle joint; plantarflexion

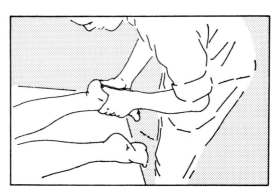

Figure 11.65 Ankle joint; plantarflexion grade III+

facing his head, and holds his right foot in both hands. She places her thumbs, pointing proximally, along the medial and lateral borders of the sole of his heel, while her fingers, meeting over the dorsum of his foot, complete the grasp from in front (Figure 11.65). The position of the fulcrum, provided by the tips of the thumbs, may be varied to emphasize the movement to any of the intertarsal or tarsometatarsal joints. To further localize the movement the therapist's fingers would be positioned firmly over the appropriate joint or immediately adjacent distally.

Method

The therapist raises the patient's leg through approximately 20° of knee flexion while partially dorsiflexing his ankle. She then drops his leg through those 20°, at the same time strongly plantar flexing his foot, timing the movement so that the drop of the leg assists the plantar flexion at the limit of range.

When it is necessary to localize the plantar flexion movement to the intertarsal joints, a different grasp of the patient's heel is required. This technique is described with other techniques related to the intertarsal joints (Figure 11.85).

Dorsiflexion***

Starting position

The patient lies prone with his knee flexed to slightly more than a right angle. The physiotherapist, standing by his right knee with her left knee on the couch to support his shin, holds his calcaneus in her right hand, with her thumb along the lateral surface and her fingers along the medial surface. She uses the web of the first interosseous space of her right hand to grip the calcaneus around its superior surface posteriorly. She places the web of the first interosseous space of her left hand across the plantar surface of his calcaneus distally and laterally, with her thumb passing laterally around his foot and her fingers medially. She directs her right elbow towards the floor and her left towards the ceiling (Figure 11.66).

Method

The oscillatory movement is gained by her forearms working in opposite directions producing a dorsifle-

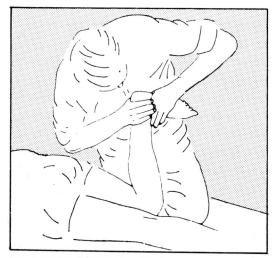

Figure 11.66 Ankle joint; dorsiflexion

xion movement about the ankle. This can be performed in any grade although the grasp described above is inadequate for stronger techniques. As the limit of the range is required, flexion of the knee beyond a right angle may be necessary to reduce tension in the gastrocnemius.

Grades III+ and IV+ *

For stronger techniques the therapist changes her left hand position to use the heel of her hand against the patient's metatarsal heads. The change of position incorporates intertarsal movement with the talocrural movement (Figure 11.67).

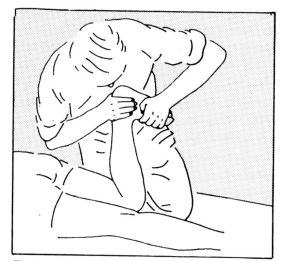

Figure 11.67 Ankle joint; dorsiflexion, grades III+ and IV+

To localize movement to the intertarsal and tarsometatarsal joints, the therapist adopts a different grasp of the patient's forefoot and heel. This technique is described with other techniques used in the treatment of intertarsal joints.

Ankle dorsiflexion/plantarflexion with compression****

This technique, both in examination and treatment, is a differentiation procedure between intra-articular and periarticular disorders.

Starting position

The patient lies prone with his left knee flexed 90°. The physiotherapist, standing approximately at the level of his knee, grasps his hind-foot in both hands and presses her chin against the back of the hand overlying the calcaneus (Figure 11.68).

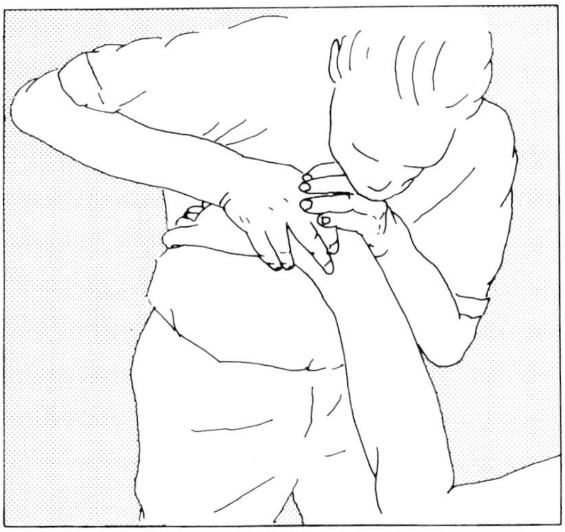

with both hands; her thumbs are adjacent to each other pointing proximally on the lateral surface while her fingers hold over the medial surface. The main grasp is between the index and middle fingers medially and the thumb laterally of each hand (Figure 11.69). With this grasp of the calcaneus the movement is isolated to the talocalcanean, the talocrural and the inferior tibiofibular joints.

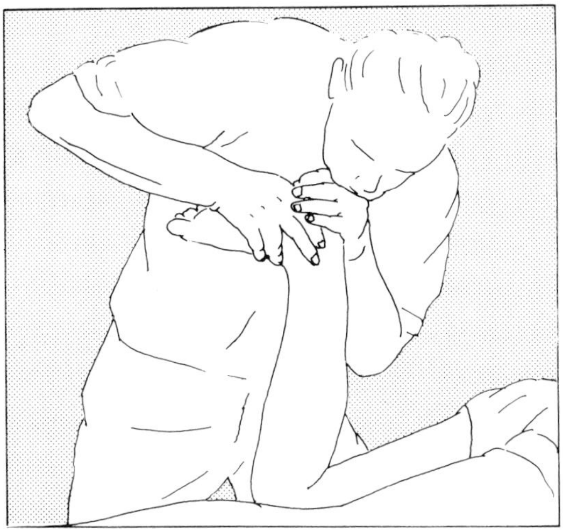

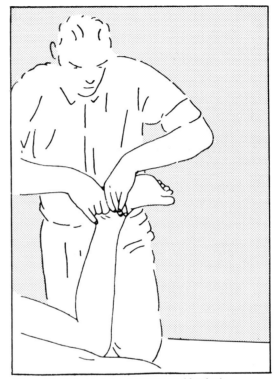

Figure 11.69 Ankle joint; inversion (adduction)

When the therapist holds around the metatarsals, which is the starting position used for a general inversion-type movement of the whole foot (see Figure 11.79), then supination (rotation) takes place at the transverse tarsal joint as well as all of the intertarsal and tarsometatarsal joints distal to the talus and calcaneus.

Method

If the technique for large-amplitude movements is described first, that for smaller amplitudes will not be necessary. To produce a grade III movement, the physiotherapist holds the patient's foot away from her and performs the movement by pulling his leg towards her while at the same time inverting (adducting) his calcaneus. The movement is performed so that the swinging movement of his leg (which is really a rotary movement of his hip

Figure 11.68 Ankle dorsiflexion/plantar flexion, with compression: (*a*) plantarflexion; (*b*) dorsiflexion

Method

She exerts pressure through his heel in line with the shaft of the tibia throughout the movement. By rocking her body from side to side, his ankle is dorsiflexed and plantarflexed alternately.

The position in the range can be varied as can the strength of the compression.

Inversion***

Starting position

The patient lies prone with his knees flexed to a right angle. The physiotherapist, standing by his knee and supporting his shin, grasps his calcaneus

(*a*)

(*b*)

through an arc of approximately 15°) assists the inversion action produced by her wrists.

When inversion is used as a treatment technique the best results are obtained when the movement is localized to the particular faulty joint. However, when a patient has an injured foot and all joints are affected, or when the most comparable joint sign is found with inversion applied through the metatarsals, then the general inversion/adduction/supination movement is the best one to use.

Eversion***

Eversion (abduction) has an identical starting position with that adopted for the inversion. The method also is similar in that eversion of the calcaneus is produced by movement of the therapist's wrists coinciding with swinging the patient's leg away from her. The swinging leg action is lateral rotation of the hip.

Posteroanterior movement**

The posteroanterior direction relates to movement of the foot on the leg.

Starting position

The patient lies with his knee flexed to a right angle. The physiotherapist stands by his knee and supports his right shin against her left thigh. She holds his calcaneus in her right hand with the heel of her hand against the posterior surface, her fingers and thumb spreading distally over and around the calcaneus. She places the heel of her supinated left hand against the anterior surface of the tibia with her fingers pointing proximally. Her medial two fingers and thumb hold around the lateral and medial surfaces respectively. She crouches over his foot to direct her forearms opposite each other parallel to the central axis of the trunk (Figure 11.70).

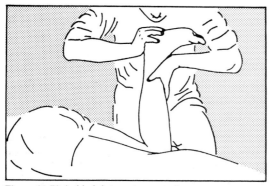

Figure 11.70 Ankle joint; posteroanterior movement

Method

A large-amplitude movement can be produced in this direction but care must be taken with two things. Firstly, the contact against the tibia must be made as cushioned as possible by cupping the thenar and hypothenar eminences, because bone-to-bone contact between the heel of the hand and the tibia is uncomfortable. Secondly, during the return part of the posteroanterior movement complete relaxation of the pressure against the heel is necessary.

Useful and effective treatment movements of grade III+ and IV+ type can be produced at the limit of the range.

Variations (more localized talocrural)

The technique described above uses the calcaneus as the bone through which the posteroanterior movement is performed. It is therefore obvious that during the technique there will be movement of the subtaloid joint as well as the ankle joint. Usually this is unimportant as the excursion of posteroanterior movement at the subtaloid joint is minimal and nearly always pain free. However, if the movement is being used as an examination technique and when performed it produces pain, then it may be necessary to produce the posteroanterior movement by direct pressure on the talus, thereby avoiding any subtaloid movement.

This localization of the posteroanterior movement is achieved while the patient is still prone with his knee flexed to 90°. The physiotherapist, standing by his knee, places the pads of both thumbs on the talus anterior to the Achilles tendon. With her fingers passing anteriorly around the malleoli to provide counterpressure on the anterior surfaces, she produces the posteroanterior movement with her arms, pushing the talus anteriorly between the malleoli.

Anteroposterior movement**
Starting position

The patient lies prone with his knee flexed to a right angle. The physiotherapist stands by his right knee, supporting his shin, and holds his leg distally from behind in her right hand with her thumb around the fibula and her fingers around the tibia. She positions her left hand with her index finger passing distal to his medial malleolus and her thumb distal to his lateral malleolus. This places the web of her first interosseous space on the neck of the talus. The therapist needs to ensure that the web is tight so that she feels she is grasping the talus around three sides with her index finger, web and thumb. She crouches over his foot and directs her forearms opposite each other, parallel to the central axis of the trunk (Figure 11.71).

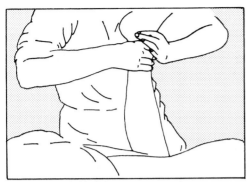

Figure 11.71 Ankle joint; anteroposterior movement

Method

There is less movement in this direction than there is with posteroanterior movement and it is a movement that is less frequently found to be painful. The movement, in any grade, is produced by an opposite action of both forearms, with the left hand creating most of the movement.

Variations (more localized talocrural)

Starting position

The patient lies supine with his hip and knee flexed and his foot resting on the couch. The physiotherapist stands beyond his foot, facing it, and places the pads of her thumbs on the talus immediately between the malleoli. It is more comfortable for the patient if the maximum area of the pads of the thumbs is used rather than the tips of the thumbs (Figure 11.72).

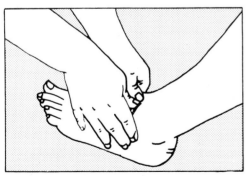

Figure 11.72 Ankle joint; localized anteroposterior movement

Method

Anteroposterior movement of the talus within the mortise is produced by the therapist's trunk and arms and it is transmitted through the talus via the pads of the thumbs. Any concentric muscle action of the thumb flexors will spoil the technique completely. It will make the technique uncomfortable for the patient and the therapist will lose all feel of movement during the technique. When the technique using the thumbs is uncomfortable it may produce discomfort which is difficult to separate from the patient's symptoms felt in the same area.

Medial rotation**

Starting position

The patient lies prone with his right knee flexed to a right angle while the physiotherapist, standing by his right knee, places her left knee on the couch to support his shin. She stabilizes his lower leg anteriorly in her left hand by holding around the medial malleolus with her fingers and placing the pad of her thumb against the anterior surface of the lateral malleolus. With her right hand she endeavours to grasp the talus posteriorly with her index finger passing medially and her thumb laterally. Her thumb and index finger must be adjacent and distal to his malleoli (Figure 11.73).

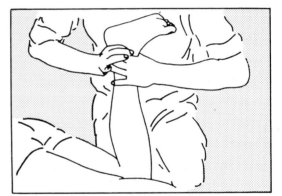

Figure 11.73 Ankle joint; medial rotation

Method

Medial rotation is a very small movement and the difficulty of the grasp results from considerable skin movement. Skin slack must be taken up before movement can be imparted. However, rotation can be produced and it can be an important technique in the mobilization of this joint. The rotation is produced by a screwing action of both arms towards each other, the right arm producing the main movement.

Lateral rotation**

Starting position

The patient lies prone with his right knee flexed to a right angle, and the physiotherapist stands by his knee holding his foot in her hands. She places her left knee on the couch to support his shin. She stabilizes his lower leg posteriorly with her right hand, hooking her fingers around the medial malleolus to grasp anteriorly while placing the pad of her thumb against the posterior surface of the lateral malleolus. With her left hand she endeavours to grasp the talus anteriorly. She places her index finger immediately adjacent and distal to the medial malleolus and her thumb adjacent and distal to the lateral malleolus (Figure 11.74).

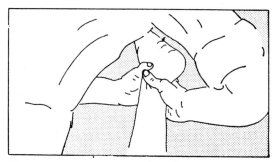

Figure 11.74 Ankle joint; lateral rotation

Method

As with medial rotation the movement is small and skin slack must be taken up first. The lateral rotation is produced by the therapist's left hand pivoting the patient's talus around the tibia and fibula which are held stabilized in her right hand.

Longitudinal movement cephalad**

Compression can be a surprisingly useful technique in the treatment of painful ankles when the movement is found to be painful or the patient experiences pain on the 'heel-strike' during walking.

Starting position

The patient lies prone with his right knee flexed to a right angle and the physiotherapist stands by his right knee and supports his shin. She holds his forefoot in her left hand to control the position of dorsiflexion of his ankle (Figure 11.75).

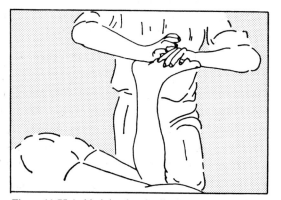

Figure 11.75 Ankle joint; longitudinal movement cephalad

Method

The therapist imparts the movement by tapping the sole of the heel between the medial and lateral processes of the calcaneus with the pisiform area of the heel of her right hand.

When this technique is used in treatment, the strength of the tap and the angle of dorsiflexion are adjusted to try to reproduce the symptoms by the tapping.

Longitudinal movement caudad*

Starting position

The patient lies prone with his knee flexed to a right angle and the physiotherapist stands by his knee. She grasps his talus in her right hand with her thumb laterally, her index finger medially, and the web of her first interosseous space stretching across the posterior process. With her left hand she holds the neck of the talus immediately anterior to the ankle joint, with her thumb crossing the lateral surface and her index finger crossing the medial surface. She then gently places her right knee across the posterior surface of his femur distally (Figure 11.76).

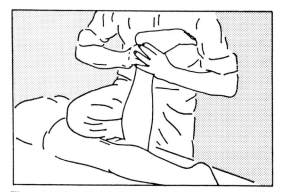

Figure 11.76 Ankle joint; longitudinal movement caudad

Method

She stabilizes his knee and lifts the talus towards the ceiling with both arms. Alternate lifting and releasing is repeated for the period of the mobilization. The technique can be performed gently or strongly in small or large-amplitudes anywhere in the range. A patient with symptoms is well aware of movement even when gentle oscillatory movements are performed.

Intertarsal movement

Movements of the foot demand different movements around different axes in different parts of the foot. The complexity of these movements needs to be understood if the best results from passive movement treatment are to be obtained. All recognized textbooks of anatomy describe the individual movements and most will concur that discrepancies in the description of movements exist. Taking the foot as a unit, inversion and eversion are separately described in this text.

From a clinical point of view, during inversion of the foot, four movements take place:

1. The heel inverts (adducts). The calcaneus inverts (adducts) at the subtalar joint, pulling the talus into a range of inversion also. This movement is really better referred to as adduction.
2. Medial rotation (supination). This is a movement of the forefoot on the hind-foot at the transverse tarsal joint, the transverse tarsal joint being between the calcaneus and talus proximally and the navicular and cuboid distally. Further medial rotation takes place between the navicular and cuneiform bones and even at the tarsometatarsal joints. (Medial rotation is better referred to as supination.)

   The forefoot, that is, that part of the foot that lies distal to the transverse tarsal joint, is made up largely of the metatarsals. However, the majority of the rotary movement takes place at the transverse tarsal joint when the movement is performed actively. If the movement of inversion is produced passively via the metatarsals then a considerable degree of supination is created between the metatarsals.
3. Forefoot adduction. This movement also takes place at the transverse tarsal joint, with the navicular bone sliding medially on the head of the talus. Although this movement is small when the foot is actively inverted, it is possible to produce passively quite a large range of adduction at the transverse tarsal joint and at the navicular cuneiform joints.
4. Plantar flexion. When inversion is performed passively and the maximum range is produced, plantar flexion occurs at three places to allow a greater amount of apparent forefoot movement. The first is at the tarsometatarsal joints, and the second part takes place at all of the forefoot joints, thus producing a maximum medial facing of the sole of the foot. When the ankle is plantar flexed a greater range of talocrural movement is possible, and it is here where a third part of plantar flexion takes place.

During eversion the reverse takes place and the total range of movement is much less.

Examination

During examination by passive movement all of the above movements can be performed. When any of them produce pain it becomes necessary to examine the movements, both physiological and accessory, that can take place at each intertarsal joint. These tests can be carried out, as described in the text that follows, and particular emphasis should be placed upon movements produced by thumb pressures on individual bones and by the gliding movements created by holding adjacent bones to each hand and forcing them to glide past each other in opposite directions.

Brief appraisal

Gait should be observed first[7]:

1. The patient should be asked to walk normally, away from and then towards the physiotherapist. He should then be asked to walk backwards, away from and then towards the physiotherapist.
2. He should be asked to walk on his toes, towards the physiotherapist and then backwards away from her.
3. He should be asked to walk forwards and backwards, away from and then towards, the physiotherapist, while on his heels and maintaining full dorsiflexion.
4. He should be asked to hop on the toes of his bad foot, and then on the heel of his bad foot keeping the ball of the foot well clear of the floor.

The patient should then be asked to squat fully, without being given any other directive. He will squat spontaneously and any abnormality of rhythm or position can be observed and noted. He should then be asked to squat, keeping his heels flat on the ground, and if the movement is full range and pain-free he should next be asked to bounce up and down in this position so as to put maximum strain onto his foot.

Special tests

The special tests used in examining the patient's foot merely require the isolating of painful and/or restricted movements to the different joints which make up the foot so as to know where to emphasize the treatment techniques.

Table 11.9 outlines the objective examination for the intertarsal joints but some points need clarification. The tendon sheaths should be examined as a source of pain by performing resisted movements through a full range, making the tendon slide within the sheath. The 'differentiating' referred to in relation to dorsiflexion, plantar flexion, inversion and eversion means that these movements are first performed as full range passive movements for the total foot. If a movement is found to be painful or stiff, the general foot movement should be broken down into its different components so as to

7. Maitland, G. D. *Gait,* Videotape No. 24 (50 mins.). Postgraduate Study Centre Hermitage, Medizinische Abteilung, Bad Ragaz, CH7310 Switzerland (1983)

Table 11.9 Intertarsal joint – objective examination

HIGHLIGHT MAIN FINDINGS WITH ASTERISKS
AS YOU GO

Observation

*Functional demonstration/tests

1. *Their* demonstration of *their* functional movements affected by *their* disorder.
2. Differentiation of *their* demonstrated functional movement(s).

Brief appraisal
Active movements (move to PAIN or move to LIMIT)

Isometric test

Other structures in 'plan'

Full active resisted movements through range for 'sheaths'.
Entrapment neuropathy.
LLTT

Passive movements
Physiological movements
Routinely
Differentiating DF, and PF, Inv., Ev.
Note range, pain, resistance, spasm and behaviour
As applicable
The injuring or aggravating movements

Accessory movements
Routinely

For foot, then differentiating for individual intertarsal joints

1. Ab, Ad (forefoot or hind-foot).
2. (↺), (↻) (axis 90° to tibia).
3. HF and HE forefoot proximally.
4. (↓), (↑), (→), (←), (↕) varying positions and angles.
5. (→), (←), (↓), (↑) subtalar.

Note range, pain, resistance, spasm and behaviour

Palpation
Include tendon sheaths
+ when 'comparable signs' ill-defined reassess 'injuring movement'

Check case records etc.

Instructions to patient

1. Warning of possible exacerbation.
2. Request to record details.
3. Instruction re 'joint care' if required.

---

determine in which joint or joints the fault lies. For example, inversion includes hind-foot adduction around a sagittal axis, forefoot adduction around a vertical axis and rotation (or supination) which takes place in all joints between the transverse tarsal joint and the tarsometatarsal joints, and finally plantar flexion at all joints. For example, it is possible to assess both range and pain caused by transverse tarsal joint rotation by grasping around the talus and calcaneus with one hand (so as to prevent them moving) while the other hand holds around the navicular and cuboid bones to rotate (supinate) them (Figure 11.77).

Similar tests are done for the remaining movements. If inversion is painful or stiff each component can be assessed separately.

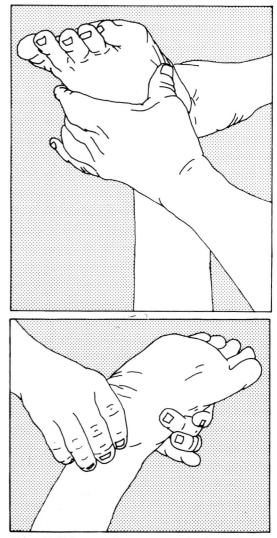

Figure 11.77 Intertarsal movement, supination localized to forefoot on hind-foot

Techniques

Inversion**

Starting position

The patient lies prone with his knee flexed to a right angle and the physiotherapist stands by his right knee with her left knee on the couch to support his right shin. When the technique is used generally for the whole foot she holds his foot with both hands from the lateral side, with her thumbs across the dorsum and her fingers across the plantar surface to reach the medial side (Figure 11.78).

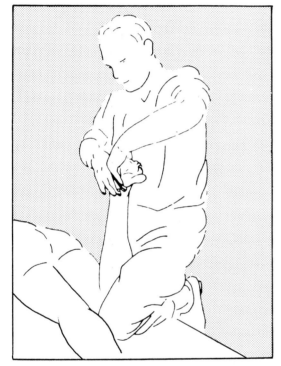

Figure 11.78 Intertarsal movement. Inversion; grades II and III−

Method

The therapist moves the patient's foot away from her by laterally rotating his hip so that his lower leg moves through an arc of 15–20°. To perform a large-amplitude inversion movement she pulls the patient's foot towards her with her arms and simultaneously inverts his foot with her hands. She times the movements so that the swing of his leg assists her reaching the limit of inversion.

The movement may be performed in varying positions of dorsiplantar flexion as dictated by the signs found on examination.

If III+ movements are required, a more economical starting position should be adopted.

Grade III+**

The technique is still being performed as a general movement for the whole foot.

Starting position

The patient lies prone with his feet near the end of the couch. The physiotherapist, standing at the foot of the couch, holds his forefoot in both hands with her thumbs and thenar eminences along the sole of the forefoot while her fingers overlap on the dorsum of the foot. She lifts his foot from the couch by flexing his knee, and places her right knee on the couch. She then lowers his leg, medially rotating his hip and inverting his foot, to rest his fully inverted foot against her thigh (Figure 11.79).

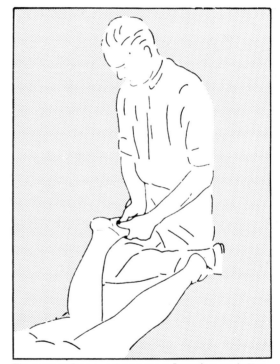

Figure 11.79 Intertarsal movement. Inversion; grade III+

Method

The movement is difficult to perform well unless care is taken. Concentration should be centred around feeling the inversion/eversion movement right up to the limit of the range. It is an extremely effective and useful treatment technique.

From the starting position described above where the patient's fully inverted foot rests against her thigh, two movements take place. Firstly, the therapist's arms move the patient's lower leg in a straight line, lifting his foot diagonally 18 inches

(45 cm) away from her knee towards his opposite
hip. This involves flexion of his knee and lateral
rotation of his hip. The second movement is
eversion of his foot combined with slight dorsiflexion, and this is performed by her hands. The return
movement is also a combination of two movements
but now they are the opposite of those described
above. The inversion and plantar flexion movement
is assisted by the drop of the lower leg and reaches
the limit of the range when his foot reaches her
thigh.

Because the therapist grasps the metatarsals and
has her thumb tips over their bases more movement
takes place distal to the transverse tarsal joint than
proximal to it. More rotation (supination) and
plantar flexion take place also.

If IV+ movements are required a completely
different technique is used.

Grade IV+***

Two positions are shown for this technique. The first
utilizes the whole foot with the emphasis on
movement distal to the transverse tarsal joint and
the second localizes the movement more to the
hind-foot, that is the talocrural and subtalar joints.

Starting position (No.1)

The patient lies on his left side with his hips and
knees comfortably flexed. His right foot extends to
the end of the couch and the physiotherapist,
standing behind his foot, places her left hand
between the medial side of his foot and the edge of
the couch to form a fulcrum for the inversion
movement. She places the heel of her right hand
directed distally, over the lateral border of the
lateral two tarsometatarsal joints with her fingers
directed distally over the plantar surface and her
thumb over the dorsal surface. If necessary she
places her left forearm against his lower leg laterally
to prevent his knee lifting during the mobilization
(Figure 11.80).

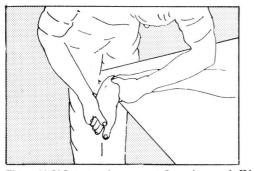

Figure 11.80 Intertarsal movement. Inversion; grade IV+
(starting position No. 1)

Method

Small-amplitude oscillations performed strongly at
the limit of the range are produced by direct
pressure against the lateral border of the patient's
foot. Small variations can be made in the position of
the therapist's hands and the direction of her
pressure to produce maximum stretch in the
appropriate direction and to localize the emphasis of
the movement to a joint or functional group of
joints.

Starting position (No.2)

To localize the inversion (or adduction) to the
talocrural and subtalar joints the therapist uses the
heel of her left hand against the lateral surface of the
calcaneus while her right hand stabilizes the
patient's metatarsals (Figure 11.81).

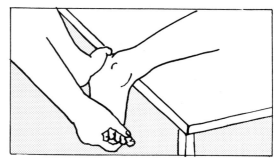

Figure 11.81 Intertarsal movement. Inversion; grade IV+
(starting position No. 2)

Method

Strong inversion can be produced by exerting
pressure through the left hand, making use of the
fingers to ensure that it is inversion that is being
produced and not a medially directed transverse
movement of the subtalar joint. This position can be
used for strong oscillatory grade IV if indicated: the
joints can be manipulated in this position.

Eversion**

As with inversion, described above, the following
describes eversion as a general mobilizing technique. It, too, can be localized in the manner
described above.

Starting position

The patient lies prone with his right knee flexed to a
right angle while the physiotherapist stands by his
knee with her left knee on the couch to support his
right shin. She holds his whole foot from the lateral

side with both hands. Her thumbs grasp over the dorsum of the foot and her fingers spread over the plantar surface reaching the medial longitudinal arch (Figure 11.82).

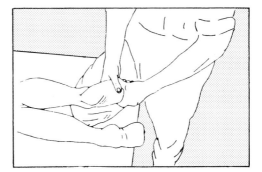

Figure 11.83 Intertarsal movement, eversion; grade III+

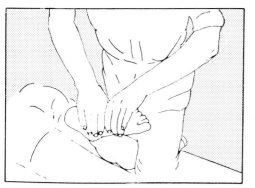

Figure 11.82 Intertarsal movement, eversion; grades II and III−

Method

The technique for eversion is the same as that described for inversion (see page 275) except that it is movement of the patient's foot away from the therapist which is the important part of the swinging action. This movement of his leg away from her needs to be carefully judged to assist the eversion of his foot performed by her hands.

If full range grade III+ type movements are required a more suitable starting position can be used.

Grade III+ **

Starting position

The patient lies prone with his feet reaching the end of the couch. The physiotherapist, standing at the foot of the couch, holds the patient's foot in both hands with her thumbs grasping over the plantar surface of the metatarsals and her fingers over the dorsal surface. She raises his foot and places her right knee on the couch near his left shin. She then lowers his foot, laterally rotating his hip and everting his foot to rest his lower leg and fully everted foot on her thigh (Figure 11.83).

Method

As was stated with the comparable technique for inversion (see page 275), though this technique is difficult to perform well, it is a very effective treatment when used in the right circumstances (through-range-symptoms). Two movements are coordinated. Firstly, the patient's knee is flexed and his hip medially rotated so that his foot traverses a straight line diagonally upwards and outwards. Secondly, the physiotherapist inverts his foot with her hands. The return movement combines dropping his leg towards her thigh, with eversion of the foot. The combined movement should be timed so that full eversion is reached when the patient's foot reaches her thigh.

When strong stretching movements are required in treatment a new position must be adopted.

Grade IV+ ***

Starting position

The patient lies on his right side with his hips and knees comfortably flexed so that the lateral surface of his lower leg lies on the couch and his foot extends over the end of the couch. The physiotherapist stands behind his foot and positions her right hand between his foot and the edge of the couch to act as a comfortable fulcrum for the movement.

If the technique is to be performed as a general eversion of the whole foot then she places her right hand between the lateral malleolus and the edge of the couch. However, if on examination, it has been possible to localize the painful or stiff joint during eversion, then she places the index finger of her right hand between that particular joint and the edge of the couch. With her left hand, if the eversion is to be performed as a general technique, she holds around the medial border of the foot around the metatarsals. If the technique is to be localized as referred to above, then she still holds around the medial border of the foot but localizes the technique by placing the heel of her left hand, through which most of the movement is transmitted, over the base of the first metatarsal, the medial cuneiform, the navicular bone or the talus.

She may need to position her right forearm across his leg to prevent it from lifting during the mobilization (Figure 11.84).

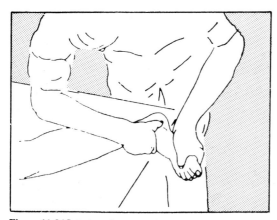

Figure 11.84 Intertarsal movement, eversion; grade IV+

Method

Small-amplitude oscillations produced firmly at the limit of the range are imparted to the foot through the therapist's left arm. During the procedure she must modify the position of her hands and his foot in relation to the fulcrum so that the leverage is economical and the direction appropriate.

Forefoot abduction***

Abduction in this instance refers to abduction of the metatarsals and intertarsal joints, about a vertical axis, and in relation to a stationary talus and calcaneus.

Starting position

The patient lies prone with his knee flexed to a right angle while the physiotherapist, standing by his knee facing his feet, places her left knee on the couch to support his shin. She holds the lateral border of his foot around the lateral border in both hands and places the pads of both thumbs over the appropriate bones (Figure 11.85).

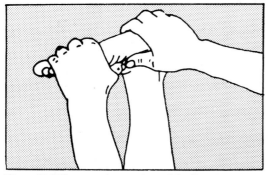

Figure 11.85 Intertarsal movement; abduction

This movement can be localized to the tarsometatarsal joint line, or the calcaneocuboid joint laterally by placing the tip of her left thumb over the tuberosity of the fifth metatarsal and the tip of her right thumb over the cuboid bone. When the movement is localized to the calcaneocuboid joint the tips of the thumbs are moved slightly proximally to overlie adjacent lateral borders of the cuboid and the calcaneus at the calcaneocuboid joint. During abduction the talocalcaneonavicular joint, the calcaneocuboid joint, the cuneonavicular joint, cuboideonavicular joint, and intercuneiform and cuneocuboid joints also move. By altering the positions of the thumb tips, the movement can be emphasized at each joint.

Method

Small-amplitude movements are produced by the therapist's arms transmitting pressure through her thumbs while her encompassing grasp holds the patient's foot firmly. The action should not be produced by the muscles of the hand but should derive from an adduction of the shoulders which approximates the elbows. It is important that the movement should not be produced by a squeezing action of the hands. To do so would make the technique uncomfortable to the patient and the therapist would lose all sense of feel of movement.

Forefoot adduction**

Adduction in this context relates to adduction of the metatarsals and tarsal bones anterior to the transverse tarsal joint around a vertical axis through the neck of the talus (Figure 11.86).

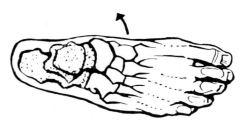

Figure 11.86 Forefoot adduction

Starting position

The patient lies prone near the edge of the couch with his right knee flexed. The physiotherapist stands by his left knee and holds his right foot from the medial aspect with both hands, placing the pads of her thumbs over the appropriate bones (Figure 11.87).

To localize or emphasize the adduction movement at the tarsometatarsal joints, the physiotherapist

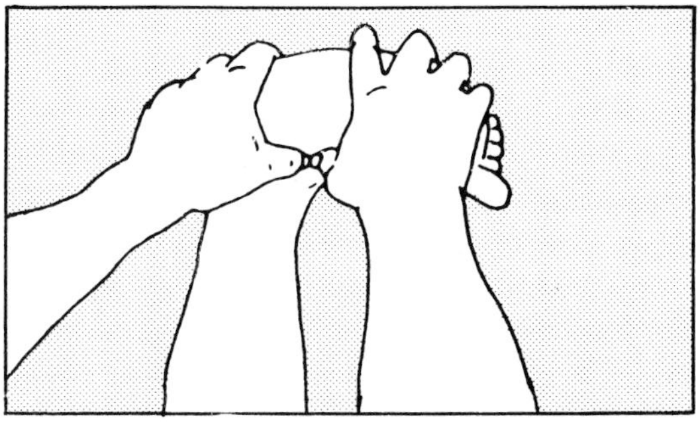

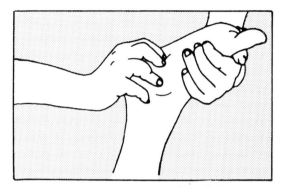

Figure 11.87 Intertarsal movement; adduction

places her right thumb over the base of the first metatarsal medially and the tip of her left thumb over the medial cuneiform bone. To localize the movement to the navicular–medial cuneiform joint the thumbs should be removed proximally to contact the navicular and medial cuneiform respectively. Similarly, to localize or emphasize the movement to the talonavicular joint the thumbs should be moved further proximally to lie over the talus and navicular immediately adjacent to the joint line. As was described with abduction, when the adduction movement is performed, movement also takes place at the other intertarsal joints distal to the transverse tarsal joint.

Method

During this technique care must be taken to prevent the foot inverting and supinating.

As with the preceding technique, adduction must be performed by arm action and not by the thumbs. It is necessary to adjust the position of the patient's foot in relation to both dorsiplantar flexion and inversion/eversion to produce the adduction movement which is stiff or painful.

Plantar flexion***

Plantar flexion of the whole ankle joint has already been described (see page 267). The intertarsal joints are also capable of plantar flexion but it is difficult to isolate them completely individually.

Starting position

The patient lies prone with his knee flexed to a right angle while the physiotherapist, standing by his knee, places her left knee on the couch to support his shin. She holds his calcaneus in her right hand with the heel of her hand posteriorly, her fingers over the plantar surface of his calcaneus and her finger tips level with the transverse tarsal joint. With her left hand she holds over the dorsal surface of his

forefoot with her fingers reaching the medial border of the foot (Figure 11.88).

To localize the movement more finely a starting position similar to that described on page 280 (Figure 11.89) may be used. The point of difference between the two starting positions is that for plantar flexion the tips of the thumbs are placed on the plantar surfaces of each bone forming one of the intertarsal joints.

Figure 11.88 Intertarsal movement; plantarflexion

Method

While she holds his heel partly dorsiflexed she plantar flexes his forefoot with her left hand around the fulcrum of her right finger tips. She times her movement so that her right index finger can apply an equal and opposite counterpressure to that exerted by her left hand.

When it is desired to localize the movement to the joint mentioned in the starting position above, the oscillatory movement is created by an ulnar deviation of both wrists combined with glenohumeral adduction. Each hand should hold its part of the foot so that it moves as a single unit. The tips of the thumbs must be made to sink gradually through the soft tissue of the plantar surface of the foot until they can feel the plantar surfaces of the respective bones. They then form the fulcrum of the plantar flexion.

Dorsiflexion***

Dorsiflexion of the ankle has already been described (see page 268) but some dorsiflexion takes place also at the intertarsal joints.

Starting position

The patient lies prone, with his right knee flexed to a right angle, while the physiotherapist stands by his knee and places her left knee on the couch to support his shin. She holds the medial side of his calcaneus and talus in her right hand so that her fingers lie anterior to his ankle with her index finger over the transverse tarsal joint. Her right thenar eminence lies across the plantar surface of his calcaneus. She holds his forefoot in her left hand so that the thenar eminence lies over the plantar surface of the metatarsals and the palmar surface of the distal two phalanges of the index finger lie over the dorsal surface of the appropriate tarsal bone or bones (Figure 11.89).

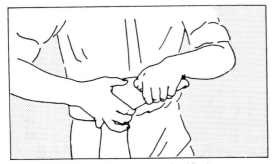

Figure 11.89 Intertarsal movement; dorsiflexion

A different starting position, similar to that described for intertarsal abduction (Figure 11.85) can be used to localize or emphasize the movement at different intertarsal joints. The tips of the thumbs can be placed on the dorsal surfaces of the talus, the navicular, the calcaneus, the cuboid and the cuneiform bones, each in turn.

Method

While the therapist's right hand holds the patient's heel plantar flexed she dorsiflexes his forefoot from a position of plantar flexion, endeavouring to apply an equal and opposite counterpressure with her right index finger.

When the technique is being used more specifically at each intertarsal joint the movement is produced by the therapist's wrists and shoulders. Her fingers and thumb encompass the bones proximal and distal

to the particular joint so that each hand and its bone moves as a single unit about the fulcrum formed by the thumbs at the intertarsal joint.

Posteroanterior and anteroposterior movements***

Only anteroposterior movement is depicted in Figure 11.90. It is unnecessary to describe posteroanterior movement as it is self-explanatory.

Starting position

The patient lies supine with his hip and knee flexed so that his foot can rest comfortably and flat on the couch. The physiotherapist stands at his feet, facing his head, and places the tips of her thumbs in the appropriate position over the dorsal surface of each tarsal bone in turn. Her fingers wrap comfortably around the foot to maintain stability (Figure 11.90).

Method

Anteroposterior movements (and posteroanterior movements) of each tarsal bone are produced by the physiotherapist's arms and trunk, and are transmitted to the bones via the tips of the thumbs. Concentric intrinsic muscle action must not be used to produce the movement as this removes all possibility of the physiotherapist appreciating the movement of one bone, say the middle cuneiform bone, in relation to the adjacent bone or bones, in this case the other two cuneiform bones, the navicular and the metatarsal bone.

It must be remembered that the direction of the anteroposterior movement (or posteroanterior movement) may be varied within a dome, that is, it can be performed in combination with medial, lateral, cephalad or caudad inclinations. It must also be remembered that the tips of the thumbs may make contact directly over the joint line, directly over the proximal bone, directly over the distal bone, or over the medial or lateral bones (see Figures 4.7–4.12).

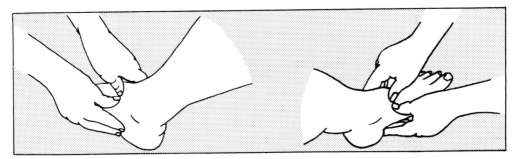

Figure 11.90 Intertarsal anteroposterior movement

Table 11.10 Tarsometatarsal joints – objective examination

HIGHLIGHT MAIN FINDINGS WITH ASTERISKS
AS YOU GO

Observation

*Functional demonstration/tests

1. *Their* demonstration of *their* functional movements
   affected by *their* disorder.
2. Differentiation of *their* demonstrated functional
   movement(s).

Brief appraisal

Active movements (move to PAIN or move to LIMIT)
Routinely (Modified as required)

Gait, walking forwards and backwards, towards and
away from you, then similarly for walking on heels and
toes, walking with feet in inversion and eversion,
forwards, backwards and sideways. Heel and toe
hopping.
Squatting on toes and flat feet.
DF, PF, Inv., Ev., toe F and E.
Note range and pain

Isometric test

Other structures in 'plan'

Full active resisted movements through range for
'sheaths'
Joint restriction cf. muscle/tendon restriction
Entrapment neuropathy & LLTT

Passive movements

Physiological movements
Routinely

F and E, foot Inv., Ev.
Note range, pain, resistance, spasm and behaviour.

Accessory movements
Routinely
(↓↑↓) (varying angles) (→ ←) (with Ab and Ad),
(⊃⊂) (with and without compression)
HF and HE (general and local)
Note range, pain, resistance, spasm and behaviour

Palpation
include tendon sheaths
+ when 'comparable signs' ill-defined reassess 'injuring
movement'

Check case records etc.

Instructions to patient

1. Warning of possible exacerbation.
2. Request to record details.
3. Instruction re 'joint care' if required.

Anteroposterior/posteroanterior movements***

These movements were described in Chapter 4 (see
Figures 4.7 and 4.8, page 43). They consist of
holding one tarsal bone between the fingers and
thumb of one hand while holding the adjacent tarsal
bone with which it forms a joint in the fingers and
thumb of the other hand. The physiotherapist then
holds one bone stationary and moves the adjacent
bone in line with the plane of the joint surface.

Tarsometatarsal joint

Flexion and extension of the big toe are the only
techniques which will be described as the remainder
are identical in principle, although the grips vary.
The 'functional demonstration' and 'brief appraisal'
tests for these joints are the same as those described
for the ankle (see page 265) and intertarsal joints
(see page 273). There are no particular 'special tests'
relevant in this area. The examination is presented
in Table 11.10.

Testing accessory movements in different end-of-
range physiological movement positions, or as
combined movements, produces the most comprehensive information, in this area.

Techniques
Flexion***
Starting position

The patient lies prone with his knee flexed to a right
angle and the physiotherapist stands by his knee.
She places her left knee on the couch to support his
shin. She holds the tarsometatarsal joint in both
hands with the thumbs on the plantar surface of the
adjacent bones at the joint and the index fingers
around the medial border of the foot to support the
joint on each side dorsally. The fingers of each hand
support the remainder of the dorsum of the foot
(Figure 11.91).

Method

The mobilization is produced by the therapist's arm
pivoting her fingers around her thumbs. As with all
techniques in which the thumbs are used to produce
movement, the thumb flexors must not be the prime
movers. This technique is very effective if care is
taken to localize the movement to the appropriate
joint. In the presence of marked tenderness a larger
area of the pad of the thumb should be used.

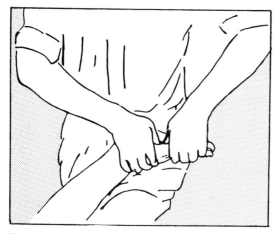

Figure 11.91 Tarsometatarsal flexion

Extension***

Starting position

The patient lies prone with his knee flexed to a right angle and the physiotherapist stands by his knee. She places her left knee on the couch to support his shin and holds his foot around the medial border in both hands placing her index fingers, pointing laterally, across the dorsal surface of the adjacent bones at the joint. Her fingers spread over the adjacent dorsum of the foot while her left palm and thenar eminence hold the ball of the foot and her right palm and thenar eminence hold the plantar surface near the heel. She places her left thenar eminence over the plantar surface of the head of the metatarsal and her right hand around the medial and plantar surfaces of the tarsal bones (Figure 11.92).

Method

The mobilization is produced by an arm action which pivots the heel of each hand (particularly that of the left hand) around the fulcrum of the index finger. The right hand provides pressure at the tarsometatarsal joint rather than providing much in the way of movement.

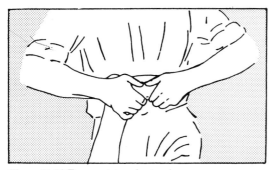

Figure 11.92 Tarsometatarsal extension

Alternative method

The patient lies supine and flexes his hip and knee so that his foot lies comfortably flat upon the couch. Extension at each tarsometatarsal joint can be produced by placing the tips of the thumbs over the adjacent bones forming each intertarsal joint and using the leverage provided by the physiotherapist's fingers on the plantar surface of the patient's foot (Figure 11.93).

This can also be done with the patient lying prone. The technique is similar to that shown in Figure 11.85.

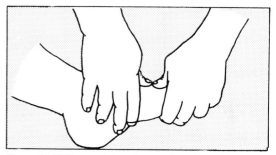

Figure 11.93 Tarsometatarsal extension; alternative method

Accessory movements

The movements now to be described are passive accessory movements which can be used both in examination and treatment. It should be appreciated that they can be combined together to produce a single accessory movement, or combined with the physiological movements of flexion or extension, and sometimes with abduction/adduction.

Transverse movement**

As was described for the carpometacarpal joints: the tips of the thumbs are placed against the base of each metatarsal to produce a transverse movement of the head of the metatarsal at the tarsometatarsal junction. The appropriate phalanges are used to assist the medial or lateral movement of the head of the metatarsal and the medial or lateral border of the foot is held by the therapist's fingers to form a stable base about which the transversely directed pressure can be applied.

Posteroanterior and anteroposterior movements**

By placing the tips of the thumbs over the base of a metatarsal, either on the dorsal surface or the plantar surface, an anteroposterior or posteroanterior movement of the base of the metatarsal in relation to its adjacent tarsal bone is produced.

Again it is pointed out that these pressures in relation to the tarsometatarsal joints may be varied in their direction throughout a global sphere, and the pressures directed through the metatarsal, the adjacent tarsal bone or the joint line.

Rotation***

Rotation is easily produced at the tarsometatarsal joints by flexing the metatarsophalangeal and interphalangeal joints of the toe and using this flexed toe to rotate the metatarsal.

Anteroposterior/posteroanterior movements***

As with other joints in the hand and foot, it is possible to produce gliding movements at the tarsometatarsal joints by holding the appropriate cuneiform or cuboid bone in one hand, and the base of the metatarsal in the other hand, then moving the adjacent bones in opposite directions in line with the plane of the joint surface.

Intermetatarsal movement

The cause of symptoms in this area is usually put down to a flattened transverse arch of the ball of the foot. However, the symptoms can often be relieved by identifying the joint(s) responsible and mobilizing them to make the movement(s) pain free.

The intermetatarsal movements are anteroposterior and posteroanterior gliding, horizontal extension which flattens the foot across the heads of the metatarsals, and horizontal flexion which increases the transverse arch of the foot. Posteroanterior and anteroposterior movements of one metatarsal in relation to its neighbour can be produced passively.

Examination

Subjective examination

The most common complaint is one of pain localized in the ball of the foot. Although it is often considered to be a general area, deeper questioning combined with palpation usually reveals a dominant area.

Objective examination

Functional demonstration/tests

The demonstrations offered by the patient usually include standing or walking and can easily be differentiated.

Brief appraisal

The only tests in this section are:

1. Gait tests as described for the ankle (see page 238) and the intertarsal area (see page 265): walking on the toes would probably be the main aspect.
2. Hopping on the toes/ball of foot.

Special tests

The two specific tests are:

1. Horizontal flexion, especially with compression.
2. Anteroposterior/posteroanterior movement with compression.

Table 11.11 lists the examination.

Techniques

Anteroposterior/posteroanterior movement***

Starting position

The patient lies prone with his feet near the end of the couch. The physiotherapist, standing at the foot of the couch, holds the distal end of the patient's metatarsals in both hands and flexes his knee

Table 11.11 Intermetatarsal movement – objective examination

HIGHLIGHT MAIN FINDINGS WITH ASTERISKS AS YOU GO

Observation

*Functional demonstration/tests

1. *Their* demonstration of *their* functional movements affected by *their* disorder.
2. Differentiation of *their* demonstrated functional movement(s).

Brief appraisal
Gait and on toes
Active movements (move to PAIN or move to LIMIT)

Isometric test (not applicable)

Other structures in 'plan'
Entrapment neuropathy

Passive movements

($\updownarrow$) individually.
HF and HE, (and individually), (heads and bases), (without and with compression), ($\uparrow$) and ($\downarrow$) of each metatarsal in relation to its neighbours, varying the directions (heads and bases).
Note range, pain, resistance, spasm and behaviour.

Palpation
Include tendon sheaths
+ when 'comparable signs' ill-defined reassess 'injuring movement'

Check case records etc.

Instructions to patient

1. Warning of possible exacerbation.
2. Request to record details.
3. Instruction re 'joint care' if required.

---

slightly. She places her thumbs, pointing proximally, side by side over the plantar surface of two adjacent metatarsals and grasps the dorsal surface of each metatarsal with each flexed index finger in order to grasp the metatarsal between the index finger and thumb of each hand. She kneels with her right knee on the couch and supports her right hand against her right thigh (Figure 11.94).

Method

Each hand should hold the individual metatarsal firmly while the movement is produced by a pushing action with one hand countered by a pulling action with the other. The same technique is used whichever pair of metatarsals is mobilized. Compression may be added.

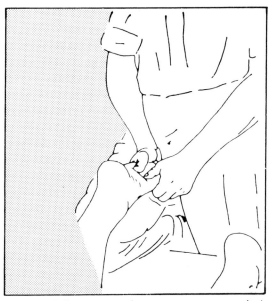

Figure 11.94 Intermetatarsal movement; anteroposterior/posteroanterior movement

Horizontal flexion*

Starting position

The patient lies prone with his feet near the end of the couch. The physiotherapist, standing at the foot of the couch, holds the patient's foot in her hands and flexes his knee slightly. By kneeling on her right knee, she can support her right hand against her thigh. She places the pads of her thumbs pointing towards each other over the plantar surface of the head of the third metatarsal while grasping around each side of the foot with her fingers. Her main finger contact is with the dorsal surface of the second and fourth metatarsals near their heads (Figure 11.95).

Method

The horizontal flexion is produced by the therapist's arms which, during adduction of the shoulders, pivot the fingers around the fulcrum of the thumbs. The examination findings may indicate that the movement should be pivoted around the second or fourth metatarsal rather than the third and this is achieved by placing the tips of the thumbs over the head of the relevant metatarsal.

Horizontal extension*

Starting position

The patient lies prone with his feet near the end of the couch. The physiotherapist, standing at the foot of the couch, holds the patient's foot in her hands and flexes his knee slightly. She places the metacarpal and phalanges of the thumb and thenar eminence of each hand, pointing towards his heel, over the plantar surface of the heads of the first and fifth metatarsals respectively. She places her fingers over the dorsum of the third metatarsal, using the pads of the fingers to make the contact more comfortable (Figure 11.96).

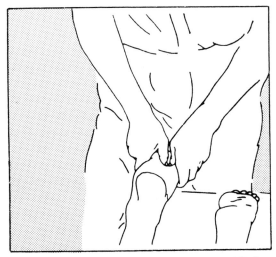

Figure 11.95 Intermetatarsal movement; horizontal flexion

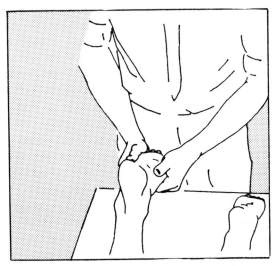

Figure 11.96 Intermetatarsal movement; horizontal extension

Table 11.12 Composite foot/ankle – objective examination

HIGHLIGHT MAIN FINDINGS WITH ASTERISKS
AS YOU GO

Observation

*Functional demonstration/tests

1. *Their* demonstration of *their* functional movements
   affected by *their* disorder.
2. Differentiation of *their* demonstrated functional
   movement(s).

Brief appraisal
Active movements (modified as required) (move to PAIN
or move to LIMIT)

Walking: forwards, backwards, on toes, on heels, all
away from and towards.
Balancing on one leg, on ball of foot.
Hopping: on flat foot, on toes, on heels.
Squatting: spontaneously, with heels on and off ground.

Isometric tests

Other structures in 'plan'
Full active resisted movements through range for sheaths
Joint restriction cf. muscle/tendon restriction
Entrapment neuropathy & LLTT

Passive movements

Prone

Inferior tibiofibular joint

($\updownarrow$) ($\updownarrow$) compression, ($\updownarrow$) with compression, ($\updownarrow$) with
compression (--) with and without compression,
talocrural rotation

Whole foot

1. DF, PF; as IV−, to IV+, to III++.
2. Inv, Ev; as IV−, to IV+, to III++.
3. ($\circlearrowright$), ($\circlearrowleft$) (axis in line with tibia) IV−, to IV+, to
   III++.
4. (--) ceph, caud, (axis in line with tibia) to III++.
5. ($\updownarrow$), ($\updownarrow$), at ankle.
6. Ab, Ad.
7. HF, FE.

Differentiating as required

1. DF and PF as IV+ at limit of range:
   (b) Ankle (DF incudes inferior tibiofibular
       movement).
   (b) Transverse tarsal joint (talocalcaneonavicular and
       calcaneocuboid).
   (c) Cuneonavicular.
   (d) Tarsometatarsal.

2. Inv. and Ev. as IV+ at limit of range.
   (a) Inferior tibiofibular joint (T/F).
   (b) Ankle (IV produces inferior T/F
       movement   } Hind-foot
   (c) Subtalar (IV produces inferior T/F
       movement
   (d) Transverse tarsal joint (talocalcaneonavicular and
       calcaneocuboid): (i) rotation i.e. Sup. and Pron.;
       (ii) Ab. and Ad.; (iii) DF and PF.
   (e) Cuneonavicular.
   (f) Intercuneiform and cuneocuboid: (i) rotation, i.e.
       Sup. and Pron.; (ii) Ab. and Ad.; (iii) DF and PF.
   (g) Tarsometatarsal: (i) rotation i.e., Sup. and Pron.;
       (ii) Ab. and Ad.; (iii) DF and PF.

3. ($\circlearrowright$) ($\circlearrowleft$) (axis in line with tibia) as IV+ at limit of
   range:
   (a) Inferior tibiofibular.
   (b) Ankle.
   (c) Subtalar.

4. (--) caud (in line with tibia) at IV+ at limit of range:
   (a) Ankle.
   (b) Subtalar (also for subtalar (--) and (--),($\updownarrow$),($\updownarrow$),
       Inv. and Ev.)
       (--) ceph (in line with tibia) as IV+ at limit of
       range.
       Various positions of ankle and subtalar joints for
       'differentiating'

5. ($\updownarrow$) ($\updownarrow$), at ankle (at right angles to tibia) as IV+ at
   limit of range:
   (a) Ankle.
   (b) Subtalar.

6. Ab. and Ad. as IV+ at limit of range:
   (a) Tarsometatarsal.
   (b) Cuneonavicular and calcaneocuboid.
   (c) Talonavicular.

7. HF and HE as IV+ at limit of range:
   (a) Intermetatarsal.
   (b) Cuneocuboid.
   (c) Cuboideonavicular.

Other test movements not included under differentiating

1. ($\updownarrow$) ($\updownarrow$), (varying angles), intertarsal and
   tarsometatarsal.
2. ($\updownarrow$) intertarsal and tarsometatarsal.
3. Tarsometatarsal ($\circlearrowright$,$\circlearrowleft$), (--, --), Ab, Ad, F and
   E.
4. Intermetatarsal ($\updownarrow$), HF, HE.

Palpation
+ when 'comparable signs' ill-defined reassess 'injuring
movement'

Check case records etc.

Instructions to patient
1. Warning of possible exacerbation.
2. Request to record details.
3. Instruction re 'joint care' if required.

Method

The horizontal extension is produced by a supination action of the therapist's forearm pivoting her
thumbs around her fingers. As with the preceding
technique, any of the metatarsals may be made the
fulcrum of the movement.

Compression***

To all of the above movements, a horizontally directed pressure can be exerted by the therapist adding a squeezing action of her two hands towards each other. Frequently, comparable signs are only found when this compression component is added to a significant movement.

Composite foot/ankle examination

Expertly assessing the behaviour of pain, resistance or muscle spasm in joints that make up the foot is an exacting exercise. Table 11.12 lists the passive movement tests to be employed when a patient complains of pain, or lacks normal function in his foot owing to joint stiffness. This table shows the sequence of tests that are applied from the inferior tibiofibular joint proximally to the tarsometatarsal joints distally.

To examine every movement of every joint from the inferior tibiofibular joint to the metatarsal area is unnecessary and would be unpractical. Though the composite foot/ankle table (Table 11.12) does list all of the major tests for each joint, it is not assumed that they are all performed. Following analysis of the 'functional demonstration/tests' the examination begins with the functional physiological movements for the 'whole foot'. If any of these produces a comparable sign then that movement is broken down to its components for the appropriate joints and these are tested and differentiated.

Chronic/minor ankle/foot symptoms

When a patient has symptoms that are chronic and probably are not much more than a nuisance, the examination passive tests are those listed below. It is only when one of those reproduces his symptoms that the investigation needs to be taken further. Differentiation tests would be used as grade IV+ movements:

1. Prone: DF & PF.
2. Inv. & Ev. (through metatarsals).
3. Ankle, rotations.
4. Ankle, longitudinal caudad.
5. Hindfoot PA & AP.
6. Inf. T/Fib PA & AP.
7. HF (may be excluded if symptoms do not extend distal to the navicular).

Test movements begin as IV− with observation for pain response. If pain-free, adequate over-pressure is applied until pain is provoked or the movement is judged 'clear'. If stronger over-pressure is required,

the following test movements should be repeated with the lower leg fully supported in the side lying position:

Side lying: Inv. & Ev., Inf. T/Fib, PA & AP with compression.

In the prone position ankle posteroanterior movement can be tested with the patient's feet over the end of the examination couch as can anteroposterior movement with the patient supine or with his hip and knee flexed and the ball of the foot supported.

When a positive pain response is provoked, that test movement may need to be differentiated to determine the specific joint at fault and/or other test movements may need to be tested so as to either exclude or incriminate other joints as contributing to the symptoms.

If all test movements prove 'clear' at first examination, they should be repeated more strongly. If still 'clear', they may prove positive when repeated at the next consultation.

Proving the ankle/foot is unaffected

The passive movement tests used here as grade IV are as follows:

1. Prone: DF/PF with compression.
2. Inv./Ev. whole complex, and with compression.
3. Rot with compression.
4. Ankle ←•→ ceph and caud.
5. Subtaloid →• and •→.
6. Inf. Tib/F ↕↓ with compression.

Treatment

The treatment of foot pain or stiffness is quickest and most successful when passive movements are localized to the precise directions of movement of the joint at fault. In most instances it is necessary to use the movements which reproduce the patient's pain or which produce a comparable pain at an appropriate joint. Although general movements, for example full inversion of the whole foot, can be used in treatment, the result will be achieved more quickly if the 'comparable sign' can be isolated to a single joint's movement and if this movement is then used as the treatment technique.

In the treatment of most joint pain problems of the foot, grade IV type movements are most commonly used to increase range or to provoke a controlled degree of the patient's pain. Alternatively, grade III movements, where the joint or joints affected are moved back and forth through a large range of movement up to the limit of the range, may be applied.

Metatarsophalangeal and interphalangeal joints

When only one toe causes trouble, it is usually the big toe and it is usually its metatarsophalangeal joint. It responds well to mobilization techniques (often requiring compression with the chosen direction of movement). In the presence of marked joint changes, though the improvement gained is useful for the patient, the end result is a compromise rather than being ideal.

The same basic principles of treatment (for pain, especially intra-articular, and for stiffness) apply as for other joints. However, when treating the metatarsophalangeal joint of the big toe treatment usually falls into one of two categories:

1. Abduction, and accessory movements at the limit of abduction for range.
2. Oscillatory through range movements of abduction or mid range rotation, frequently with compression.

Examination

Objective examination

Brief appraisal

Table 11.13 lists the examination for these joints. The appraisal tests are again squatting, gait tests and hopping as listed in Table 11.8).

The movements that can be performed at the metatarsophalangeal and interphalangeal joints are identical with those of the fingers described on pages 213–217. Compression is an important component which, as a 'special test' is added to any test movement of the metatarsophalangeal and interphalangeal movements.

Techniques

All techniques for the toes are the same as those described for the fingers, therefore they are not repeated here. The big toe is not as different as is the thumb. However, bunion and hallux valgus are peculiar to the foot. For the former laterally directed pressures, both oscillatory and sustained, against the thickened tissues, assist in relieving symptoms, especially when the tissues are spongy and painful.

Abduction**

Abduction of the metatarsophalangeal joint of the big toe is shown in Figure 11.97. It is often of value in the treatment of hallux valgus. Under these circumstances abduction is used as grade IV and grade III− movements.

Table 11.13 Metatarsophalangeal and interphalanageal joints – objective examination

---

HIGHLIGHT MAIN FINDINGS WITH ASTERISKS AS YOU GO

Observation

*Functional demonstration/tests

1. *Their* demonstration of *their* functional movements affected by *their* disorder.
2. Differentiation of *their* demonstrated functional movement(s).

Brief appraisal

Active movements (modified as required) (move to PAIN or move to LIMIT)
Gait, walking on toes forwards and backwards, hopping, squatting on heels and toes

As applicable

The injuring or aggravating movements

Isometric test

Other structures in 'plan'

Joint restriction cf. muscle/tendon restriction
Entrapment neuropathy & LLTT

Passive movements

Physiological movements
Routinely
F and E of toes
Note range, pain, resistance, spasm and behaviour

Accessory movements
Routinely

1. (↑), (↓), (→), (←), Ab, Ad, (↻), (↺) (with and without compression) (↔ ceph and caud).
2. Above techniques combined in varying sequences.
3. For metatarsophalangeal joints add HF and HE, general and localized.
Note range, pain, resistance, spasm and behaviour

Palpation
Include tendon sheaths
+ when 'comparable signs' ill-defined reassess 'injuring movement'

Check case records etc.

Instructions to patient

1. Warning of possible exacerbation.
2. Request to record details.
3. Instruction re 'joint care' if required.

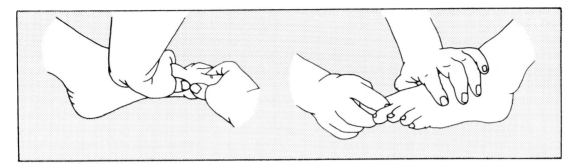

Figure 11.97 Metatarsophalangeal abduction of the big toe

Treatment

The big toe frequently requires mobilizing in many or all directions and compression is very often required in conjunction with such movements as abduction or rotation. The techniques can be carried out with the patient supine or prone.

The metatarsophalangeal joints of one or more toes are very frequently the source of what is diagnosed as 'metatarsalgia'. Localized mobilizing techniques of the joint and/or the intermetatarsal heads are very effective as well as producing quick results.

12

Other joints and structures

Costal joints and intercostal movement

Symptoms arising from musculo-skeletal structures of the thoracic area frequently have a traumatic origin. The symptoms are only felt locally at the site of the disorder unless intercostal nerves, the nerve root, or the posterior primary ramus are affected. Under these latter circumstances diminished sensory awareness can be found. Passive movement treatment can often be used with good effect.

Synovial joints exist in the costochondral, interchondral and sternocostal articulations. Even though there are no intercostal joints, the movement between the ribs can be restricted and painful. The direction of movement produced by thumb pressures can be varied in the way as is done for the sternoclavicular joint (see page 161), to suit the findings on examination. The 'special test' consists of maximum inspiration (and expiration) and inspiration performed at maximum speed (Table 12.1).

Movement in only one direction will be described but reference will be made to movement in other directions.

Technique
Anteroposterior movement***
Starting position

The physiotherapist stands by the patient's right shoulder, facing across his trunk. To increase intercostal movement she places the pads of her thumbs side by side across the joint to be mobilized with her fingers spreading in a fan to provide stability. As much of the pad as possible is used to make the contact more comfortable. The thumbs are more stable in this position than when directed along the shaft of the rib. She must position her shoulders directly above her hands and keep the base of her thumbs close together (Figure 12.1).

When symptoms can be attributed to abnormal movement between adjacent ribs the thumbs are placed along the line of the rib to spread the pressure area on the ribs. The physiotherapist directs her arms cephalad or caudad so that the movement will stretch the restriction or reproduce the symptoms.

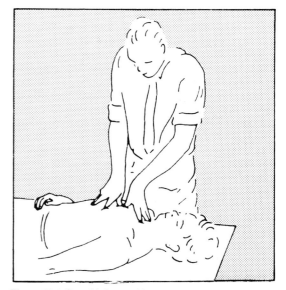

Figure 12.1 Costal joints and intercostal movement; anteroposterior movement

Table 12.1 Costal joints and intercostal movement – objective examination

---

Thoracic intervertebral joints should form part of the examination.

HIGHLIGHT MAIN FINDINGS WITH ASTERISKS AS YOU GO

Observation

*Functional demonstration/tests

1. *Their* demonstration of *their* functional movements affected by *their* disorder.
2. Differentiation of *their* demonstrated functional movement(s).

Brief appraisal

Active movements (move to PAIN or move to LIMIT)

Routinely

Inspiration and expiration, to maximum, quickly.
Trunk F, E, LF, Rotn in F and E.
Full scapulohumeral F through F & Ab.
Side-lying arm through abduction to full flexion position.
Note range, pain and behaviour.

As applicable

The injuring or aggravating movements

Isometric tests (not applicable)

Other structures in 'plan'

Passive movements
Physiological movements
Routinely

As for 'routine active movements' above, with over pressure and localizing
Accessory movements

(↕) (↕) (↔) (↔), adding ceph and caud and other varying angles. Note range, pain, resistance, spasm and behaviour

Palpation
For intercostal and thoracic interspinous spacing, prominence and thickening + when 'comparable signs' ill-defined reassess 'injuring movement'

Check case records etc.

Instructions to patient

1. Warning of possible exacerbation.
2. Request to record details.
3. Instruction re 'joint care' if required.

Method

As with all other techniques affecting the use of the thumbs, the anteroposterior movement must be produced by trunk and arm movements rather than by the thumb flexors.

The mobilization may be directed towards the patient's feet by applying pressure against the upper border of the rib. The therapist then stands alongside the patient's head. If the movement is to be directed in an upward direction with the contact against the lower border of the rib, she must stand by the patient's right side at waist level. In both of these positions the thumbs may be directed along the shaft of the rib.

Laryngeal and hyoid joints

Synovial joints occur in pairs between the inferior cornua of the thyroid cartilage and the sides of the cricoid cartilage and also between the facets on the lateral surfaces of the upper border of the lamina of the cricoid cartilage and the base of the arytenoid cartilage. Occasionally there is a synovial joint between the less cornua and the greater cornua in the hyoid bone. It is not common for pain to arise from these joints but as they are synovial joints and are supported by ligaments they can, and in fact occasionally do, give rise to symptoms.

Examination
Subjective examination

Symptoms are localized to the affected structures, but is felt to be deep.

Objective examination

Intervertebral structures should form part of the examination.

Brief appraisal

Coughing, swallowing and talking are tests that can guide the examination and assessment.

Musicians who play wind instruments may develop symptoms under circumstances of fatigue and 'over-use'.

The passive movement test consists in holding the adjacent cartilages with the index finger and thumb of each hand so as to be able to produce transverse and rotary movements (Table 12.2).

Technique
Starting position*

The patient lies supine without a pillow so that neither his head nor his neck are flexed. The

Table 12.2 Thyroid area – objective examination

Synovial joints are present and related to movement of hyoid, cricoid, arytenoid and thyroid cartilages and bones.
The cervical spine should also form part of the examination.

HIGHLIGHT MAIN FINDINGS WITH ASTERISKS AS YOU GO

Observation

*Functional demonstration/tests

1. *Their* demonstration of *their* functional movements affected by *their* disorder.
2. Differentiation of *their* demonstrated functional movement(s).

Brief appraisal
Active movements
Routinely

Swallow.
Cough.
Speak (volume) sing.
Blow (resisted).

Isometric tests

Other structures in 'plan'

Passive movements
$(\rightarrow)$, $(\leftarrow)$, $(\dagger)$, $(\dagger)$, $(\circlearrowright)$, $(\circlearrowleft)$, (ζ), $(\rangle)$
cervical F, E, LF, Rotn.

Palpation
When 'comparable signs' ill-defined reassess 'injuring movement' (wind instrument player, singer)
+ thickening
Cervical $(\lfloor\_)$ $(\_\rfloor)$

Check case records etc.

Instructions to patient

1. Warning of possible exacerbation.
2. Request to record details.
3. Instruction re 'joint care' if required.

physiotherapist loosely grasps the upper and lower margins of the thyroid cartilage between the index finger and thumb of her left and right hands respectively. Her fingers spread forward over the adjacent neck, chest and face with her little fingers making the firmest contact (Figure 12.2).

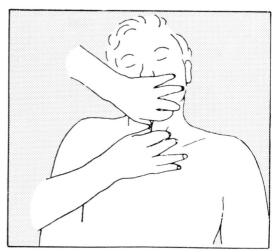

Figure 12.2 Thyroid cartilage movement

Method

Movement of the thyroid cartilage away from the therapist is produced by pressure through the thumbs. The little fingers form a pivot about which the thumb movement takes place. To make the pressure as comfortable as possible the movement should be produced by glenohumeral adduction and slight elbow extension rather than by the thumb flexors.

Movement of the thyroid cartilage towards the therapist is produced by the opposite movement of her arms acting through her index fingers. A rotary movement can also be performed.

Movement of the hyoid bone in relation to the mandible and thyroid cartilage can be produced by holding the hyoid bone between the index finger and thumb of the left hand while stabilizing the thyroid cartilage with the right hand.

Temporomandibular joint

Movements of the jaw include depression, elevation, protraction, retraction, lateral movements of the chin, and, more importantly, the accessory posteroanterior movement, transverse movements, longitudinal movement cephalad and caudad.

Alignment of teeth during opening and closing of the mouth is important to watch as is the occlusal position.

Examination

Subjective examination

Symptoms can refer into:

1. The face.
2. The head.
3. In the ear.
4. Behind the ear.

As well as locally within the joint.

Chewing and yawning are two common subjective complaints.

Objective examination

Brief appraisal

Opening the mouth as widely as possible and clenching the teeth tightly are two tests that can guide the remainder of the examination.

The full passive movement examination, which includes examination of the cervical spine, is given in Table 12.3.

Techniques

One of the greatest difficulties encountered when passively mobilizing the jaw is the patient's inability to relax his jaw completely. This may be one of the reasons why mobilization using pressure against the head of the mandible is much more successful in the treatment of jaw pain than techniques that use large movements of the mandible. The accessory movements will be described first.

Transverse movement medially***

Starting position

The patient lies with his head turned to the left, resting on a pillow, or lies on his left side. The physiotherapist stands behind his head and places the pads of her thumbs pointing towards each other over the head of the mandible.

She spreads her fingers comfortably around her

Table 12.3 Temporomandibular joint – objective examination

Cervical spine should form part of the examination.

HIGHLIGHT MAIN FINDINGS WITH ASTERISKS AS YOU GO

Observation

*Functional demonstration/tests

1. *Their* demonstration of *their* functional movements affected by *their* disorder.
2. Differentiation of *their* demonstrated functional movement(s).

Brief appraisal
Active movements (move to PAIN or move to LIMIT)
Routinely
Note occlusal position.
Depression, elevation, protraction, retraction, note range and teeth alignment; lateral movement.
Note range and pain for all movements.
Muscle power.

As applicable
Upper cervical spine

Isometric tests

Other structures in 'plan'

Passive movements
Routinely
Depression, elevation, protraction, retraction and lateral mandibular movements.
($\uparrow$)($\downarrow$)($\rightarrow$)($\leftarrow$) (with and without compression).
($\leftrightarrow$) ceph and caudad.
Note range, pain, resistance, spasm and behaviour.
Note alignment during movement.
Upper cervical spine.

Palpation

Capsular thickening T/M joint.
Cervical spine.
+ when 'comparable signs' ill-defined reassess 'injuring movement' (wind instrument player, singer).

Check case records etc.

Instructions to patient

1. Warning of possible exacerbation.
2. Request to record details.
3. Instruction re 'joint care' if required.

thumbs to provide stability (and may position the backs of her thumbs close together). Her arms must be directed in line with the transverse movement of the joint (Figure 12.3).

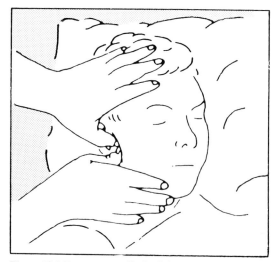

Figure 12.3 Temporomandibular joint; transverse movement medially

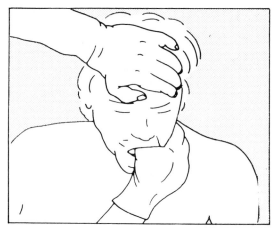

Figure 12.4 Temporomandibular joint; transverse movement laterally

range of lateral movement will be readily discernible.

Method

Small-amplitude oscillatory mobilizations are produced by her arms acting through her thumbs. Very little pressure is required to produce quite a lot of movement. Care must be exercised to make the technique as comfortable as possible.

Transverse movement laterally***
Starting position

The patient lies supine and the physiotherapist stabilizes his head with her left hand. She then places the pad of her right thumb, facing laterally against the medial surface of the ramus of the mandible, close to or against the head of the mandible (Figure 12.4).

Method

Gentle oscillatory pressures are applied to the medial surface of the mandible so as to produce lateral movement of the head of the mandible in the mandibular fossa of the temporal bone. The therapist holds the ramus between her thumb, within the patient's mouth, and her fingers, outside the mouth on the lateral surface of the ramus. With this grasp the movement is produced by the action of the therapist's arm, care being taken not to use the thumb flexors concentrically, but rather, eccentrically. If the technique is not performed in this manner the pressure on the medial surface of the ramus will be most uncomfortable.

The therapist should also place the pad of one finger over the temporomandibular joint so that the

Posteroanterior movement***
Starting position

The patient lies with his head turned to the left, resting on a pillow, or lies on his left side. The physiotherapist stands by his right shoulder and places the pads of her thumbs, pointing towards each other, against the posterior surface of the head of the mandible, behind the lobe of the ear, with the backs of her thumbs close together. Her fingers rest comfortably over the head and jaw. She directs her forearms in line with the posteroanterior movement of the joint (Figure 12.5).

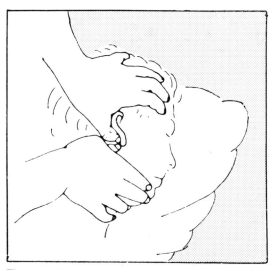

Figure 12.5 Temporomandibular joint; posteroanterior movement

Method

Mobilization in this direction is produced by the therapist's arms acting through her thumbs. As this area is normally tender, it is necessary to position the thumbs carefully and produce movement with the arms and not the thumb flexors.

Protraction**

Starting position

The patient lies with his head resting comfortably on a pillow. The physiotherapist stands beyond his head, facing his feet. She holds his mandible by placing her thumbs in his mouth with the medial border of her thumbs against the inner surface of his lower incisors and the posterolateral surface of the interphalangeal joints against the outer surface of his upper incisors. Her fingers grasp comfortably under either side of the mandible (Figure 12.6).

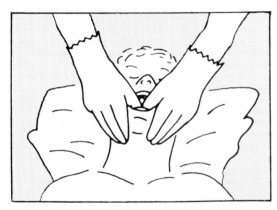

Figure 12.6 Temporomandibular joint; protraction

Method

Oscillatory protraction movements are produced by pivoting the tips of the thumbs against the lower teeth around the fulcrum of the interphalangeal joint against the upper teeth. This action should be produced by the therapist's hand and forearm and not by the thumb flexors.

Retraction*

Starting position

The patient lies with his head resting on a pillow. The physiotherapist stands beyond his head, facing his feet. She places the pads of her thumbs, pointing towards his feet, against the anterior margin of the ramus of the mandible while her fingers reach

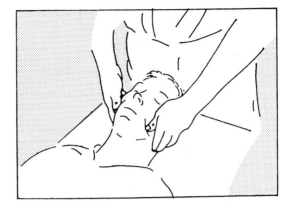

Figure 12.7 Temporomandibular joint; retraction

comfortably around the side of his head. The base of the pad of her thumb makes the main contact, not the tip (Figure 12.7).

Method

The retraction is produced by the therapist's arms acting through the base of her thumbs. Care must be taken to prevent the thumbs sliding laterally off the ramus by directing some pressure medially.

Lateral chin movement***

Starting position

The patient lies with his head turned to the left, resting on a pillow, while the physiotherapist stands behind his head. She places her left hand over the left zygomatic arch to stabilize his head, preventing it from rotating further to the left during the mobilization. She adopts a particular grasp of the right side of the mandible with her right hand so that she will be able to protract the right temporomandibular joint and displace the chin to the left. She places her index finger and thumb along the line of the jaw laterally and her middle finger beneath the jaw so that she can grasp it to control the opened or closed position of the mouth. Her ring and little fingers are flexed at the metacarpophalangeal and proximal interphalangeal joints so that the lateral border of the ring finger can be placed behind the angle of the jaw. The little finger reinforces the ring finger (Figure 12.8).

Method

With the patient's mouth slightly open and his jaw held firmly in the physiotherapist's right hand she produces movement of the jaw with her right hand. She should endeavour to pivot the right half of the jaw around the left temporomandibular joint.

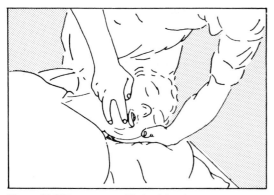

Figure 12.8 Temporomandibular joint; lateral chin movement

Depression**

Starting position

The patient rests his head on a pillow while the physiotherapist stands by his right upper arm facing his head. She holds each side of his mandible in her hands so that the pads of her middle and ring fingers contact the posterior surface of the ramus of the mandible near the head. The metacarpophalangeal joint of the thumb and thenar eminence are placed against the superior margin of the body of the mandible near the chin. Care must be taken to use as much of the pads of the fingers as possible to make the contact comfortable (Figure 12.9).

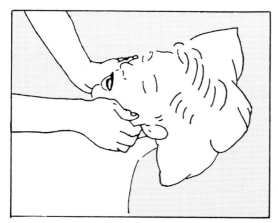

Figure 12.9 Temporomandibular joint; depression

Method

This movement must be produced by the therapist's wrists and arms while her hands move with his jaw as a single unit. She can control the depression to encourage protraction of the head of the mandible or backward movement of the angle of the jaw. This

is achieved by increasing the work performed through the fingers or that performed through the base of the thumbs because patients find relaxation so difficult. This is the most difficult of the techniques described for the jaw. However, by performing the movements smoothly and encouraging relaxation a finely controlled movement can be performed.

Alternative technique

Starting position

The patient lies supine and the physiotherapist places two fingers of each hand into his mouth so as to grasp over the upper and lower incisors (Figure 12.10).

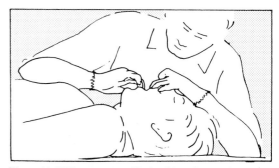

Figure 12.10 Temporomandibular joint; depression. Alternative technique

Method

The therapist stabilizes his maxilla with her left hand and applies oscillatory movements (usually at the limit of the range of depression) holding firmly with the fingers of her right hand while producing the movement with her right arm.

Longitudinal movement caudad**

Starting position

The patient lies supine and the physiotherapist places her right thumb in his mouth with the pad of her thumb facing caudad and braced against his lower left molars. She then stabilizes his head with her left hand (Figure 12.11).

Method

While stabilizing the patient's head with her left hand, the therapist exerts pressure against his left lower molars so as to distract the temporomandibular joint. This is best produced as an oscillatory

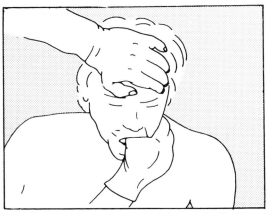

Figure 12.11 Temporomandibular joint; longitudinal movement caudad

Longitudinal movement cephalad*

Starting position

The patient lies supine and the physiotherapist stabilizes his head between her right hand and her thorax. She places the heel of her left hand on the inferior margin of the angle of the mandible.

Method

The technique is one of pushing cephalad to jam the head of the mandible against the articular disc and mandibular fossa. Movements may be incorporated with the compression.

movement at the limit of the range, with the therapist feeling the extent of the joint movement by placing one finger of her right hand over the lateral surface of the temporomandibular joint.

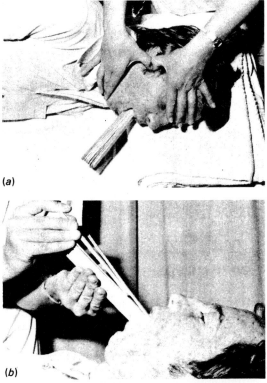

Figure 12.12 (*a*) Transverse accessory movement at the limit of mandibular depression. (*b*) Inserting spatulas following mobilizing and contract/relax techniques (Reproduced by kind permission of P. H. Trott[8].)

Treatment

When a temporomandibular joint is locked, with the mouth fixed in the open position, the best technique is one that combines caudad longitudinal movement with repeated oscillatory depression and elevation rocking close to the point of limited elevation. An alternative procedure, also performed while the temporomandibular joint is held distracted, is either to rock the head of the mandible in an anteroposterior to posteroanterior direction or to rock it medially and laterally.

For the most part, patients seek treatment because they have pain in the region of their temporomandibular joint when chewing, biting with a widely opened mouth, or yawning. This pain usually responds very readily to medial transverse oscillatory movements (see Figure 12.3).

The third common disorder of this joint is one of very limited depression which prevents the patient from eating normally. The passive movement technique effecting depression has been described but if the condition is chronic, or the limitation of mandibular movement is severe, then the use of spatulas is necessary to maintain the range gained passively and to exercise the muscles producing depression by 'contract/relax' techniques. The complete treatment for this problem is described fully by Trott[8]. Figure 12.12 (a) shows transverse pressure mobilizing being administered with the mouth opened at its maximum range by the use of spatulas. Figure 12.12 (b) shows more spatulas being inserted following the mobilization described above and 'contract/relax' procedures.

This is a perfect example of the use of accessory movements at the limit of the range when treating joint stiffness.

8. Trott, P. H. *Temporomandibular Myofascial Pain Dysfunction Syndrome.* Thesis for graduate diploma in manipulative therapy (1976)

Appendix 1

Movement diagram theory and compiling a movement diagram

> 'Geography would be incomprehensible without maps. They've reduced a tremendous muddle of facts into something you can read at a glance. Now I suspect . . . *economics* [read passive movement] is fundamentally no more difficult than geography except it's about things in motion. If only somebody would invent a dynamic map.'[1]

The movement diagram: A teaching aid, a means of communication and self-learning

The movement diagram is intended solely as a teaching aid and a means of communication. When examining, say, posteroanterior movement of the acromio-clavicular joint produced by pressure on the clavicle (see Figure 10.51) newcomers to this method of examination will find it difficult to know what they are feeling. However, the movement diagram makes them analyse the movement in terms of range, pain, resistance and muscle spasm. Also, it makes them analyse the *manner* in which these factors interact to affect the movement.

The movement diagram (and also the grades of movement) are not necessarily essential to using passive movement as a form of treatment. However, they are essential to understanding the relationship that the various grades of movement have to a patient's abnormal joint signs. Therefore, although they are not essential for a person to be a good manipulator, they are essential if the teaching of the whole concept of manipulative treatment is to be done at the highest level.

Movement diagrams are essential when trying to separate the different components that can be felt when a movement is examined. They therefore become essential for either teaching other people, or for teaching one's self and thereby progressing one's own analysis and understanding of treatment techniques and their effect on symptoms and signs.

The components considered in the diagram are *pain, spasm-free resistance* (i.e. stiffness) and *muscle spasm* found on joint examination, their relative strength and behaviour in all parts of the available range and in relation to each other. Thus the response of the joint to movement is shown in a very detailed way. The theory of the movement diagram is described in this appendix by discussing each component separately at first. The practical compilation of a diagram for one direction of movement of one joint in a particular patient follows on page 307.

Each of the above components is an extensive subject in itself and it should be realized that discussion in this appendix is deliberately limited in the following ways. The spasm referred to is protective muscle spasm secondary to joint disorder; spasticity caused by upper motor neurone disease and the voluntary contraction of muscles is excluded.

1. Snow, C. P. *Strangers and Brothers*, Penguin Books, London, p. 67 (1965)

Frequently this voluntary contraction is out of all proportion to the pain experienced yet in very direct proportion to the patient's apprehension about the examiner's handling of the joint. Careless handling will provoke such a reaction and thereby obscure the real clinical findings. Resistance (stiffness) free of muscle spasm is discussed only from the clinical point of view; that is, discussion about the pathology causing the stiffness is excluded.

A movement diagram is compiled by drawing graphs for the behaviour of pain, physical resistance and muscle spasm, depicting the position in the range at which each is felt (this is shown on the horizontal line AB) and the intensity, nature or quality of each (which is shown on the vertical line AC) (Figure A1.1).

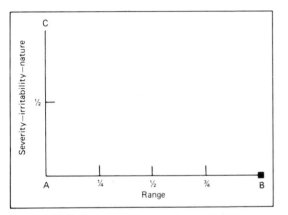

Figure A1.1 Beginning a movement diagram

The base line AB represents any range of movement from a starting position at A to the limit of the average normal passive range at B, remembering that when examining a patient's movement of any joint, it is only considered normal if firm proportionate over-pressure may be applied without pain (see page 40). It makes no difference whether the movement depicted is small or large, whether it involves one joint or a group of joints working together, or whether it represents 2 mm of posteroanterior movement or 180° of shoulder flexion.

Because of soft-tissue compliance, the end of range of *any* joint (even 'bone to bone') will have some soft-tissue component, physiological or pathological. Thus the range of the 'end of range', B, will be a movable point, or have a depth of position on the range line. To locate half way through the range of the 'end of range' as a grade IV and fit in either side of it a plus sign (+) and a minus sign (−) allows the depiction of the force with which this 'end of range' point is approached (Edwards, A., unpublished observations).

Point A, the starting position of the movement, is also variable: its position may be the extreme of range opposite B or somewhere in mid-range, whichever is most suitable for the diagram. For example, if shoulder flexion is the movement being represented and the pain or limitation occurs only in the last 10° of the range, the diagram will more clearly demonstrate the behaviour of the three factors if the base line represents the last 20° rather than 90° of flexion. For the purpose of clarity, position A is defined by stating the range represented by the base line AB. In the above example, if the base line represents 90°, A must be at about 90°; and similarly, if the base line represents 20° position A is with the arm 20° short of full flexion (assuming of course that the range of flexion is 180°).

As the movement diagram is used to depict what can be felt when examining passive movement, it must be clearly understood that point B represents the extreme of PASSIVE MOVEMENT, and that this lies variably, but very importantly, beyond the extreme of active movement.

The vertical axis AC represents the quality, nature or intensity of the factors being plotted; point A represents complete absence of the factor and point C represents the maximum quality, nature or intensity of the factor to which the examiner is prepared to subject the person. The word 'maximum' in relation to 'intensity' is obvious: it means point C is the maximum intensity of pain the examiner is prepared to provoke. 'Maximum' in relation to 'quality' and 'nature' refers to two other essential parts. They are:

1. *Irritability* – When the examiner would stop the testing movement when the pain was not necessarily intense but when she assessed that if she continued the movement into greater pain there would be an exacerbation or latent reaction.
2. *Nature* – When P_1 represents the onset of say scapular pain, but as the movement is continued the pain spreads down the arm. The examiner may decide to stop when the provoked pain reaches the forearm.

This meaning of 'maximum' in relation to each component is discussed again later.

The basic diagram is completed by vertical and horizontal lines drawn from B and C to meet at D (Figure A.1.2).

Other variations of the base line AB are described on page 311.

Pain
P_1

The initial fact to be established is whether the patient has any pain at all; and if he has pain whether it is present at rest or only on movement.

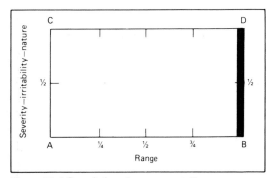

Figure A1.2 Completion of a movement diagram

To begin the exercise it is assumed he only has pain on movement.

The first step is to move the joint slowly and carefully into the range being tested, asking the patient to report immediately when he feels any discomfort at all. The position at which this is first felt is noted.

The second step consists of several small oscillatory movements in different parts of the pain-free range, gradually moving further into the range up to the point where pain is first felt, thus establishing the exact position of the onset of the pain. There is no danger of exacerbation if (a) sufficient care is used and (b) if the examiner bears in mind that it is the very first provocation of pain that is being sought. The point at which this occurs is called P_1 and is marked on the base line of the diagram (Figure A1.3).

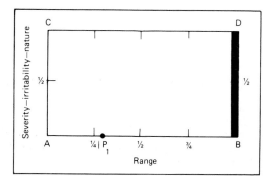

Figure A1.3 Onset of pain

Thus there are two steps to establishing P_1:

1. A single slow movement first.
2. Small oscillatory movements.

If the pain is reasonably severe then the point found with the first single slow movement will be deeper in the range than that found with oscillatory movements. Having thus found where the pain is first felt

with a slow movement, the oscillatory test movements will be carried out in a part of the range that will not provoke exacerbation.

L (1 of 3) where (L = limit of range)

The next step is to determine the available range of movement. This is done by slowly moving the joint beyond P_1 until the limit of the range is reached. This point is marked on the base line as **L** (Figure A1.4).

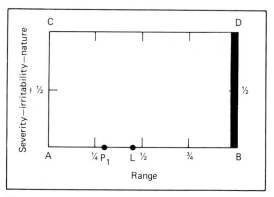

Figure A1.4 Limit of the range

L (2 of 3) what

The next step is to determine what component it is that prevents or inhibits further movement. As we are only discussing pain at this stage, P_2 is then marked vertically above L at maximum quality, nature or intensity (Figure A1.5). The intensity or quality of pain in any one position is assessed as lying somewhere on the vertical axis of the graph (i.e. between A and C) between no pain at all (i.e.

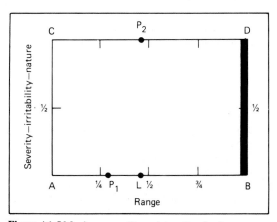

Figure A1.5 Maximum quality or intensity of pain

A) and the limit (i.e. C). It is important to realize that maximum intensity or quality of pain in the diagram represents the maximum the physiotherapist is prepared to provoke. This point is well within, and quite different from, a level representing intolerable pain for the patient. Estimation of 'maximum' in this way is, of course, entirely subjective, and varies from person to person. Though this may seem to some readers a grave weakness of the movement diagram, YET IT IS IN FACT ITS STRENGTH. When the student compares her 'L', 'P_2' with her instructor's, the differences that may exist will teach her that she has been too heavy handed or too 'kind-and-gentle'.

L (3 of 3) qualify

Having decided to stop the movement at L because of the pain's 'maximum "quality or intensity"' and therefore drawn in point P_2 on the line CD, it becomes necessary to qualify what P_2 represents: if it is the intensity of the pain that is the reason for stopping at L, then P_2 should be qualified thus: 'P_2 (intensity)'.

If, however, the examiner believes that there may be some latent reaction if she moves the joint further even though the pain is not severe, then P_2 should be qualified thus: 'P_2 (latent)' (Figure A1.6).

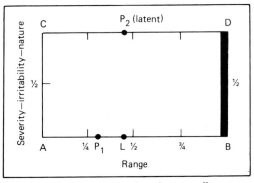

Figure A1.6 Latent reaction of maximum quality or intensity of pain

P_1P_2

The next step is to depict the behaviour of the pain during the movement between P_1 and P_2. If pain increases evenly with movement into the painful range the line joining P_1 and P_2 is a straight line (Figure A1.7). However, pain may not increase evenly in this way. Its build-up may be irregular, calling for a graph that is curved or angular. Pain may be first felt at about quarter range and may

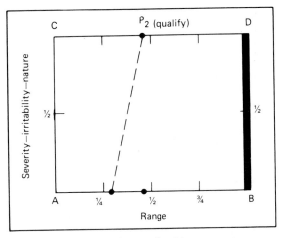

Figure A1.7 Pain increasing evenly with movement.
— — — — — = Pain

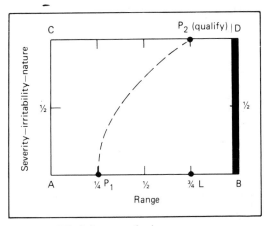

Figure A1.8 Early increase of pain

initially change quickly, then the movement can be taken further until a limit at three-quarter range is reached (Figure A1.8).

In another example, pain may be first felt at quarter range and remain at a low level until suddenly it changes, reaching P_2 at three-quarter range (Figure A1.9).

The examples given demonstrate pain that prevents a full range of movement of the joint, but there are instances where pain may never reach a limiting intensity. Figure A1.10 is an example where a little pain may be felt at half range but the pain scarcely changes beyond this point in the range and the end of normal range may be reached without provoking anything approaching a limit to full range of movement. There is thus no point L, and P′ (P′ means P prime) appears on the vertical line BD to

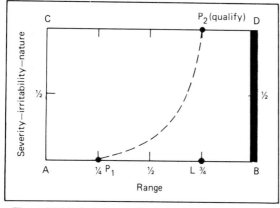

Figure A1.9 Later increase of pain reaching a maximum at three-quarter range

indicate the relative significance of the pain at that point (Figure A1.10). The mathematical use of 'prime' in this context is that it represents 'a numerical value which has itself and unity as its only factors' (*Concise Oxford Dictionary*).

If we now return to an example where the joint is painful at rest, mentioned at the beginning of this appendix, an estimate must be made of the amount or quality of pain present at rest, and this appears as P on the vertical axis AC (Figure A1.11). Movement is then begun slowly and carefully until the original level of pain begins to increase (P_1 in Figure A1.12). The behaviour of pain beyond this point is plotted in the manner already described, and an example of such a graph is given in Figure A1.13. When the joint is painful at rest the symptoms are easily exacerbated by poor handling. However, if examination is carried out with care and skill, no difficulty is encountered.

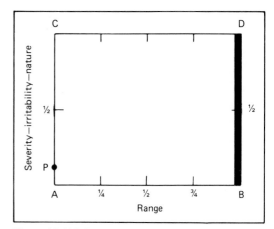

Figure A1.11 Pain at rest

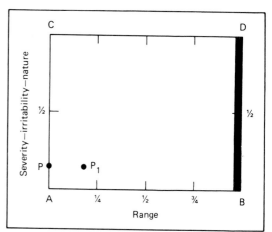

Figure A1.12 Level where pain begins to increase

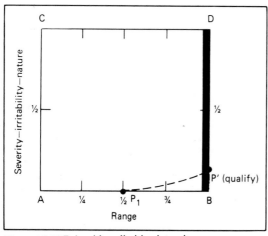

Figure A1.10 Pain with no limiting intensity

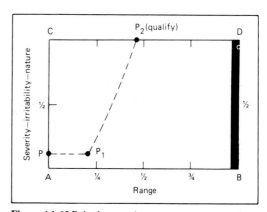

Figure A1.13 Pain due to subsequent movement

Again it must be emphasized that this evaluation of pain is purely subjective. Nevertheless, it presents an invaluable method whereby students can learn to perceive different behaviours of pain, and their appreciation of these variations of pain patterns will mature as this type of assessment is practised from patient to patient and checked against the judgement of a more experienced physiotherapist.

An arc of pain provoked on passive movement might be depicted as shown in Figure A1.14.

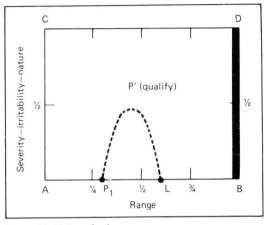

Figure A1.14 Arc of pain

Resistance (free of muscle spasm)

These resistances may be due to adaptive shortening of muscles or capsules, scar tissue, arthritic joint changes and many other non-muscle-spasm situations.

A normal joint, when completely relaxed and moved passively, has the feel of being well oiled and friction free[2]. It can be likened to wet soap sliding on wet glass. It is important for the physiotherapist using passive movement as a form of treatment to appreciate the difference between a free-running, friction-free movement and one that, although being full range, has minor resistance within the range of movement. A strong recommendation is made for therapists to feel the movements suggested in the article[2].

When depicting a compliance diagram of the forces applied to stretching a ligament from start to breaking point, the graph includes a 'toe region', a 'linear region' and a 'plastic region'; the plastic region ends at the 'break point' (Figure A.1.15).

When a physiotherapist assesses abnormal resistance present in joint movement, physical laws state that there must be a degree of resistance, at the

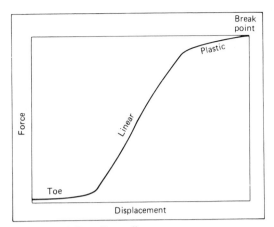

Figure A1.15 Compliance diagram

immediate moment that movement commences. The resistance is in the opposite direction to the direction of movement being assessed, and it may be so minimal as to be imperceptible to the physiotherapist. This is the 'toe region' of the compliance diagram, and it is omitted from the movement diagram as used by the manipulative physiotherapist.

The section of the compliance graph that forms the movement diagram represents the clinical findings of the behaviour of resistance when examining a patient's movement in the linear region only (Figure A1.16).

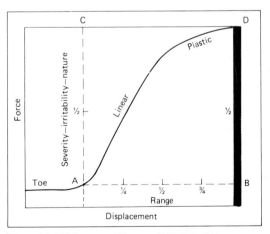

Figure A1.16 Movement diagram (ABCD) within compliance diagram. The dotted rectangular area (ABCD) is that part of the compliance diagram that is the basis of the movement diagram used for representing abnormal resistance ($R_1 R_2$ or $R_1 R'$)

2. Maitland, G. D. The hypothesis of adding compression when examining and treating synovial joints. *Journal of Orthopaedic and Sports Physical Therapy*, **2**, 7–14 (1980)

R_1

When assessing for resistance, the best way to appreciate the free running of a joint is to support and hold around the joint with one hand while the other hand produces an oscillatory movement back and forth through a chosen path of the range. If this movement is felt to be friction free then the oscillatory movement can be moved more deeply into the range. In this way the total available range can be assessed. With experience, by comparing two patients, and also comparing a patient's right side with his left side, the physiotherapist will quickly learn to appreciate minor resistance to movement. Point R_1 is then established and marked on the base line AB (Figure A1.17).

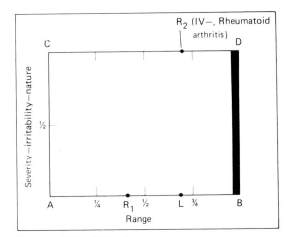

Figure A1.18 Qualifying R_2

$R_1 R_2$

The next step is to determine the behaviour of the resistance between R_1 and L, that is between R_1 and R_2. The behaviour of the resistance between R_1 and R_2 is assessed by movements back and forth in the range between R_1 and L, and the line depicting the behaviour of the resistance is drawn on the diagram (Figure A1.19). As with pain, resistance can vary in its behaviour, and examples are shown in Figure A1.19.

The foregoing resistances have been related to extra-articular structures. However, if the joint is held in such a way as to compress the surfaces, intra-articular resistance may be felt. Such resistance might be depicted as in Figure A1.20.

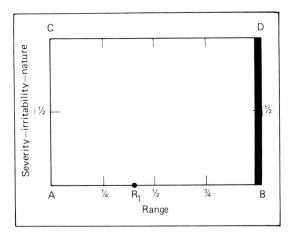

Figure A1.17 Positioning of R_1

L – where, L – what

The joint movement is then taken to the limit of the range. If resistance limits movement, the range is assessed and marked by L on the base line. Vertically above L, R_2 is drawn on CD to indicate that it is resistance that limited the range. R_2 does not necessarily mean that the physiotherapist is too weak to push any harder; it represents the strength of the resistance beyond which the physiotherapist is not prepared to push. There may be factors such as rheumatoid arthritis, which will limit the strength represented by R_2 to being moderately gentle. Therefore, as with P_2, R_2 needs to be qualified. The qualification needs to be of two kinds if it is gentle (e.g. R_2(IV−, RA)), the first indicating its strength and the second indicating the reason why the movement is stopped even though the strength is weak (Figure A1.18). When R_2 is a strong resistance (e.g. R_2(IV++)), its strength only needs to be indicated (Figure A1.18).

Muscle spasm

There are only two kinds of muscle spasm that will be considered here; one that always limits range and occupies a small part of it, and the other that occurs as a quick contraction to prevent a painful movement.

Whether it is spasm, or stiffness, that is limiting the range can frequently only be accurately assessed by (1) repeated movement taken somewhat beyond the point at which resistance is first encountered and (2) performed at different speeds. Muscle spasm shows a power of active recoil. In contrast, resistance that is free of muscle activity does not have this quality; rather it is constant in strength at any given point in the range.

The following examples may help to clarify the point. If a resistance to passive movement is felt between Z_1 and Z_2 on the base line AB of the movement diagram (Figure A1.21) and if this resistance is 'resistance free of muscle spasm', then at point 'O', between Z_1 and Z_2 (Figure A1.22), the

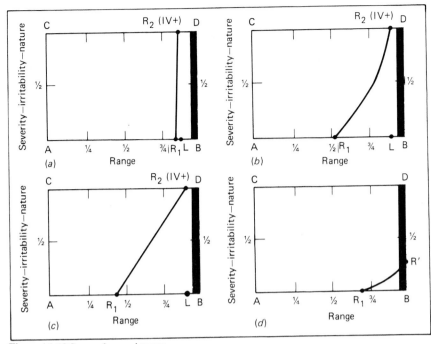

Figure A1.19 Spasm-free resistance

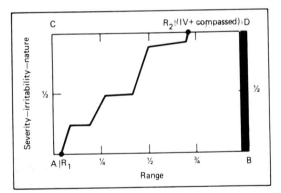

Figure A1.20 Crepitus

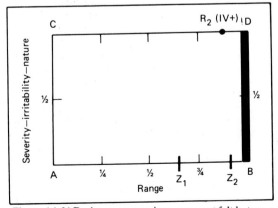

Figure A1.21 Resistance to passive movement felt between
Z_1 and Z_2

strength of the resistance will be exactly the same
irrespective of how fast or slowly a movement is
oscillated up to it. Also, any increase in strength will
be directly proportional to the depth in range,
regardless of the speed with which the movement is
carried out; that is, the resistance felt at one point in
movement will always be less than that felt at a point
deeper in the range. However, if the block is a
muscle spasm and test movements are taken up to a
point 'O' at different speeds, the strength of the
resistance will be greater, with increases in speed.

The first of the two kinds of muscle spasm will feel
like spring steel and will push back against the
testing movement, particularly if the test movement
is varied in speed and in position in the range.

S_1

Testing this kind of spasm is done by moving the
joint slowly to the point at which spasm is first
elicited, and this point is noted on the base line as S.

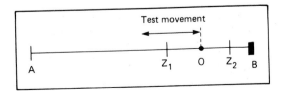

Figure A1.22 Differentiating resistance from spasm

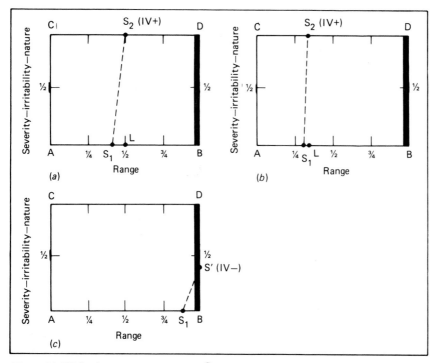

Figure A1.23 Muscle spasm. — — — — = Spasm

L – where, L – what

This limit is noted by L on the base line and S_2 is marked vertically above L on the line CD. As with P_2 and R_2, S_2 needs to be qualified in terms of strength and quality e.g. S_2 (IV−, very sharp).

$S_1 S_2$

The graph for the behaviour of spasm is plotted between S_1 and S_2 (Figure A1.23). When muscle spasm limits range it always reaches its maximum quickly, and thus occupies only a small part of the range. Therefore, it will always be depicted as a near-vertical line (Figure A1.23(a) and (b)). In some cases when the joint disorder is less severe, a little spasm that increases slightly but never prohibits full movement may be felt just before the end of range (Figure A1.23(c)).

The second kind of muscle spasm is directly proportional to the severity of the patient's pain: movement of the joint in varying parts of the range causes sharply limiting muscular contractions. This usually occurs when a very painful joint is moved without adequate care and can be completely avoided if the joint is well supported and moved gently. This spasm is reflex in type, coming into action very rapidly during the test movement. A very similar kind of muscular contraction can occur as a voluntary action by the patient, indicating a sharp increase in pain. If the physiotherapist varies the speed of her test movements she will be able to distinguish quickly between the reflex spasm and the voluntary spasm by the speed with which the spasm occurs – reflex spasm occurs more quickly in response to a provoking movement than does voluntary spasm. This second kind of spasm, which does not limit a range of movement, can usually be avoided by careful handling during the test.

To represent this kind of spasm, a near-vertical line is drawn from above the base line; its height and position on the base line will signify whether the spasm is easy to provoke and will also give some indication of its strength. Two examples are drawn of the extremes that may be found (Figure A1.24(a) and (b)).

Modification

There is a modification of the base line AB which can be used when the significant range to be

Further movement is then attempted. If maximum intensity is reached before the end of range, spasm thus becomes a limiting factor.

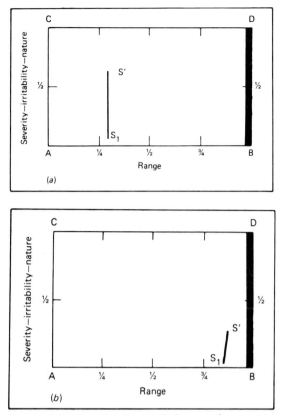

(a)

(b)

Figure A1.24 Spasm that does not limit range of movement

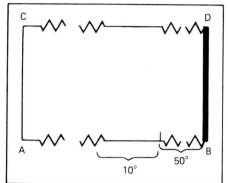

Figure A1.25 Modified movement diagram

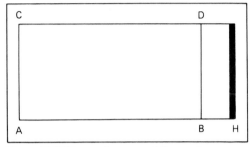

Figure A1.26 Frame of movement diagram for hypermobile joint

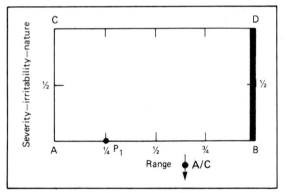

Figure A1.27 Point at which pain is first felt

depicted occupies only say 10° yet it is 50° short of B. The movement diagram would be as shown in Figure A1.25, and when used to depict a movement, the range between 'L' and 'B' must be stated.

The base line AB for the hypermobile joint movement to be depicted would be the same as that shown earlier where grades of movement are discussed, and the frame of the movement diagram would be as in Figure A1.26.

Having discussed at length the graphing of the separate elements of a movement diagram, it is now necessary to put them together as a whole.

Compiling a movement diagram

This book places great emphasis on the kinds and behaviours of pain as they present with the different movements of disordered joints. Pain is of major importance to the patient and therefore takes priority in the examination of joint movement. The following demonstrates how the diagram is formulated. When testing the acromio-clavicular (A/C) joint by posteroanterior pressure on the clavicle (for example) the routine is as follows.

Step 1. P_1

Gentle, increasing pressure is applied very slowly to the clavicle in a posteroanterior direction and the patient is asked to report when he first feels pain. This point in the range is noted and the physiotherapist then releases some of the pressure from the clavicle and performs small oscillatory movements. Again she asks the patient if he feels any pain. If he does not, the oscillation should then be carried out slightly deeper into the range. Conversely, if he does feel pain, the oscillatory movement should be withdrawn in the range. By these oscillatory movements in different parts of the range, the point at which pain is first felt with movements can be identified and is then recorded on the base line of the movement diagram as P_1 (Figure A1.27). The estimation of the position in the range of P_1 is best achieved by performing the oscillations at what the physiotherapist feels is ¼ range, then at ⅓ range and then at ½ range. By this means, P_1 can be very accurately assessed. Therefore these are the two steps to establishing P_1:

1. A single slow movement.
2. Small oscillatory movements.

Step 2. L – where

Having found P_1 the physiotherapist should continue further into the range with the posteroanterior movements until she reaches the limit of the range. She identifies where that position is in relation to the normal range and records it on the base line of the movement diagram as point L (Figure A1.28).

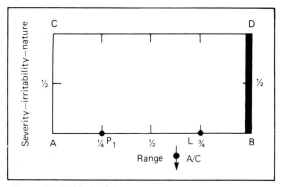

Figure A1.28 Limit of the range

Step 3. L – what

For the hypomobile joint the next step is to decide *why* the movement was stopped at point L. This means that the examiner has moved the joint as far as she is willing to go but she has not made it reach 'B'. Having decided WHERE 'L' is, the examiner has to decide why she chose to stop at L; WHAT was it that prevented her reaching 'B'. Assume, for the purpose of this example, that it was physical resistance, free of muscle spasm, that prevented movement beyond L. Where the vertical line above L meets the horizontal projection CD, it is marked as R_2 (Figure A1.29). The R_2 needs to be qualified using words or symbols to indicate what it was about

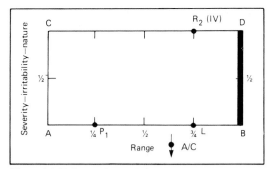

Figure A1.29 Spasm-free resistance limiting movement

the resistance that prevented the examiner stretching it further; for example the patient may have rheumatoid arthritis and she may not be prepared to go further (see Figure A1.18), or she may not be prepared to push harder than Grade IV (Figure A1.29).

Step 4. P′ and defined

The physiotherapist then decides the quality, nature or the intensity of the pain at the limit of the range. This can be estimated in relation to two values: (1) what maximum would feel like, and (2) what half way (50%) between no pain and maximum would feel like. By this means the intensity of the pain is fairly easily decided thus enabling the physiotherapist to put P′ on the vertical above L in its accurately estimated position (Figure A1.30).

If the limiting factor at L were P_2, then Step 4 would be estimating the quality or intensity of R′ and defining it (Figure A1.31).

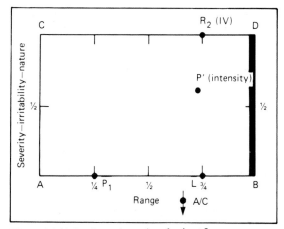

Figure A1.30 Quality or intensity of pain at L

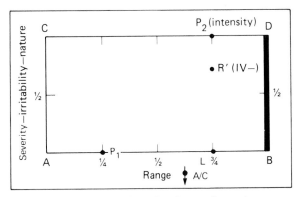

Figure A1.31 Quality or intensity of spasm-free resistance

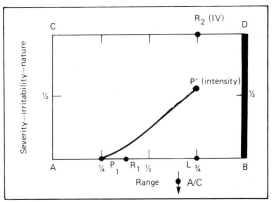

Figure A1.33 Commencement of resistance

Step 5. *Behaviour of pain P_1 P_2 or P_1P'*

The A/C joint is then moved in a posteroanterior direction between P_1 and L to determine, by watching the patient's hands and face, and also by asking him how the pain behaves between P_1 and P_2 or between P_1 and P': in fact it is better to think of pain between P_1 and L because at L, pain is going to be represented as P_2 or P'. The line representing the behaviour of pain is then drawn on the movement diagram; that is, the line P_1 P_2 or between P_1 and P', is completed (Figure A1.32).

Step 7. *Behaviour of resistance R_1 R_2*

By moving the joint between R_1 and L the behaviour of the resistance can be determined and plotted on the graph between the points R_1 and R_2 (Figure A1.34).

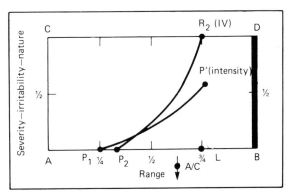

Figure A1.34 Behaviour of resistance

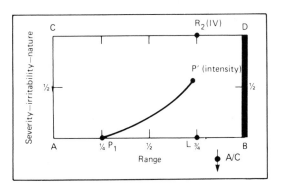

Figure A1.32 Behaviour of the pain

Step 6. *R_1*

Having completed the representation of pain, resistance must be considered. This is achieved by receding further back in the range than P_1, where, with carefully applied and carefully felt oscillatory movements, the presence or not of any resistance is ascertained. Where it commences is noted and marked on the base line AB as R_1 (Figure A1.33).

Step 8. *S_1S'*

If no muscle spasm has been felt during this examination and if the patient's pain is not excessive, the physiotherapist should continue the oscillatory posteroanterior movements, but perform them more sharply and quicker to determine whether any spasm can be provoked. If no spasm can be provoked, then there is nothing to record on the movement diagram. However, if with quick sharper movements a reflex type of muscle spasm is elicited to protect the movement, this should be drawn on the movement diagram in a manner that will indicate how easy or difficult it is to provoke (i.e. by placing the spasm line towards A if it is easy to provoke, and towards B if it is difficult to provoke). The strength of the spasm so provoked is indicated by the height of the spasm line, S_1S' (Figure A1.35).

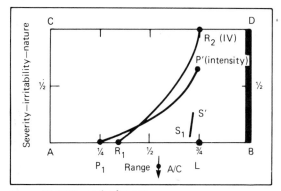

Figure A1.35 Strength of spasm

Thus the diagram for that movement is compiled showing the behaviour of all elements. It is then possible to assess any relationships between the factors found on the examination. The relationships give a distinct guide as to the treatment that should be given, particularly in relation to the 'grade' of the treatment movements; that is, whether 'pain' is going to be treated or whether the treatment will be directed at the resistance.

Summary of steps

Compiling a movement diagram may seem complicated, but it is not. It is a very important part of training in manipulative physiotherapy because it forces the physiotherapist to understand clearly what it is she is feeling when moving the joint passively. Committing those thoughts to paper thwarts any guesswork, or any 'hit-and-miss' approach to treatment. Table A1.1 summarizes the steps taken in compiling a movement diagram where resistance limits movement, and the steps when pain limits movement.

Modified diagram base line

When either the limit of available range is very restricted (i.e. L is a long way from B), or when the elements of the movement diagram occupy only a very small percentage of the full range, the basis of the movement diagram needs modification. This is achieved by breaking the base line as in Figure A1.36. The centre section can then be identified to represent any length, in any part of the minimal full

Table A1.1 Steps taken in compiling a movement diagram

Where resistance limits movement	*Where pain limits movement*
1. P_1 (a) slow (b) oscillatory	1. P_1 (a) slow (b) oscillatory
2. L – where	2. L – where
3. L – what (and define) R_2	3. L – what (and define) P_2
4. P' (define)	4. $P_1 P_2$ (behaviour)
5. $P_1 P'$ (behaviour)	5. R_1
6. R_1	6. R' (and define)
7. $R_1 R_2$ (behaviour)	7. $R_1 R'$ (behaviour)
8. S (defined)	8. S (defined)

1. Snow, C. P. *Strangers and Brothers*, Penguin Books, London, p. 67 (1965)
2. Maitland, G. D. The hypothesis of adding compression when examining and treating synovial joints. *Journal of Orthopaedic and Sports Physical Therapy*, **2**, 7–14 (1980)

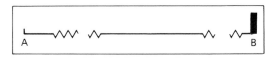

Figure A1.36 Modified diagram base line

range. When the examination findings are only to be found in the last, say 5° of a full range, point A in the range is changed and the line AB is suitably identified as in Figure A1.37. This example demonstrates that from A to B is 8°, and A to ¼ is 2°, and so on.

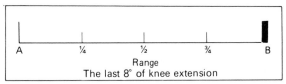

Figure A1.37 The last 8° of knee extension

Example – range limited by 50%

Marked stiffness, with 'L' a large distance before 'B', necessitates a modified format of the movement diagram. The example will be restricted knee flexion, a long-standing condition following a fracture.

The first element is R_1, and the distance between R_1 and L is only 12°. Pain is provoked only by stretching (Figure A1.38). If the movement diagram were drawn on an unmodified format it would be as in Figure A1.39. Figure A1.39 clearly wastes considerable diagram space, and it is difficult to interpret. With the same joint movement findings represented on the modified format of the movement diagram it becomes clearer and much more

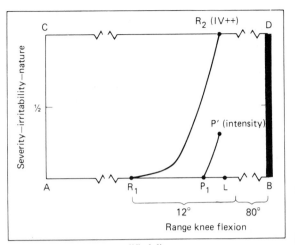

Figure A1.38 Using a modified diagram

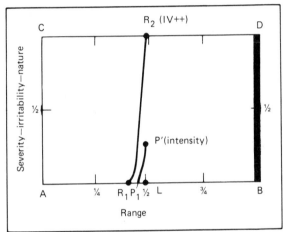

Figure A1.39 Range limited by 50%, shown on an unmodified diagram (160° knee flexion)

useful. The modified format of the base line of the diagram (Figure A1.38) requires only two extra measurements to be stated:

1. The measurement between L and B.
2. The measurement between R_1 and L.

Knowing that R_1 to L equals 12° makes it easy to see that R_1 is approximately 7° before P_1. Because of the increased space allowed to represent the elements of the movement, the behaviour also is far easier to demonstrate.

Clinical example – hypermobility

This example is included for the express purpose of clarifying the misconceptions that exist about hypermobility and the direct influence that some

authors and practitioners afford it in restricting passive movement treatment.

If the movement (using the same acromioclavicular joint being tested with posteroanterior movements), before having become painful, were hypermobile, the basic format of the movement diagram would be as shown in Figure A1.40.

If it becomes painful and requires treatment the movement diagram could be found to be as follows.

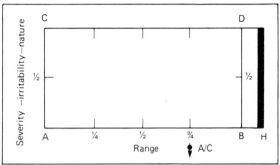

Figure A1.40 Movement diagram for hypermobile range

Step 1. P_1

The method is the same as in example 1; see also Figure A1.41.

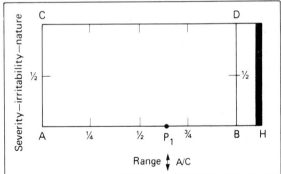

Figure A1.41 P_1 hypermobile joint

Step 2. L – where

The method is the same as in Example 1 (page 312); see Figure A1.42.

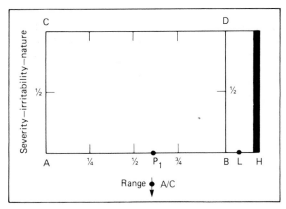

Figure A1.42 L – 'where;' hypermobile joint

Step 3. L – what (and define)

The method is the same as in Example 1; see also Figure A1.43.

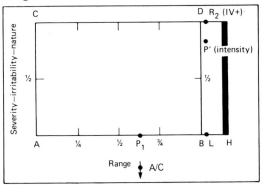

Figure A1.43 L – 'what' (and define), hypermobile joint

Step 4. P' define (Figure A1.44)

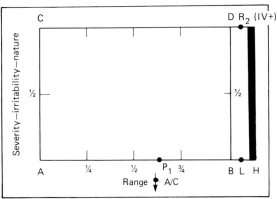

Figure A1.44 P' – 'define', hypermobile joint

Step 5. P₁ P' behaviour (Figure A1.45)

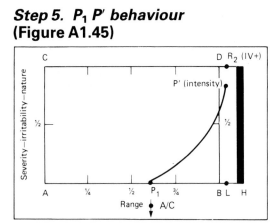

Figure A1.45 P₁ P' behaviour, hypermobile joint

Step 6. R₁ (Figure A1.46)

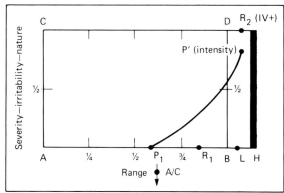

Figure A1.46 R₁, hypermobile joint

Step 7. R₁R₂ behaviour (Figure A1.47)

Step 7. R₁R₂ behaviour (Figure A2.8)

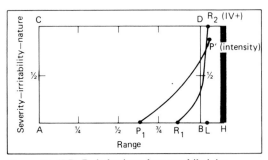

Figure A1.47 R₁ R₂ behaviour, hypermobile joint

Treatment

Hypermobility is not a contraindication to manipulation. Most patients with hypermobile joints, one of which becomes painful, have a hypomobile situation at that joint. They are therefore treated on the same basis as is used for hypomobility. It makes no difference whether the limit (L) of the range, on examination, is found to be beyond the end of the average-normal range (as in the example above, L being beyond B) or before it (L being on the side of B). Proof of the hypomobility is validated by assessment at the end of successful treatment.

References

Aichroth, P. M., Scott, R. A. P. and Nott, M. Changes in bone marrow pressure on walking in patients with osteoarthritis of the hip. *Journal of Bone & Joint Surgery,* **57B**, 246 (1975)

Akison, W. H., Woo, S. L. Y., Amiel, D., Coutts, R. D. and Daniel, D. The connective tissue response to immobility: biochemical changes in periarticular connective tissue of the immobilized rabbit knee. *Clinical Orthopaedics,* **93**, 356–422 (1973)

Apley, A. G. and Solomon, L. *Apley's System of Orthopaedics and Fractures,* 6th ed. Butterworths, London (1982)

Argyle, M. *Bodily communication,* Methuen, London (1975)

Barnett, C. H. Wear and tear in joints: an experimental study. *Journal of Bone & Joint Surgery,* **38B**, 567–575 (1956)

Beighton, P., Grahame, R. and Bird, H. *Hypermobility of joints.* Springer-Verlag, Berlin (1983)

Bohler, L. cited by Platt, H. Orthopaedics in Continental Europe 1900–1950. *Journal of Bone & Joint Surgery,* **32B**, 574–584 (1950)

Broderick, P. A., Corvese, N., Pierik, M. G., Pike, R. F. and Mariorenzi, A. L. Exfoliative cytology interpretation of synovial fluid in joint disease. *Journal of Bone & Joint Surgery,* **58A**, 396–399 (1976)

Butler, D. S. *Mobilization of the Nervous System.* Churchill Livingstone, London (1990)

Catersen, B. and Lowther, D. A. Changes in the metabolism of the porteoglycan from sheep articular cartilage in response to mechanical stress. *Biochimica et Biophysica Acta,* **540**, 412–422 (1978)

Charnley, J. Communication to a symposium on biomechanics, Institution of Mechanical Engineers, London (1959). In *Gray's Anatomy,* 35th edn. Longman, London, p. 193 (1973)

Clarke, I. C. Friction and wear of articular cartilage – a pendulum/SES system. *Journal of Bone & Joint Surgery,* **57A**, (1975)

Corrigan, B. and Maitland, G. D. *Practical Orthopaedic Medicine,* Butterworths, London (1983)

Critchley, M. (ed.) *Butterworths Medical Dictionary,* 2nd ed. Butterworths, London (1978)

Cyriax, J. H. and Cyriax, P. J. *Illustrated Manual of Orthopaedic Medicine,* Butterworths, London, pp. 51–98 (1983)

Cyriax, J. *Textbook of Orthopaedic Medicine,* 7th ed. Vol. II, Baillière Tindall, London (1965)

Dalrymple, J. *Costing Not Less Than Everything.* Darton, Longman and Todd, London, p. 93 (1975)

Delbet, L. C. cited by Platt, H. Orthopaedics in Continental Europe 1900–1950. *Journal of Bone & Joint Surgery,* **32B**, 574–584 (1950)

Edwards, B. C. Combined movements of the lumbar spine. *Australian Journal of Physiotherapy,* **25**, 4 (1979)

Ekholm, R. Nutrition of articular cartilage. *Acta Anatomica,* **12**, 77 (1955)

Elvey, R. L. Brachial plexus tension tests and the pathogenic origin of arm pain. In *Proceedings of Multidisciplinary International Conference on Manipulative Therapy,* Melbourne, pp. 105–111 (1979)

Flint, M. H. The role of environmental factors in connective tissue ultrastructure. In The *Ultrastructure of Collagen,* C. C. Thomas, Springfield, Ill., pp. 60–66 (1976)

Fry, H. J. H. Overuse syndrome in musicians: prevention and management. *Lancet,* **ii**, 728–731 (1986)

Gillard, G. C., Merrilees, M. J., Bell-Booth, P. G., Reilly, H. C. and Flint, M. H. The proteoglycan content and the axial periodicity of collagen in tendon. *Biochemistry Journal,* **163**, 145–151 (1977)

Goodfellow, J., Hungerford, D. S. and Woods, C. Patello-femoral joint mechanics and pathology. *Journal of Bone & Joint Surgery,* **58B**, 291–299 (1976)

Gowers, E. *The Complete Plain Words,* 3rd ed. Penguin Books, Harmondsworth (1987)

Hassler, C. R., Rybicki, E. F., Diegle, R. B. and Clark, L. C. Studies of enhanced bone healing via electrical stimuli. *Clinical Orthopaedic and Related Research,* **124**, 5–9 (1977)

Hickling, J. and Maitland, G. D. Abnormalities in passive movement: diagrammatic representation. *Journal of the Chartered Society of Physiotherapists,* **56**, 105 (1970)

Hickling, J. and Maitland, G. D. Abnormalities in passive movement: diagrammatic representation. *Australian Journal of Physiotherapy,* **XVI**, 13 (1970)

Joint Motion: Method of Measuring and Recording. American Academy of Orthopaedic Surgeons (1976)

Jull, G. The role of passive mobilization in the immediate management of the fractured neck of humerus. *Australian Journal of Physiotherapy,* **25**, 107–114 (1979)

Keele, K. E. Discussion on research into pain. *Practitioner,* **198**, 287 (1967)

Lowther, D. A. The effect of compression and tension on the behaviour of connective tissues. In *Aspects of Manipulative Therapy,* 2nd ed., G. D. Maitland, Churchill Livingstone, Melbourne, pp. 16–22 (1985)

Lowther, D. A. The effect of mechanical stress on the behaviour of connective tissue. *Australian Journal of Physiotherapy,* **29**, 181 (1983)

Ludlum, R. *The Aquitaine Progression,* Granada Publishing, London (1984)

McDevitt, C. and Muir, H. An experimental model of osteoarthritis: early morphological and biochemical changes. *Journal of Bone & Joint Surgery,* **59B**, 24–35 (1977)

MacDonald, R. *Black Money,* Collins Fontana Books, London (1970)

McNair, J. and Maitland, G. D. The role of passive mobilization in the treatment of a non-uniting fracture site – a case study. *International Conference on Manipulation Therapy* (1983)

Maitland, G. D. The importance of adding compression when examining and treating synovial joints. *Aspects of Manipulative Therapy,* 2nd ed. Churchill Livingstone, Melbourne, pp. 109–115 (1985)

Maitland, G. D. *Vertebral Manipulation,* 5th ed. Butterworths, London (1968)

Maitland, G. D. *Mrs. E.: Demonstration of patient I: Shoulder manipulation* (50 mins) and *Demonstration of a patient: Mrs. E. II and III* (55 mins). Videotape numbers 17 and 18. Postgraduate Teaching Centre, Hermitage, Medizinische Abteilung, Bad Ragaz, Switzerland CH7310 (1978)

Maitland, G. D. *Shoulder quadrant, hip flexion/adduction,* Video number 6 (42 mins). Postgraduate Teaching Centre, Hermitage, Medizinische Abteilung, Bad Ragaz, Switzerland CH7310 (1978)

Maitland, G. D. *Mrs. E.: Demonstration of a patient – (1) Shoulder manipulation.* Videotape numbers 17 (50 mins), 18 (2) and (3) 55 mins. Postgraduate Teaching

Centre, Hermitage, Medizinische Abteilung, Bad Ragaz, Switzerland CH7310 (1980)

Maitland, G. D. *Elbow, Knee, Shoulder.* Videotape number 13 (32 mins). Postgraduate Teaching Centre, Hermitage, Medizinische Abteilung, Bad Ragaz, Switzerland CH7310 (1978)

Maitland, G. D. *The foot: differentiation.* Videotape number 25 (45 mins). Postgraduate Teaching Centre, Hermitage, Medizinische Abteilung, Bad Ragaz, Switzerland CH7310 (1982)

Maitland, G. D. *Gait.* Videotape number 24 (50 mins) Postgraduate Teaching Centre, Hermitage, Medizinische Abteilung, Bad Ragaz, Switzerland CH7310 (1983)

Maitland, G. D. The hypothesis of adding compression when examining and treating synovial joints. *Journal of Orthopaedic and Sports Physical Therapy,* **2**, 7–14 (1980)

Mennell, J. *Science and Art of Joint Manipulation,* Vol. II. Churchill Livingstone, London (1952)

Mennell, J. McM. *Joint Pain.* Churchill Livingstone, London; Little Brown & Co., Boston (1964)

Malcolm, L. L., Fung, Y. C., Woo, S. L. Y., Akeson, W. H. and Amiel, D. Steady-state dynamic functional properties of cartilage–cartilage inferfaces. *Journal of Bone & Joint Surgery,* **57A**, 567 (1975)

Maroudas, A., Bullough, P., Swanson, S. A. V. and Freeman, M. A. R. The permeability of articular cartilage. *Journal of Bone and Joint Surgery,* **50B**, 166–177 (1968)

Miller, M. R. and Kasahara, M. Observations on the innervation of human long bones. *Anatomical Record,* **145**, 13–23 (1963)

Mow, Van C. and Kuei, C. K. The effect of visco-elasticity on the squeeze film action of lubrication of synovial joints. *Journal of Bone & Joint Surgery,* **57A** (1975)

Panjabi, M. M., White, A. A. and Wolf, W. W. Jr. A biochemical comparison of the effects of constant and cyclic compression on fracture healing in rabbit long-bones. *Acta Orthopaedica Scandinavica,* **50**, 653–661 (1979)

Peacock, E. E. and van Winkle, W. *Wound repair,* 2nd ed. W. B. Saunders, Philadelphia (1976)

Peters, E. *Monk's Hood,* Future Publications, London, p. 18 (1984)

Reimann, I. and Christensen, S. Bach. A histological demonstration on nerves in sub-chondral bone. *Acta Orthopaedica Scandinavica,* **48**, 345–352 (1977)

Salter, R. B., Simmonds, D. F., Malcolm, B. W., Rumble, E. J. and MacMichael, D. The effects of continuous passive motion on the healing of articular cartilage defects – an experimental investigation in rabbits. *Journal of Bone & Joint Surgery,* **57A**, 570–571 (1975)

Salter, R. B. Presidential address. *Journal of Bone & Joint Surgery,* **64B**, 251–254 (1982)

Salter, R. B. Motion versus rest: why immobilize joints? *Proceedings of the Manipulative Therapists Association of Australia, Brisbane,* 1–11 (1985)

Salter, R. B., Simmonds, D. F., Malcolm, B. W., Rumble, E. J., Macmichael, D. and Clements, N. D. The biological effects of continuous passive motion on the healing of full-thickness defects in articular cartilage. *Journal of Bone & Joint Surgery,* **62A**, 1232–1251 (1980)

Snow, C. P. *Strangers and Brothers.* Penguin Books, Harmondsworth (1965)

Thomas, H. O. cited by Osmond-Clarke, H. Half a century of orthopaedic progress in Great Britain. *Journal of Bone & Joint Surgery,* **32B**, 622–623 (1950)

Trott, P. H. *Temporomandibular Myofascial Pain Dysfunction Syndrome.* Thesis for graduate diploma in manipulative therapy (1976)

Williams, P. L. and Warwick, R. *Gray's Anatomy,* 36th ed. Churchill Livingstone, London (1980)

Index

Note: Page entries that include illustrations are entered in *italics*.